SPEECH CORRECTION

An Introduction to Speech Pathology and Audiology

NINTH EDITION

CHARLES VAN RIPER

Late of Western Michigan University

ROBERT L. ERICKSON

Western Michigan University

Allyn and Bacon

Boston ■ London ■ Toronto ■ Sydney ■ Tokyo ■ Singapore

Series Editor: Kris Farnsworth
Editorial Assistant: Christine Svitila
Senior Marketing Manager: Kathy Hunter
Editorial-Production Administrator: Joe Sweeney
Editorial-Production Service: Walsh Associates
Composition Buyer: Linda Cox
Manufacturing Buyer: Megan Cochran
Cover Administrator: Linda Knowles

Copyright © 1996, 1990, 1984 by Allyn & Bacon
A Simon & Schuster Company
Needham Heights, MA 02194

Library of Congress Cataloging-in-Publication Data

Van Riper, Charles
    Speech correction : an introduction to speech pathology and audiology / Charles Van Riper, Robert L. Erickson. — 9th ed.
      p. cm.
    Includes bibliographical references and index.
    ISBN 0-13-825142-8
    1. Speech disorders. 2. Speech therapy. 3. Audiology.
  I. Erickson, Robert L. II. Title.
    [DNLM: 1. Speech Disorders. 2. Voice Disorders. 3. Speech Therapy. WM 475 V274s 1995]
    RC423.V35 1995
    616.85′5—dc20
    DNLM/DLC
    for Library of Congress   95–41718
                                    CIP

Printed in the United States of America

10 9 8 7 6 5 4 3 2 1   00 99 98 97 96 95

To Catharine Hull Van Riper, aka Katy, "The Earth Mother"
(1909–1984)

to Jackie, Doug, Chuck, and Deanna,

to our clients, and to our students and their future clients, and

to the memory of Charles "Cully" Gage Van Riper,

the man from Michigan's Upper Peninsula who, following the completion of his doctoral studies at the University of Iowa, came to Western State Normal College in 1936 to begin a speech clinic and to establish one of the country's earliest educational programs for the preparation of "speech correctionists." For decades to follow, Charles Van Riper played a pioneering and dominant role in the developing profession of speech-language pathology.

Doctor Van Riper was destined to become part of the very fiber of generations of students and practitioners throughout the world, even as he also was to become a source of strength, hope, inspiration, understanding, and help for countless persons with communication disabilities.

"Doctor Van" lived, and urged his students and his colleagues to live, in ways intended to have positive and enduring effects. He sought to teach us that, "although we are specks at the intersection of the two infinities of time and space," we are able to erect a perpendicular at that point. "Every time you help a person to have a better life," he reminds us still, "and every time you've made this earth a bit more beautiful, you add another unit to your perpendicular." Through word and deed he impacted in many ways on myriad lives. He relished the notion thus of "playing billiards with eternity."

It is in his spirit, and now in remembrance of him, that you are invited to explore in these pages the miracle of human speech and hearing, the devastations wrought by their malfunctions, and the still-evolving professions of speech-language pathology and audiology.

CONTENTS

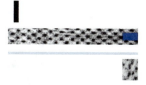
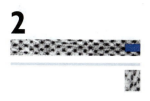
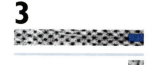

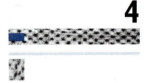
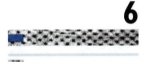

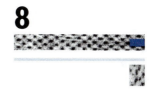

Fluency Disorders 253

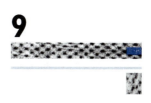

Voice Disorders 303

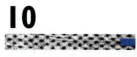
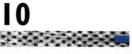

Cleft Palate 343

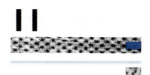

Aphasia and Related Disorders 375

12 Cerebral Palsy and Other Neuropathologies   403

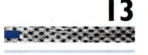

13 Hearing and Hearing Impairment   423

14 The Speech and Hearing Professions   472

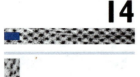

PREFACE

As were its eight previous editions, this book is intended primarily for undergraduate students of human communication sciences and disorders; however, it also should be of interest to students of elementary and pre-primary education, music therapy, nursing, occupational therapy, physical therapy, special education, psychology, and social work. Predentistry and premedicine students also may find in this text useful overviews of many of the disability types that they eventually will encounter in their practices.

In an introductory textbook it is impossible, of course, to reflect adequately the ever-expanding roles and responsibilities of today's speech-language pathologists and audiologists, so students who plan to enter either of these professions will be well advised to supplement their studies with readings from current journals and specialized texts. Toward that end we have suggested various sources of more detailed information when our own discussion necessarily is foreshortened.

In this ninth edition we have maintained the clinical focus that has helped to make the book uniquely readable, relevant, and informative for many generations of students. As in previous editions, we have used actual client examples to illustrate and clarify text material. However, some of the detailed discussions of specific therapy procedures found in earlier editions have been either condensed or eliminated. Chapter 8 is an exception in this regard, representing as it does the senior author's final writings on the treatment of stuttering.

In addition to updating information, we have included far more comprehensive coverage of normal communication processes, and we have expanded considerably our consideration of hearing problems and audiology. Some materials have been reorganized (for example, emotional problems associated with speech disorders are discussed in a separate chapter, and alaryngeal speech has been combined with voice disorders in a single chapter); and materials related to professional ethics and scopes of practice have been added as appendices. Among the other new features of this edition are the inclusion of study questions in each chapter and the marginal definition of highlighted glossary terms throughout the book. We trust that such changes as well as the improved layout of this edition will enhance its usefulness to students and instructors alike.

ACKNOWLEDGMENTS

Thank you to the reviewers of various versions of this edition—Donald Fucci, Ohio University; Nancy K. O'Hare, Ph.D., James Madison University; Arthur M. Guilford, Ph.D., University of South Florida; and Bonnie Lucido, Brigham Young University—and to the many faculty colleagues at Western Michigan University have provided generous advice and other forms of assistance during the preparation of this revision. Among those at WMU, Harold L. Bate, James M. Hillenbrand, Gary D. Lawson, Donna B. Oas, and Karen K. Seelig were particularly helpful. Their interest and support have been very much appreciated. Gratitude also is extended to John M. Hanley for having afforded me sufficient workload flexibility to ensure completion of the project. Kris Farnsworth of Allyn and Bacon has been especially patient, considerate, and persistent in bringing this edition to closure. I am most grateful for her assistance and unfailing encouragement. Finally, I wish also to acknowledge my long-standing indebtedness to John Wiley, whose gentle wisdom and understanding guidance so greatly influenced the early career decisions that led me eventually to Kalamazoo.

Robert L. Erickson

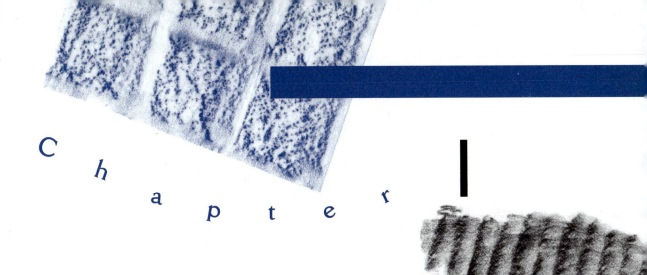

Chapter 1

Introduction

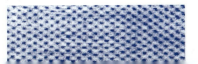

Students take the introductory course in communication disorders for various reasons. Some plan to enter one or the other of the new and rapidly growing professions of audiology or speech-language pathology. Some who seek careers in music therapy, occupational therapy, physical therapy, or in counseling, know they will have patients with communication disabilities. Others, majoring in special education or classroom teaching, will have students with impaired speech or hearing. Some of you have family members or friends who stutter or have hearing losses or other kinds of speech or voice disorders. And, of course, there are students who need an elective course in a convenient time slot. Whatever your motivation, we welcome you. We are delighted to be your guides because we know that those who have been deprived of that most fundamental of all human traits, the ability to communicate, need all the help and understanding they can get.

Many of you, too, may be searching for a way to make your lives meaningful, for a basic philosophy of living. You may have realized that in terms of the immensities of time and space we are only microscopic specks. Should you spend your lives seeking possessions or fame? That doesn't really make much sense. Fame is for fruitflies. You will not be remembered for long. Should you spend your life acquiring things, houses, and land? Your senior author has eighty acres and a big old farm house, but when he went over them in a hot air balloon they were so small he could barely see them. Yes, we are specks at the intersection of the two infinities of time and space, but one can erect a perpendicular at that point—the perpendicular pronoun "**I**"(Figure 1-1).

We believe that the units of that perpendicular of significance are built of impact. Every time you help a person to have a better life and every time you've made this earth of ours a bit more beautiful, you add another unit to your perpendicular. And every time you hurt another person or pollute your nest you lose some of your life's meaning. Those of us in the helping and healing professions may have more opportunity for growth than others but all of us have impact. No, we needn't be specks.

This is a book about people troubled by the way in which they communicate, about children and adults who stutter, who cannot utter a sound because they have lost their vocal folds, who possess some other speech disorder, who have hearing losses, or who have suffered strokes. At first glance, it might seem as though its contents could have no bearing on this generation's compelling need to make the world a fit place for men and women to fulfill their infinite potential for something other than evil. But there are many kinds of pollution, and some of the worst are those that reflect people's inhumanity to one another.

Perhaps all other evils flow from this befouled spring. If so, the study of speech pathology[1] and audiology should help us to discern what must be done. It is important to realize that speech is the unique fea-

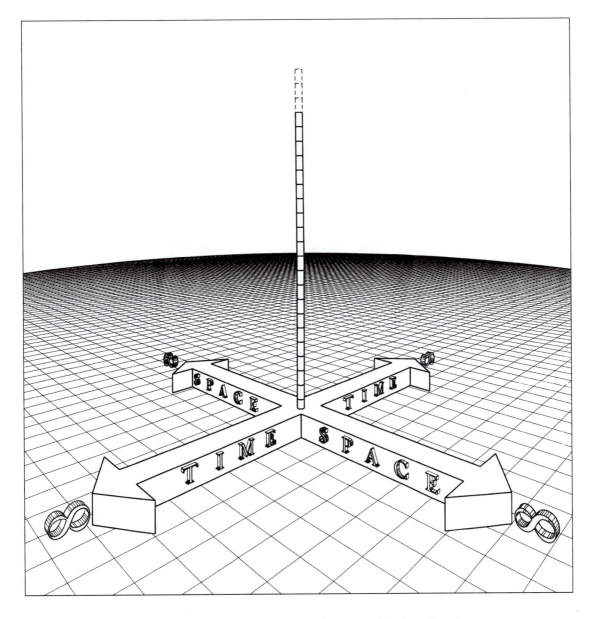

 FIGURE 1-1 The Perpendicular of Significance *(Courtesy of Andrew Amor)*

ture that distinguishes human from animal. If we had not heard, we would not speak. Had we not talked, we would still be in Eden or the cave. In the dark mirror of communication disorders we may find reflected the fears, the frustrations, the shame, and the way a person is treated by others; but the professions of speech pathology and audiology also provide us hope that somehow, someday, we can solve such problems.

Sometimes it seems that there are so many human ills and evils that those who dedicate their lives to their diminishing are dooming themselves to lives of futility and frustration. We have not found it so. Although our individual efforts may seem at times to have no more effect than those of an ant carrying a grain of sand away from the seashore, we have before us the example of atomic fission in which one active particle triggers those about it, and these then fire others until incredible forces are released. Each human being has a host of opportunities to trigger forces for good or evil that lie latent in others. We believe that it is therefore possible for any one of us to start chain reactions that may finally result in the kind of world and the kind of people we hope for. It is through the fragile miracle of interpersonal communication that we can initiate this chain of reactions for human betterment.

But where to begin? The possibilities to relieve human distress are everywhere. We who have chosen to direct our energies toward helping those who have communication disorders are fortunate in that we often can see the results much sooner than those who deal with such other problems as poverty, crime, or environmental pollution. It is very good to know that we have helped people lost in the swamp of despair gain or regain their human birthright—the ability to communicate. It is good to know that you have freed them from the penalties and frustrations that are their lot and from the anxieties, guilt, and frustration that too often are their daily fare.

People who cannot communicate effectively are sorely handicapped, so to understand their burdens we present a brief history of how society has treated the disabled and the handicapped in the past.

In this text we occasionally use the word *handicap* as well as *disability* to refer to those individuals who, through no fault of their own, have differences that make living difficult. Blindness, deafness, or any other physical or mental impairment that substantially limits one or more of the major life activities are examples of handicaps or disabilities. We are quite aware of the many objections to the word "handicapped." That term comes from the past when persons with many kinds of deformities or impairments would beg with cap in hand. It is now well recognized, of course, that such people have the same rights as any other citizens and that they neither need· nor wish to be pitied.

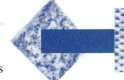

HISTORY OF THE DISABLED

There are times, when we survey the extent of human distress, that this dream of creating a better world is so unrealistic that it would be foolish to try to do anything to make it come true. Why seek to make one's life meaningful in this way when there is such an immense amount of misfortune all about us? Why pick up a few beer cans when millions are discarded each day? Why try to help those who are less fortunate than we are when the forces of our own culture keep generating more unhappiness? Is there any hope for humankind?

The history of the way society has treated the handicapped, sad as it is, may give us the glimmerings of that hope. Although we have some way to go before we can call ourselves civilized, the contrast between the present and past treatments of people who are retarded, deaf, blind, crippled, insane, or poor, and of those who cannot talk normally shows very clearly that we have made gains. We find in this cultural history a hopeful progression from considering handicapped persons as intolerable nuisances, then as objects of mirth, then as pitiful beggars, then as challenging problems, and now as individuals who are challenged. Today, persons with disabilities are increasingly recognized as persons, and as persons who also have abilities. But clearly it was not always so.

Rejection

Primitive society tolerated no weakness. Tribes struggled hard for survival, and those members who could not aid materially were quickly rejected. The younger men killed the leaders when they had lost their teeth or their energies had abated. The inhabitants of ancient India cast crippled people into the Ganges; the Spartans hurled theirs from a precipice. The Aztecs regularly sacrificed deformed persons in times of famine or when one of their leaders died. The Melanesians had a simple solution for the problem of the handicapped: They buried them alive. Among the earlier Romans, twins were considered so abnormal that one of them was always put to death, and frequently both were killed. They left their malformed children on the highways or in the forests. If the children survived they were often picked up by those who always prey upon the handicapped and were carried to the marketplace to be trained as beggars. They were not even valuable enough to be slaves.

The Bible clearly reflects these early rejection attitudes. Remember Job? The prevailing belief in Old Testament times was that people's physical states were determined by their good or bad relationship with a deity. Disabilities were regarded as divine punishment for sin. A normal person could invoke similar punishment merely by associating with those who had thus incurred the wrath of God. Consequently, the blind and the crippled wailed with the lepers outside the city wall.

During the Middle Ages the physically disabled were frequently considered to be possessed by evil spirits. They were confined to their own homes. They dared not walk to the marketplace lest they be stoned. Even in this century, elimination of the handicapped has been practiced. Just a few decades ago in our own country the sterilization of mentally impaired people was sometimes practiced. The Kalfir tribes in South Africa clubbed sickly or deformed children. The Nazis kept only the best of their civilian prisoners for slaves; the others died in the gas chamber. And the abandonment of physically deformed infants occurs even today in some parts of our world.

Today in this country the person who killed a disabled child might be executed. We have come far in our journey toward civilization, but perhaps not far enough. Rejection takes many other forms. Spirits, too, can be killed.

How many of those reading this book would accept unhesitatingly an invitation to a dance or dinner if it were tendered by a person whose physical disability was obvious and severe?

Humor

It did not take promoters long to discover that the handicapped provided a rewarding source of humor. One history of the subject states that before 1000 B.C. the fool or buffoon became a necessary part of feast-making and "won the laughter of the guests by his idiocy or his deformity." In Homer's *Odyssey,* comic relief from tragedy was illustrated by the vain effort of the one-eyed Polyphemus to pursue his tormentors after they had blinded him. For a thousand years thereafter every court had its crippled buffoons, it dwarf jesters, its stuttering fools. Attila the Hun held banquets at which "a Moorish and Scythian buffoon successively excited the mirth of the rude spectators by their deformed figures, ridiculous dress, antic gestures, and absurd speech." Cages along the Appian Way displayed various grotesque human disabilities, including "Balbus Blaesus" the stutterer, who would attempt to talk when a coin was flung through the bars. In Shakespeare's *Timon of Athens,* Caphis says, "Here comes the fool; let's ha' some sport with 'im." Often this sport consisted of physical abuse or exposure of the twisted limb. These unfortunate individuals accepted and even expected ridicule. At least it provided a means of survival, a livelihood, and it represented an advance in civilized living.

Gradually, the use of people with disabilities to provoke mirth became less popular in continental Europe, and the more enterprising had to migrate to less culturally advanced areas to make a living. At one time Peter the Great had so many that he found it necessary to classify them for different occasions. When Cortez conquered Mexico he discovered deformed creatures of all kinds at the court of Montezuma. On the same continents today you may find them used to provoke laughter only in the circus sideshows, in the movies, on the radio and television and in every schoolyard.

Pity

Religion is doubtless responsible for the development of true pity as a cultural reaction to handicaps. James Joyce said that pity is the feeling that arrests the mind in the presence of whatsoever is grave and constant in human suffering and unites it with the human sufferer. It was this spontaneous feeling that prompted religious leaders to give the handicapped shelter and protection. Before 200 B.C. Asoka, a Buddhist, created a ministry for the care of unfortunates and appointed officers to supervise charitable works. Confucius said, "With whom should I associate but with suffering men?" Jesus preached compassion for all the disabled and made all men their brothers' keepers. In the seventh century after Jesus's death the Moslem religion proposed a society free from cruelty and social oppression and insisted on kindliness and consideration for all men. A few hundred years later Saint Francis of Assisi devoted his life to the care of the sick and the disabled. Following this, the "Mad Priest of Kent," John Ball, was so aroused by the plight of the crippled and needy left in the wake of the Black Death that he publicly pleaded their cause, often at the risk of his own life. With the rise of the middle class, pity for the handicapped became more commonplace. The oppression that the merchants and serfs had suffered left them more sympathetic to others who were ill used. The doctrine of the equality of man did much for the disabled as well as for the economically downtrodden.

However, many crimes have been committed in the name of charity. The halt and the blind began to acquire commercial value as beggars. Legs and backs of children were broken and twisted by their exploiters. Soon the commercialization of pity became so universal that it became a community nuisance. Alms became a conventional gesture to buy relief from the piteous whining that dominated every public place. True pity was lost in revulsion. Recognizing this unhappy trend, Hyperious of Ypres advocated that beggars be classified so that work could be provided according to their capacities. His own motives were humanitarian, but he cleverly won support for his cause by pointing out that other citizens "would be freed of clamor, of fear of outrage, or the sight of ugly bodies." His appeal was successful; and asylums and homes for the handicapped began to appear, if only to isolate the occupants so that the public need not be reminded of their distress. Another motive that improved the position of the handicapped was the belief that one could purchase his way into heaven or out of hell by charity. The thrown coin has been impelled by many motives: the longing for religious security, the heightening of one's own superiority by comparison with the unfortunate, the social prestige of philanthropy, and the desire to be freed from embarrassment. Pseudopity has accomplished much, but true compassion would have ended the tragedy.

HOW THE DISABLED PERSON REACTS

Thus far we have been describing how society has reacted to people with handicaps. Now let us consider how disabled persons have reacted to the penalties and frustration that too often are their lot. The basic emotional responses are those of *anxiety, shame,* and *hostility.* Having to live with the expectation that you will be rejected because of your disability adds to your burden. Mockery and playground teasing have warped many a child's life by coloring it with shame. Of course they resent the mistreatment. So would you. People with communication disorders suffer the same hurts experienced by people with other disabilities, and in Chapter 5 we will describe their emotional reactions more fully and how we cope with them.

CURRENT ATTITUDES TOWARD DISABILITY

In the senior author's lifetime, he has seen a dramatic improvement in the way people with disabilities are treated. It is ironic that this change was due in part to World Wars I and II, and to the Great Depression of 1929 and the early thirties. These experiences, with their resulting injuries and miseries, gave rise to universal feelings of concern and compassion for the unfortunate members of our society. The old practices of rejection and neglect no longer seemed tolerable.

Accordingly, with the support of governmental agencies, we began to assist the elderly, the impoverished, and the impaired through social security, Medicare, and Medicaid. Programs in special education and speech correction sprang up all over the country in one school system after another. Charitable agencies flourished. The positive change was revolutionary, and the process is continuing. Employers receiving any type of federal support have been forbidden since 1973 to refuse services or jobs to qualified persons because of handicaps. In 1975, Public Law 94–142, the *Education of the Handicapped Act* (later retitled as the *Individuals with Disabilities Education Act*), mandated free and appropriate educations for disabled students from ages 5 to 21. Later amendments added appropriate services for infants, toddlers, and preschoolers as well. Public Law 101–336, the landmark *Americans with Disabilities Act,* enacted in 1990, provides civil rights protection to all individuals with disabilities in the areas of employment, state and local government services, telecommunications, and public accommodations.

Facilities and services now must be provided so that individuals who have physical, visual, hearing, speech, and other disabilities can have access. Just to cite a few examples, hotels must provide rooms that would enable a disabled person to use the bathroom facilities as well as having doors through which a wheelchair can pass. Auditory signals must be added to visual signs so that the blind can know when an elevator door is open for entry. Restaurants must provide picture menus (implemented by McDonald's, for example, as shown in Figure 1-2). Assistive devices such as amplifiers must be available, and the list goes on.

"The ADA is not just about opening doors, opening jobs, and opening telephone lines for the approximately 43 million Americans with disabilities, including those with hearing, speech, or language disabilities. It is also about opening minds." (Carey, 1992) That message is clear. We no longer will make it difficult for the disabled to have a good life; instead, we are committed to seeing that they live well. Yes, finally we gradually are becoming a bit more civilized.

COMMUNICATING WITH THE COMMUNICATIVELY IMPAIRED

Being more civilized means, first and foremost, that we respond to the *person* rather than—as some have tended to do—concentrating on the person's *disability*. We must not allow the disability to become the focal point of social interaction, for this inevitably limits the style and scope of interaction and, of course, thereby magnifies the effect of any disability. Nevertheless, it is easy to feel at least a vague sense of doubt or discomfort when interacting with an individual who has a disability. How should we act? What should we say?

Here are some guidelines that we have found helpful in talking with a person who has trouble communicating. Some are equally applicable to individuals with other impairments or disabilities.

1. The most important thing is to acknowledge your uncertainty and fear, and then try to relax. Focus on the person rather than on your own nervousness. Remember, despite the speech, language, or hearing disorder, the individual is a person just like you; and he or she has many attributes besides the communication disorder.
2. Maintain eye contact with the person. This is a basic nonverbal way in which we bond with others—it shows that we are "open for business."
3. Give the person enough time and opportunity to talk. It may take longer for the individual to transmit a message. Speech is not an option for all persons who have communication disorders. There are

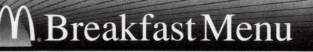

M.Breakfast Menu

THIS PROGRAM ENDORSED BY AMERICAN SPEECH, LANGUAGE AND HEARING ASSOCIATION, ROCKVILLE, MD.

EGG McMUFFIN

SAUSAGE McMUFFIN WITH EGG

SAUSAGE BISCUIT

SAUSAGE BISCUIT WITH EGG

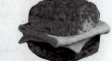

BACON, EGG AND CHEESE BISCUIT

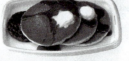

HOTCAKES AND SAUSAGE

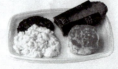

BIG BREAKFAST

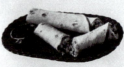

BREAKFAST BURRITO
(One Per Order)

HASH BROWNS

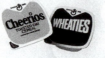

CEREAL: CHEERIOS, WHEATIES

APPLE BRAN MUFFIN

BREAKFAST DANISH

COFFEE: REGULAR AND DECAF
Large, Medium, Small

1% LOWFAT MILK

ORANGE JUICE
Large, Medium, Small

HOT TEA

HOT CHOCOLATE
(Seasonal)

The following trademarks are owned by McDonald's Corporation: Egg McMuffin, Sausage McMuffin, Big Breakfast. Wheaties and Cheerios are trademarks of General Mills, Inc.
©1991 McDonald's Corporation McD 1-1635   Printed on McGlove™ McDonald's recycled paper.

FIGURE 1-2   McDonald's Convenience Breakfast Menu for the Disabled *(Courtesy of McDonald's Corporation)*

other systems (signs, symbol boards, electronic devices) to assist in communication.

4. You may have to listen more carefully than you usually do. Be aware that this requires more effort—listening closely is hard work.

5. Focus on *what* the person is saying rather than *how* he or she is saying it. The message is what is important, not its form. In fact, it is sometimes helpful to rephrase what was said so that the speaker knows the intended message has been transmitted.

6. If you don't understand what the person is trying to say, tell him or her. Don't pretend that you understand when you don't. Ask the person to repeat if necessary.

7. Never fill in a word or assist an individual unless he or she asks for help. Offering assistance before it is requested—simply assuming that help is needed—can be demeaning and frustrating.

8. Speak directly to the person, not to a companion, even if the individual is using an interpreter. Never, under any circumstances, talk about the person in his or her presence.

9. In some instances, it may be helpful if you talk more slowly and more simply. But don't talk down to the person or adopt a patronizing manner. It may also help to use gestures along with your verbal message.

10. Finally, let your language affirm the entire person, not just the communication disorder. Put the person first, not the disability. The way we refer to individuals with disabilities may shape our images of them—they become lispers, aphasics, or clutterers.

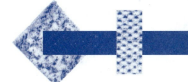

A BRIEF LOOK AT THE PROFESSIONS

As we have mentioned, basic changes in our earlier attitudes toward people with disabilities resulted in two new professions being born, speech pathology and audiology. No longer do people who cannot hear or speak normally need to live in desperation and without hope. You may or may not choose to enter either of these still young professions, but you should know the kinds of services they provide. You or your family or friends may need them one day.

Some of our former students now practicing their professions have shared with us the following brief descriptions of what they had done in a typical day. Our first account comes from a young speech clinician who works in the public schools.

Today was an especially good one and I felt refreshed reviewing what happened as I drove home. First, in the morning, I had a conference with Sara's mother. Sara has a language problem—she confuses pronouns and mixes up tense and plurals, and her sentence structure is immature. Her mother was very open and amenable to some suggestions for work at home. Some parents are not, despite all my attempts to include them in preparing an Individualized Educational Plan. Then I worked with two groups of children who are in the carryover stage of therapy for their sound errors. At noon I drove to my other school. I saw Mark alone at 1:00. He is eleven years old and stutters quite severely. He has long silent blocks. I have been trying to show him how to stutter in an easier fashion, to let the words slide out instead of fighting himself. He seems to be catching on now. But my big success today was with Terri: She finally was able to make a good *r* sound. She has been in my caseload now for two years; she could tell the error from the correct production in my speech, but, until today, all her efforts to say the sound were faulty. We were experimenting with some scary false teeth (next week is Halloween) and they must have pushed her tongue up and back a bit. All I know is she said it clearly. She blinked and I didn't move. Casually, I asked her to say the *r* sound again in a whisper. Then she said it out loud. When she left the therapy room she was saying simple words like run, ran, and rain very slowly and her face was radiant. So was mine.

Among the many evidences that speech pathology and audiology are rapidly growing professions is the continuing growth of community speech and hearing centers. These often are partially funded by charitable agencies such as the United Way and are usually supported in part by fees. Here is the report of a worker in such a center.

My duties are varied and depend upon the particular caseload we have at any one time. At present I usually have one or two diagnostic sessions each morning or application interviews with parents. Then I may see a stutterer or an aphasic for therapy. In the afternoon, most of my work is with small groups. One of these consists of preschool deaf children, but the one I enjoy most is the group of three **laryngectomees.**[2] One of them, Mr. J., was diagnosed with **laryngeal** cancer about a year ago and has had quite a lot of radiation, both before and after the surgeon removed his **larynx.** Anyway, he has the best **esophageal speech** of any of them. Very intelligible! Yesterday he managed to say a thirteen-syllable sentence with good intensity. He's working mainly on trying to get more loudness and more inflections. The second man is Mr. F., who is just beginning to string a series of words into phrases without having to stop and gulp before every syllable. Our third member is a fifty-year-old woman who is having a very hard time. She wrote me a note saying that she hates the sound of the burp, that it sounds vulgar, ugly. Mrs. W. is very depressed most of the time, and until we put her with the two men I was pretty sure she'd quit. But they've really helped her, Mr. J. especially, for he's so upbeat and a fine example. And he's a pretty good teacher of esophageal speech, too. Even better than I am, though I'm much better than when you coached me a few years ago. When I demonstrate, they kid me about my larynx getting in the way.

Laryngectomee. Person whose larynx has been surgically removed, typically because of laryngeal cancer.

Laryngeal. Pertaining to the larynx.

Larynx. Cartilaginous structure in neck between trachea and pharynx; includes vocal folds and muscles that control their tension and positioning; the "voice box."

Esophageal speech. Speech of laryngectomized persons produced by air pulses ejected from the esophagus.

Here's the report from a speech pathologist in another kind of job setting.

This is my third year working at the Child Guidance Clinic. I never dreamed that my days could be so filled with varied and interesting activities. Our clientele consists mainly of children with severe emotional problems and I work closely with our psychiatrists, social workers, and psychologists. Today we did a lengthy evaluation of a child referred to the clinic as autistic. Joel is three years old, has no speech, does not attend to messages directed to him, and rejects any attempt to touch or hold him. His play consisted of repetitive rituals. He flicked his fingers in front of his face and spun around while staring at the ceiling light. At the staffing conference, the parents told us that Joel insists upon keeping everything the same at home; he becomes enraged if the family takes a different route into town or if the household furniture is rearranged. They are worried also that the child doesn't seem to feel pain or recognize danger; he will bang his head repeatedly or run full tilt into a table, bounce off, and not cry at all. We are going to work out a multidisciplinary program for Joel in conjunction with the special education program in the school system and our agency.

In the afternoon I had a session with a nine-year-old child with a severe voice problem. Gary is extremely **hoarse** due to vocal abuse. He has been examined by a physician who observed reddening and thickening of both vocal folds. The doctor recommended therapy because she felt that the youngster must learn more about vocal hygiene and how to use his voice in a more conservative and relaxed manner. Gary talks loudly and constantly; and when he is not talking, he is making motorcycle or animal noises. We did some role playing to show him how to use a soft, medium, and loud voice. Then we prepared a "shouting graph" so we can tally the number of episodes of vocal abuse Gary has each day.

The last thing I did was work on my presentation for the local Rotary Club. Several of us are going to the meeting tonight in conjunction with our annual fund raising drive.

Many speech-language pathologists also work in hospital clinics. This is how one described her work (Figure 1-3).

You asked for a description of my professional activities on a typical day, but there seem to be no typical days. They all are very different: Each new one brings new problems, which is why I like working in the medical setting of a hospital speech and hearing clinic. That, and the chance to work closely with physicians, nurses, physical therapists, occupational therapists, and even with our medical social worker. There are so many different kinds of patients and so many disorders that I have never seen before.

But the bulk of my cases are stroke patients or patients whose **aphasia** resulted from **traumatic brain injuries** that required neurosurgery. Besides doing therapy with them, I also have to do repeated assessment of their speech and language to provide the attending physician with the

Hoarseness.
Voice quality often defined as a combination of *breathiness* and *harshness*.

Aphasia.
Impairment in the use of meaningful symbols due to brain injury.

Traumatic brain injury (TBI).
Damage to brain or nervous system caused by externally induced head injury; also called *closed head injury*.

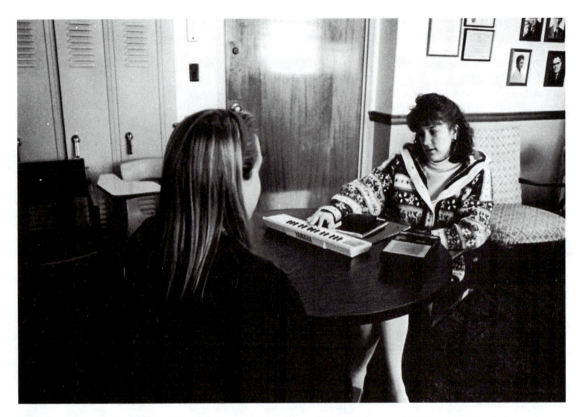

 FIGURE 1-3   Client in Voice Therapy *(Van Riper Clinic, Western Michigan University)*

information he or she needs about their progress or lack of it. I've found that the usual formal tests for aphasia must be supplemented by a lot of informal observation and interaction with these patients because they tire so fast or get so emotional when they fail a test item. In the testing situation they rarely show how much speech and language ability they really possess.

This afternoon one of the nurses complimented me on my "bedside manner" after hearing a young male patient laugh for the first time in many weeks. The man had been in a deep depression and with plenty of reasons for it. He'd been in an automobile wreck that killed his wife and child and left him a **hemiplegic.** When he did try to talk, all that came out was compulsive **jargon.** Not all aphasics know when they talk gibberish but he did and it devastated him. Almost every time he tries to talk, he starts crying and does not seem to be able to stop. But today I got him to count aloud up to twenty with only one mistake. Trying to establish some imitation, I got him to mimic gestures like nodding

Hemiplegia.
Paralysis or neurological involvement of one side of the body.

Jargon.
Continuous but unintelligible speech.

yes and head shaking for no and then trying to read my lips and mimic them silently.

After some of this I then began to count aloud and so did he. It shocked him to hear himself saying those numbers, and that's when the nurse heard him laugh. Of course, when he started laughing, he couldn't stop and then he was laughing and crying at the same time. Took me a long time to calm him down and he didn't want me to leave, so I had to make sure he understood that I'd be back tomorrow at the same time. Pretty hard to do because my words didn't seem to sink in; so I acted out my leaving the room and then returning, pointing to the clock and then a calendar and saying something like this over and over again with plenty of pauses: "Miss Peterson (pointing to myself) go now . . . Miss Peterson come back (turning one page of my calendar). Miss Peterson (pointing) see John (pointing) tomorrow . . . this time (I showed him the time on the clock). John eat . . . (pointed to five o'clock feeding time). Then John sleep (I acted out sleeping as I pointed to ten o'clock)" and so on. Somehow, something got through and I feel he understood I'd be back, for he waved the fingers of his nonparalyzed hand to indicate goodbye and smiled when I left. For the first time John and I have a tiny ray of hope, but I've still got my fingers crossed.

Still another facet of the field is the opportunity for private practice. Those who undertake to set up a private clinical practice have to be very competent, experienced, and able to establish close relationships with medical and other related professionals. And they must be prepared to undergo an initial period of financial uncertainty. Even so, their numbers have increased continuously and we submit this portion of a letter from one of them.

At the present time I do most of my private practice in conjunction with a local organization called Visiting Nurses. Through this agency I have many contacts with the medical profession, and from them I get most of my referrals. I do some therapy in the agency office, some in my home, and, in a few instances, in homes of clients. Let me tell you about three clients.

Two are stroke victims. Miss H. is only forty-seven, a librarian, and has mild expressive aphasia. Reading and using numbers, though, are very difficult for her. Even making change in a store is almost impossible. She is withdrawn and depressed. Most of my work with her has been on practical skills: writing checks, adding and subtracting, reading advertisements to find bargains. She is improving, but progress is slow. The other is sixty-eight. Mr. B. is paralyzed on the right side and has global aphasia. Even though he can only utter a word or two, he is always in good humor. I am working on a communication board so that he can express his needs by pointing to the appropriate picture. My third client is a new **laryngectomy** patient. I am working with Mr. L. three days a week, trying to help him learn to inject air into the top of his **esophagus** and then quickly push it back out. He gets frustrated pretty easily, and his language

Laryngectomy.
The surgical removal of the larynx.

Esophagus.
The tube leading from the throat to the stomach.

is sure salty at times, but he really tries hard. I've found that when people have to pay me directly for my services they work harder and, heaven knows, so do I.

My latest project involves a plan to provide services to geriatric patients. I am negotiating with the administrators of two nursing homes. In one of the homes I found a man with Parkinson's disease, another with severe **dysarthria** following surgery for oral cancer, and three aphasics. Many of the residents are severely hard-of-hearing, and I will see that they are tested and treated. I think more university graduate programs should emphasize the potential benefits of speech therapy with elderly persons. In my judgment, communication is one of the keys to a healthy and happy old age, and professionals in our field certainly know more about communication than most other professionals working with the elderly.

Several former students, after gaining experience in other settings, now serve as practicum supervisors in university speech and hearing programs. Here is how one of these graduates described her work.

I have the best job in the whole world! Sometimes I feel guilty on payday because I am having so much fun doing what I do. Today, for instance, I met a group of students for breakfast. We are planning an intensive treatment program for an adult stutterer. It is a real joy to see their teamwork and sense the group support when a number of clinicians combine forces. It takes a lot of planning, though, to come off well.

Then I gave a lecture to a class on therapy methods. We had a lively discussion about behavior modification versus a more authentic communication approach. Next I supervised a student working with a preschool language delayed child, wrote some reports, and previewed a film to show during practicum meeting.

I miss having a caseload of my own, so I do as much demonstration therapy as I can. This afternoon I had a session with a student from Cambodia to improve his **articulation** of English speech sounds. I also work twice a week with an adolescent boy who has a repaired cleft palate. I accepted him as a challenge: He has had several operations on his mouth, countless evaluations, and many years of speech therapy. He is still **hypernasal,** and his motivation is very low. Instead of voice therapy for the nasality, I am concentrating on his articulation of **plosive** sounds. His progress is slow, and he is always testing me in therapy, but I think we are getting somewhere.

The best part of my role at the university, though, is the relationships I have with students. Their enthusiasm, fresh perspectives, and energy are contagious.

Here is an account of a day well spent by a speech pathologist who works with patients who have little or no speech.

I am employed by a large city hospital and my duties are mainly with patients who have great difficulty in communicating at all. Among them

---

Dysarthria.
Group of motor speech impairments that stem from neuromotor damage; may disturb respiration, phonation, articulation, resonance, and prosody.

Articulation.
The utterance of the individual speech sounds.

Hypernasality (Rhinolalia aperta).
Excessively nasal voice quality.

Plosive.
A speech sound characterized by the sudden release of a puff of air. Examples are /p/, /t/, and /g/.

are stroke patients with aphasia or **apraxia,** parkinsonism, dysarthria due to **cerebral palsy** and other neurological disorders.

Although much of my caseload is made up of patients in the hospital, I also make some homecalls and work closely with physical and occupational therapists and other health professionals as we try to provide some way so these persons can communicate. Some have no speech at all; most are unintelligible. Basically, what I do is to teach these patients a way to communicate without talking.

You asked for a sample day's work. Well, first this morning I saw a patient whose recent head injury has left him hemiplegic and unable to produce anything but jargon although he seems to understand some of what we say if we speak very slowly and simply. To give him some way to cope I brought in a simple communication board and taught him to point to the Yes and No displays with his good left hand, always saying the words when he did so. This was more difficult than it sounds because he had been nodding his head sideways for yes and vertically for no, and the nurses were confused. After some training he was able to respond appropriately when I asked him if he wanted a heavy blanket (which I was sure he didn't, because it was hot in there). I then brought out a more complicated picture board but he was too tired to try it. Not much, but at least a beginning.

My next patient was a severely disabled man with cerebral palsy who is strapped in a wheelchair because of the uncontrollable movements of his arms and legs. He has some language but the involuntary movements of his head and tongue make him almost impossible to understand. I am a member of a team consisting of a physical therapist and an occupational therapist, and our mission was to try to determine whether braces could be constructed that would stabilize one of his extremities so he could point or activate a switching mechanism that would allow him to select an item on a communication board. We'll continue to work on that.

The rest of the morning I spent with a laryngectomy patient trying to improve his use of the electrolarynx. Because he has been unable to learn esophageal speech and is very depressed, I concentrated mainly on teaching him how to articulate more carefully and to simplify his utterances.

Well, that was my morning. This afternoon I must familiarize myself with a computerized communication aid the hospital has just purchased. I'm also scheduled for some additional **dysphagia** training so we'll be able to provide better help for patients who are having swallowing difficulties. I guess this is going to be one of my rough days, but most of them are very good and there's always a new challenge.

These brief pictures of the field of speech pathology just sketch the surface of the topography. You have seen just a few of the many opportunities that exist within its boundaries and only a few of the many kinds of communication disorders that need help. Some members of the profession continue their education in doctoral programs where they are able to become even more highly specialized clinicians or perhaps to prepare for

Apraxia.
Loss of ability to make voluntary movements such as producing speech sounds, while involuntary movements remain intact; caused by neurologic damage.

Cerebral palsy.
A group of disorders due to brain injury in which the motor coordinations are especially affected. Most common forms are athetosis, spasticity, and ataxia.

Dysphagia.
Disorder of swallowing due to neck or mouth injury or to a neurological condition.

academic faculty positions. Others seek the doctorate as preparation for research careers in university or other laboratory settings where communication disorders or basic communication sciences are studied. Moreover, for some workers, the profession provides an initial stepping stone to other fields of service.

Public school clinicians, because they come into close contact with many teachers and principals, and because they work with so many children with other handicaps, may end up administering programs in special education. Because such persons often are qualified also as classroom teachers, they may shift into that occupation. Since much of their work in clinical settings involves testing and diagnosis as well as individual and family counseling, some speech pathologists also go into clinical psychology. Still others have become health care managers.

Many individuals, including some whose initial interests were directed toward speech pathology, pursue careers in the profession of audiology. The decision to focus on audiology typically occurs during undergraduate studies, although most of the specialized courses and practicum experiences usually have been available only at the graduate level. Much of the undergraduate coursework in basic communication processes—for example, anatomy and physiology, acoustics, and speech science—is applicable to both professions, of course. And all speech-language pathologists must take some courses concerned with problems of deafness and hearing impairment, just as all audiologists must have some preparation related to speech and language disorders.

Like speech pathologists, audiologists work in a variety of settings. Some are employed in school system positions, others in hospitals and free-standing clinics, community speech and hearing centers, or university clinics. Audiologists often are associated with otology practices, working closely with physicians who specialize in the diagnosis and treatment of ear and hearing problems. Some audiologists are involved directly with the fitting and dispensing of hearing aids, increasingly as the owners of private corporations. The audiologist also is found in industry trying to prevent noise-induced hearing loss, conducting noise surveys to assess noise pollution, and documenting the status of employees' hearing. One of our former students, an audiologist in a hospital speech and hearing department, gives this picture of his professional day.

I spent the eight o'clock hour on correspondence and reports of yesterday's testing. Then at nine o'clock I examined a patient with otosclerosis referred by the **otologist** who is considering performing a **stapedectomy.** For various reasons, this took longer than I expected and I was late for my next appointment with a patient I had previously tested and who was ready for hearing aid selection and orientation. She found it very hard to decide on the aid that seemed to help her the most. She said they all sounded "too noisy." She's had a hearing loss for so long, she's forgotten what the world of sound is like. And I guess she expected,

Otologist.
Physician who specializes in hearing disorders and diseases; typically an *otorhinolaryngologist (ENT).*

Stapedectomy.
Surgical removal of the stapes and implantation of a prosthesis; used in treatment of otosclerosis.

like most of my clients, that the hearing aid would not be just an aid but would restore her hearing completely. Took a lot of delicate counseling. Then in the early afternoon I conducted an aural rehabilitation session. Next I tested a man who had been in an industrial accident and claimed it had deafened him totally. It hadn't; he was **malingering.** Then I examined the eardrum of a teenager with a complaint of fullness in her ear and ended my day by calibrating one of our audiometers. Every day is different, but that's the way this one went.

Another audiologist told us of her day in the schools.

I am one of five specialists for the hearing impaired who serve Kalamazoo County. As such I travel from school to school helping deaf and hearing-impaired students. My caseload consists of twenty-four youngsters. The first thing I did this morning was to check the auditory amplification equipment at Amberly school to be sure it was working properly. Then I saw one of my students who has been doing poorly in her school work, finding that she has not been wearing her hearing aid because it makes her feel conspicuous. She has long hair but combs it straight back, so I showed her a new hairdo that would cover the aid and make her more attractive, too. I also arranged for preferential seating in her classroom and discovered that her teacher did not know she had a hearing loss.

Next, I spent an hour with a fourth-grade boy to improve his lip-reading skills. From there I traveled to Vicksburg and conferred with the parents of a boy who had been evaluated recently at the Constance Brown Hearing and Speech Center. Jim has otitis media and needs medical attention, but his parents said they could not afford it. I explained the seriousness of the problem to them and arranged for them to talk with a caseworker at Social Services about obtaining help. I'm sure they'll follow through, but I will make a point of checking back next week.

I then met with a school psychologist about a high-school girl with a moderate bilateral loss who has been refusing to recite in class and even refused to talk to him. I made an appointment to see her on my rounds next week. She may just need to talk to someone who understands the stress she is under.

At Edison school after lunch I helped a deaf girl prepare for a speech she has to give tomorrow in her social studies class on "Sign Language." She had been very worried about it, but after some suggestions and two rehearsals she felt much better.

Then I did audiological screening tests on three kindergarten children referred to me by their teachers. I found that one of them will need to be seen for more thorough testing. Finally, I returned to my office, wrote reports, made a few phone calls and updated my files. Every day has its own challenges, and I always find the work varied and interesting. A good job.

In recent years, we must note, the scope of professional activities in which some audiologists are engaged has been undergoing a rapid and

Malingering.
The conscious
simulation of a disorder.

Aural.
Pertaining to hearing.

Cochlear implant.
Surgically implanted device that directly stimulates the auditory nerve when an externally worn component receives sound input; used only with severely hearing impaired individuals who are unable to benefit from a hearing aid.

dynamic expansion that is not adequately reflected in our two reports. Beyond the administration and interpretation of traditional hearing tests of various types (Figure 1-4), and in addition to **aural** rehabilitation and environmental and occupational hearing conservation, audiologists also may be involved with electrophysiological assessment of balance as well as auditory systems. They also are called upon to evaluate assistive listening equipment and, in some settings, to be knowledgeable about such devices as **cochlear implants.** These changes have led to reexamination of the academic and clinical preparation appropriate for entering the profession and in the foreseeable future may dictate changes in the minimum qualifications expected of beginning practitioners.

Many of you who read this book are not planning to become professional speech pathologists or audiologists, but all of you are certain to encounter adults and children who cannot speak normally or who are hearing impaired, for there are at least 42 million such persons (not all persons with these impairments are regarded, in legal terms, as having disabilities) in our country alone (National Deafness and Other Commu-

 FIGURE 1-4
Traditional Pure Tone Hearing Testing *(Van Riper Clinic, Western Michigan University)*

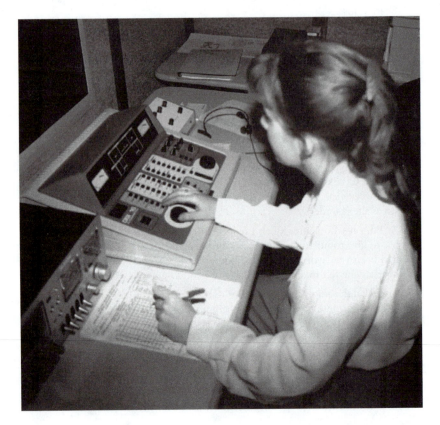

nication Disorders Advisory Board, 1991). And with the growing population of older citizens, the number with communication disorders also will grow. Will you turn away from their need for help and understanding? Will you add one more rejection to the many they have already endured? Or will you do what you can? Here is an excerpt from a letter written us by a former student who eventually became an elementary classroom teacher.

> Although I only had the introductory course in speech pathology I've often been able to help a few children with speech problems right in my classroom. I've been teaching third grade now for three years and love it. Wouldn't do anything else. I've steered clear of the severe speech disorders because we have a speech therapist who visits our school twice each week and who knows a lot more than I do, but I've been able to help the gains she gets become more permanent by following her suggestions with my children who **lisp** or cannot pronounce their *r* or *l* sounds. We also consult quite often about improving the communication skills of students in general.
>
> Well, anyway, at lunch hour I asked her why she didn't take Joe for therapy. Joe's a very bad stutterer when he recites, which is seldom. Her answer was that Joe's mother had refused permission to let him have any speech help this year, so her hands were tied. She said that Joe's mother was a mild stutterer herself and perhaps that was why, though it didn't make sense. I told the therapist that Joe never volunteered in class and usually answered my questions in as few words as possible or said he didn't know when I was pretty sure he did. And when I told her too that Joe rarely went out with the other children to play at recess time, the therapist asked me to find out why. So today, when he stayed in again, I asked Joe about it when we were by ourselves. Tears came in his eyes and he said it was because he "talked funny" and the other kids teased him. And he even asked me if I would teach him to talk better. Of course I said yes and we made a date to begin after school tomorrow. I put in a frantic call to the speech therapist and she will coach me and help out indirectly. She said that there was lots that I could do and I'm sure there is. At least I can make it easier for him. Poor little kid! I was really touched when, just before he left to get on the bus, he came up to my desk and shyly touched my hand. That's all—just a touch, and then he ran out.

As you can see from these few brief glimpses, speech pathologists and audiologists work in a variety of settings and serve a wide range of clients. But what they share in common are enthusiasm for their professions and a very personal dedication to the welfare of individuals with speech, language, and hearing disorders. They are concerned about the unfortunate; they devote their lives to the relief of human distress. But there is something more—and it is difficult to put into words. When we deal with communication disorders, we deal with the essence of humankind. Only human beings have mastered speech. It sets us apart from all other species.

Lisp.
An articulatory disorder characterized by defective sibilant sounds such as the /s/ and /z/.

Because we can speak, we can think symbolically; and it is this that has enabled us to survive and usually thrive, to begin to understand our earth, and even to begin to explore outer space. Dimly we believe, or at least hope, that someday it may enable us to master ourselves.

STUDY QUESTIONS

1. What is the origin of the word "handicapped"? What term(s) other than "handicap" are often preferred, and why?
2. What historic examples do the authors provide to illustrate the cruelty and rejection encountered over the years by persons with deformities and disabilities?
3. What current examples can you cite, from the movies or from television, where an abnormality or disability has been portrayed in a way intended somehow to be humorous?
4. Certain events in the early to mid-1900s helped to promote more compassionate attitudes toward people with disabilities. What were these events, and for what reasons might they have led many people to be a bit more sensitive and caring?
5. The past four decades have seen the enactment of laws and regulations designed to help ensure that the rights of people with disabilities are recognized and protected. Describe the major types of legislation which have focused on this issue.
6. What advice can you give to a friend who is worried about how he or she should behave while communicating with a classmate who stutters? How should you alter your own speech when talking, for example, with a person who has become aphasic following a stroke?
7. With what other professionals do speech pathologists and audiologists work to ensure that their clients' needs are served?
8. In what types of settings are we likely to find audiologists or speech-language pathologists employed?
9. For what reasons do some audiologists urge that the minimum qualifications for their profession be made more rigorous?
10. What basic similarities and common interests are shared by audiologists and speech-language pathologists?

ENDNOTES

[1]The terms *speech pathologist* and *speech clinician* are used interchangeably in this text rather than *speech therapist,* because the latter term tends to imply an auxiliary service to the medical profession. Another current but somewhat cumber-

some title for workers in this profession is *speech-language pathologist* or *speech-language clinician.*

[2]Words in boldface print are among the terms you will find defined in the Glossary.

REFERENCES

Carey, A. (1992). Americans with Disabilities Act and you. *Asha, 34,* 7–8.

National Deafness and Other Communication Disorders Advisory Board. (1991). *Research in human communication* (NIH Publication No. 92-3317). Bethesda, MD: National Institute on Deafness and Other Communication Disorders.

SUGGESTED READINGS

These sources can provide additionally informative insights for the curious student.

American Speech-Language-Hearing Association. (1992). Report on professional education in audiology. *Asha, 34,* 58–63.

Emerick, L. (1984). *Speaking for ourselves: Self-portraits of the speech or hearing handicapped.* Danville, IL: Interstate Publishers.

Helm-Estabrooks, N., et al. (1994). Speech-language pathology: Moving toward the 21st century. *American Journal of Speech-Language Pathology, 3 (3),* 23–47.

Keller, H. (1954). *The story of my life.* New York: Doubleday.

Roush, J. (1991). Early intervention: Expanding the audiologist's role. *Asha, 33,* 47–49.

Sarachan-Deily, A. (1992). Beyond the one-room schoolhouse. *Asha, 34,* 34–37.

Shapiro, J. (1993). *No pity.* New York: Times Books.

Basic Components of Speech and Language

In the beginning there was communication. The ongoing exchange of messages, in one form or another, connects all living creatures in a never-ending circle. Brontosauri did it, birds do it, even honey bees do it; but it is only in humans that we find language being used as a most remarkably facile means of sharing information. And, although other modalities also are utilized, speech is the most common and important way in which we use language to communicate.

Those of us who seek to understand and help individuals who have communication disorders should first understand as thoroughly as possible the nature of communication, language, and speech and how they are related. In this chapter we will take a few steps along the path toward these understandings.

The act of communication is a process, not an entity. In its simplest form it consists of the *transfer of a message from a sender to a receiver.* The message may be verbal, nonverbal, chemical, electromagnetic, and so on. In the case of humans, the basic unit of communication typically involves a speaker and one or more listeners. We listen, too, when we speak, of course, and sometimes we talk aloud to ourselves when we are uncertain or trying to accomplish a very difficult task, such as assembling a complex toy on Christmas Eve. The flow of messages is reflexive; when a listener has processed the information, he generally lets the speaker know what impact it has had (**feedback**).

Before we begin to describe the ways in which speech pathologists treat the various communication disorders, it is necessary to provide you with some essential information about the speech mechanism, the types of speech sounds, the basic structure of our language, and how we shape sound waves into speech. When you are acquainted with how oral communication is organized and regulated, you will be in a much better position to understand a malfunction of the system and what needs to be done to correct it. An understanding of abnormality most logically stems from an appreciation of the normal. Although the act of talking is extremely complex, probably the most intricate of all human behaviors, in this introductory text we present only its most salient features. Our discussion begins with an overview of the interrelationships among communication, language, and speech.

While all living creatures communicate, only humans exchange information using a code that we call language. Only the human species has devised an *elaborate system of shared symbols and procedures for combining them into meaningful units.* The key words in the definition are that there is a *system,* which implies an order or regularity in the supply of symbols; that these symbols are *shared* or hold common meanings for a group of persons; and that there are *procedures* or rules concerning how to array or join the symbols into messages.

During your first few years, you and a million other babies accomplished something that you could not possibly do now, not even if you

Feedback.
The backflow of information concerning the output of a motor system. Auditory feedback refers to self-hearing; kinesthetic feedback to the self-perception of one's movements.

spent the rest of your life at the task. You learned to understand a strange new language and to speak it like a native. Moreover, you learned that language easily. Without any formal instruction you perfected your pronunciation of its sounds, acquired a large number of meaningful words, and mastered the hidden linguistic rules that appropriately link these words together in phrases and sentences of incredible variety.

Present linguistic theory holds that this incredibly difficult achievement is possible only due to an inborn trait of all human beings—the capacity for language acquisition. Attempts to explain the phenomenal rapidity of that acquisition solely in terms of learning theory have not been very satisfactory, although learning, of course, must be involved. Otherwise, some of us wouldn't be speaking English while others are talking Swahili. Linguists distinguish language *competence* from language *performance,* the former referring to the knowledge of the features and structure of language and the latter to its use in communication. They speak of a "universal language competence" as being innate in all human beings and a "particular language competence," which reflects how well a person knows a particular language such as Spanish or Thai or English.

Performance is assessed by observing how a person actually uses language when **encoding** (speaking, writing, using signs) or decoding (listening, reading) in a typical day-to-day situation. When we ask a client to distinguish sentences from nonsentences or to recognize an ambiguous statement, we are evaluating language competence (Figure 2-1).

Although it is possible to teach a parrot or a child who is mentally retarded to echo "Polly wants a cracker," the bird will not have any true language and the child may have very little. Without competence one cannot generate new sentences. Although the parrot may have said that one sentence a thousand times, it could never transform it into such an utterance as "Polly wants a drink" no matter how thirsty it was. Nor could the child express a desire for water if his teachers had merely asked him to repeat that same utterance about crackers over and over again. He needs language, not just the facsimile of speech. Some of the most difficult clients

Encoding.
Process of converting an idea into an audible or visual signal.

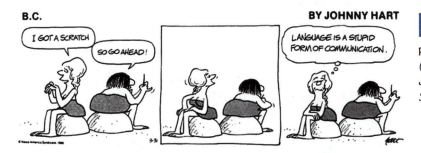

B.C.   BY JOHNNY HART

FIGURE 2-1
Language is powerful—but also fragile
(Used by permission of Johnny Hart and Creators Syndicate, Inc.)

with whom the speech clinician must work are those with **echolalia.** These children parrot the speech of others, often with remarkable fidelity, but they do not know what they are saying and they cannot communicate their wants. They lack the particular language competence they need. They can "speak," but they cannot speak our language, for they have not discovered the basic structure of that language.

The clinician also works with some clients (for example, persons with severe cerebral palsy, or aphasia, or with traumatic brain injuries, or persons in the early stages of a degenerative neurological disease) who may be unable to use language in a conventional manner. In such instances, a system may be devised whereby the individual can express messages by pointing to, or otherwise selecting, pictures or symbols or printed words or letters. Alternatively, signing or some simplified system of manual gestures might be used. In some cases a computer or other electronic device may be used to generate audible or visible signals. The essential objective, of course, is to establish (or re-establish) a communicative link between the client and other persons.

We are not sure how a human infant acquires his or her competence in a particular language. Certainly he or she must be exposed to it. Kaspar Hauser, imprisoned when a child and isolated for sixteen years, acquired no speech at all and remained almost mute despite intensive training by the best teachers of his time. Kamala, the Wolf Girl of India, Victor, the Wild Boy of Aveyron, and Lucas, the Baboon Boy of Africa, were physically normal but not one of these abandoned children raised by animals ever acquired meaningful speech. Evidently the propensity of human beings to acquire language (universal competence) must be triggered by close contact with other humans

Moreover, the contact must be a significant, meaningful one. A child exposed only to the constant chatter of a radio or a television screen would not master our language although she might be able to repeat a few commercials. *She must be spoken to by someone important to her and encouraged to respond.* There must be both models and involvement. There must be identification both ways. When a speech pathologist finds a child with very deficient language ability, he knows that somehow he must provide for that child another involved human being with whom the child can identify. Usually that person is the clinician himself.

Communication, language, speech—and the greatest of these is communication, for if there is no communication, there is nothing but isolation and despair. The need to exchange messages, in some form, is critical to being human.

"If Duane could only speak," the parents of a child with profound retardation told us recently, "he would be . . . more normal." It was difficult for them to understand, as it has been for many parents of language-delayed children, that without symbols a youngster does not have much to say. Most laypersons tend to confuse language and speech.

Echolalia.
The automatic involuntary repetition of heard phrases and sentences.

Perhaps an analogy will help. When an orchestra is playing a tune, the music (language) is being performed (speech) by the various instruments. Without the music of Mozart, Rogers, or Dylan, a tuba, guitar, or French horn would only produce meaningless noise; without language, speech would only be jargon. Speech is a language-dependent behavior: A person can talk only to the level of his language ability.

We define speech, then, as the *audible manifestation of language*. By a complex, and still rather mysterious, process called encoding, a speaker converts an idea in his mind into a stream of sounds; moving his lips, tongue, and jaws in swift, precise gestures, he transmits information in orderly audible segments. When a listener decodes the signal back into an idea in his mind—the same idea, it is hoped, that the speaker intended!—the act of oral communication is completed (see Figure 2-2).

The human miracle—the acquisition of speech and language—becomes even more astounding when we consider the complexity of the task. Even the instrument that the infant must master if he is to speak a language is so complicated in its structure and manipulation that it seems impossible that a baby could ever learn to play it at all, let alone be required to become a virtuoso. If you were given a trumpet and told to play the overture to Wagner's *Tannhäuser*, you'd be in a similar situation. Let us examine the human instrument.

you must be able to understand the lang.- word + sent. formation in order to speak it!

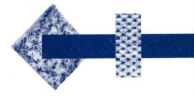

THE SPEECH MECHANISM

In Figure 2-3 we see the instrument all of us must learn to play if we are to speak. The structures detailed in our upper drawing include those that you probably would first consider if asked to define the speech mechanism. The lower drawing places the upper one in perspective and reminds us that the entire respiratory system also is part of this elegant instrument. Actually, of course, we also would need to depict the auditory system and

FIGURE 2-2   The Speech Chain: The process of talking connects speaker and listener (P. Denes and E. Pinson, *The Speech Chain*. New York: Doubleday, 1973)

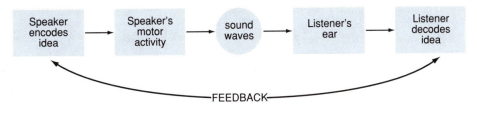

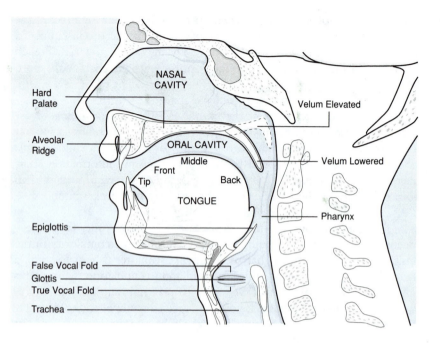

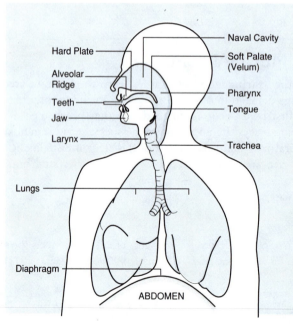

FIGURE 2-3
The speech
mechanism and
respiratory tract

the central and peripheral nervous systems in order to represent more fully the complete speech mechanism. And, indeed, we will return shortly to a discussion of these latter systems.

Even in simplified terms, however, the speech mechanism is more complicated (and more versatile) than any instrument to be found in a symphony orchestra. It seems almost impossible that a child could master it, but most babies do so with relatively little difficulty. This accomplishment seems even more amazing when we realize that these structures actually serve other fundamental life-sustaining functions.[1]

The primary function of the lungs is not for speaking but for oxygenating the blood; the larynx (pronounced "lair-inks") is basically a valve to keep foreign material from entering the lungs; and the throat, tongue, teeth, and lips are for the intake and chewing and swallowing of food. Accordingly, speech is said to be a *secondary* or *overlaid* function of these structures. Even when we are "scared speechless" we continue to breathe.

Respiration

When we inhale we use our muscles to lift and slightly rotate our ribs, thereby expanding our chest **(thorax),** in which the lungs are situated. Simultaneously, the **diaphragm** (which forms the muscular floor of the chest cavity) is lowered, further expanding the thorax (and compressing the contents of the abdomen). This thoracic expansion creates a negative pressure, or vacuum, inside the chest cavity. As a result, air flows in through the mouth and nose, down through the throat **(pharynx),** between the vocal folds in the larynx, on downward through the **trachea** and bronchial tubes, finally reaching and inflating the lungs. In addition to the diaphragm and the external intercostal muscles of the chest, many other muscles will have been actively contracted during this inspiratory part of the respiratory cycle.

In order for us to exhale, on the other hand, all that actually must occur is that we relax the contraction of inspiratory muscles. Thus, during ongoing breathing for life, *inhalation is an active process,* while *exhalation is passive.* Relaxing the contracted muscles of inhalation allows the rib cage to return to its resting position and allows the compressed abdominal contents to expand. Our chest cavity begins to lose its expansion, and air begins its exit from the lungs. Gravity also exerts a downward pull on the elevated ribs; and, due to their elasticity, the lungs themselves will recoil toward a resting size (just as an inflated balloon will recoil toward its deflated state when its neck is released). All of these passive forces combine to force out of our lungs the air that we just inhaled. This inhalation-exhalation cycle is repeated regularly several times per minute in relaxed "vegetative" breathing, and the amount of air we exchange during each cycle (in an adult, about half a quart, on the average) is known as our *tidal volume.*

Thorax.
Chest.

Diaphragm.
Sheet of muscle separating the thorax from the abdomen; contraction expands the thorax for inhalation of air.

Pharynx.
The throat cavity.

Trachea.
The windpipe.

Tidal volume.
The amount of air inhaled or exhaled during one cycle of quiet relaxed breathing.

When we are breathing for speech the respiratory system works differently than it does when merely oxygenating our blood in relaxed tidal breathing. Typically, we inhale much more quickly and a bit more deeply while we are speaking. Moreover, we do not now immediately relax the muscles of inhalation as we begin to speak. Instead, after inhalation we must control the exhalation of air very precisely in order to maintain just the right rate of airflow and the amount of pressure needed to "drive" the speech mechanism. We achieve this controlled (and prolonged) exhalation by "checking," or restraining, the relaxation of inspiratory muscles. If we did not do so, the air would come flowing out too rapidly and too forcefully for normal speech (a condition that we sometimes observe, by the way, in the speech of individuals with certain neuromuscular disorders). As our exhalation continues, we reach a level of lung volume where the passive expiratory forces are no longer so great, but this "relaxation pressure" still may be sufficient for speaking purposes. Then, if we continue to speak without taking in another supply of air, the relaxation pressure will become negligible and we will need to contract some of our abdominal and thoracic muscles of expiration to maintain the requisite driving force.

Already we can understand that speaking involves complex respiratory adjustments, and we've only just begun. As you might expect, such factors as speaking rate, loudness, and pitch further complicate these adjustments. And, as you would anticipate, a variety of medical conditions such as emphysema and asthma, in addition to muscle and nerve disorders, can impact significantly on speech breathing.

Phonation

The larynx, a delicate and very important part of the speech mechanism, is suspended in our neck beneath the hyoid bone (the only bone in our body that does not articulate with any other bone) and above the trachea (or windpipe). The sound of the human voice **(phonation)** is produced by paired vocal folds, one on the left and one on the right, which lie within the major cartilage of the larynx, the **thyroid cartilage.** The vocal folds are joined together at the front of the larynx where they attach to the thyroid cartilage just below and behind the "Adam's apple." From this attachment they extend horizontally backward to attach to the right and left arytenoid cartilages, respectively.

Each vocal fold is a relatively thick shelf of tissue consisting of layers of muscle and ligament covered by **epithelium.** Although they sometimes have been called vocal *cords,* they actually have no resemblance to cords or strings. They are thicker in men than in women and thicker in adults than in children (which accounts for the pitch differences which we hear), but they are never very long, averaging something less than one inch in length even in the large larynx of an adult male.

Phonation.
Voice.

Thyroid cartilage.
The major cartilage of the larynx; notch of the thyroid is often called the "Adam's apple."

Epithelium.
Cellular tissue that forms a lining for body cavities and covers body surface.

When the vocal folds are relaxed, as they are when we are engaged in silent tidal breathing, they are positioned much as we see them in Figure 2-4, with an opening between them called the **glottis.** In this drawing we are looking downward from the very back of the mouth, and at the top of our drawing (the front of the throat), we barely see just a bit of the base of the tongue. Looking between the vocal folds and down through the glottis, we can even see a few of the uppermost cartilaginous rings of the trachea.

If we were to observe this same larynx from the same point while its owner was breathing rapidly and deeply (during strenuous exercise, for example), we would find the arytenoid cartilages, hence also the vocal folds, more widely separated. This increased size of the space between the folds is necessary to permit more rapid passage of air in and out of the lungs during forceful breathing. In contrast, if we could observe the scene during a swallow we would see the arytenoids and vocal folds being drawn tightly together in the midline, closing the glottis completely in order to help ensure that food or liquid does not enter the airway. The **epiglottis,** just in front of and above the vocal folds, also tilts backward to assist in this protection of the airway.

As we prepare to phonate, we begin to draw the arytenoids and vocal folds together to close the glottis. Then, as air pressure from the lungs begins to build up beneath the vocal folds, the *front* membranous portion (but not the back cartilaginous portion) of the glottis is forced to open. The opening is small and brief, and the vocal folds come back together quickly as the air pressure subsides. For as long as voicing continues, this cycle of glottal opening and closing repeats itself over and over, very rapidly (up to several hundred times per second when a soprano is singing a very high-pitched tone). A tiny puff of air passes through the glottis each time it opens. These air puffs set into vibration the column of air above the larynx, producing voice in much the way tones are produced in a pipe organ.

Glottis.
The space between the vocal cords when they are not brought together.

Epiglottis.
The shieldlike cartilage that hovers over the front of the larynx.

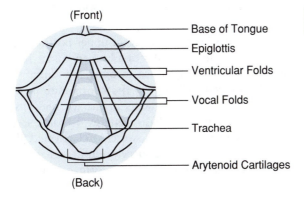

 FIGURE 2-4   Vocal folds seen from above

(Front)
— Base of Tongue
— Epiglottis
— Ventricular Folds
— Vocal Folds
— Trachea
— Arytenoid Cartilages
(Back)

We hear slow vibrations as low-pitched phonation. More rapid vibrations are perceived as being higher in pitch. The perceived loudness of a voice is determined basically by how much air pressure is built up beneath the vocal folds, how tightly the glottis is closed, and how widely the folds are blown apart during vibration.

Before we leave the larynx, we should note that each of us possesses another pair of membranous folds that are situated directly above the vocal folds. These are called **ventricular folds,** sometimes known as **false vocal folds.** The ventricular folds also can be drawn together to close off the airway, but this usually will happen only during swallowing, defecating, or grunting, or during a brief exertion of strong physical effort. Sometimes, when a person habitually uses excessive laryngeal tension during phonation, the ventricular folds may be squeezed closely enough together that they mask any view of the true vocal folds from above. The voice then may sound very tense and strained, but it still is being produced by the true (albeit hyperfunctioning) vocal folds. However, there are some individuals who use their ventricular folds to produce voice. The extremely strained, harsh sound heard in such cases is called *ventricular* **dysphonia.** This disorder occurs very rarely, and usually only when the true vocal folds have been damaged.

Resonation

The sound produced by our vibrating vocal folds is a complex periodic tone consisting of a fundamental frequency—the rate at which vibration is occurring, measured in *cycles per second (cps)* or, more commonly, in **Hertz (Hz)**—and many overtones, or harmonics, at frequencies that are multiples of the fundamental. In some voices, energy also is present at other frequencies in the form of noise. All voices have sound energy present over a very wide range of frequencies. Normally there are greater amounts of energy present in the fundamental and lower frequency **harmonics** than in the higher frequencies. In any event, if you could hear this tone at the level of the larynx you would never recognize it as being a voice. Heard at its source, the voice would sound more like a buzzing tone than like anything human.

Only when a laryngeal tone has been resonated in upper portions of the vocal tract do we recognize its sound as that of a human voice. This process of resonation also enables us to produce recognizably different vowel (and some consonant) sounds. By altering the configurations of our throat and mouth cavities through movements of the tongue, lips, and jaw, we create resonators that will emphasize energy at some frequencies and suppress energy at others. In brief, we can selectively "filter" our laryngeal tones and thereby produce a speech output signal that has been shaped in ways which will convey essential information to the listener.

Ventricular folds. Folds of tissue immediately above the true vocal folds; also known as *false vocal folds.*

False vocal folds. Folds of tissue immediately above the true vocal folds; also known as *ventricular folds.*

Dysphonia. Disorder of voice.

Hertz (Hz). Unit of measurement of rate of vibration of sound source; same as *cycles per second.*

Harmonics. Vibrations that occur at whole number multiples of the fundamental frequency.

Above the pharynx and oral cavities is the nasal cavity, a resonating chamber that also can add to (or subtract from) the original character of the glottal tone. In producing the nasal consonants (*m*, *n*, and *ng*), of course, nasal resonance is an essential and distinguishing feature. During the production of several other of the sounds of our language, however, the addition of nasal resonance can be detrimental. In the extreme (when it could be labelled as hypernasality), it can interfere significantly with our ability to understand the speaker's message. Lesser degrees of nasalization might only be mildly distracting or, in some circumstances, might sound quite normal to the listener.

Fortunately, unless structural or functional limitations are present, we generally are able to control nasalization of the laryngeal tone by adjusting the muscular soft palate (or **velum**) and the pharyngeal walls surrounding it. We can tense and elevate the velum, as well as contract the pharynx, and virtually disconnect the nasal cavity from the rest of the vocal tract. Alternatively, we typically also can permit nasal resonance to occur, when appropriate, by relaxing the muscles of the velum and upper pharynx.

As we shall see in later chapters, not everyone is able to make the rapid and precise adjustments required to avoid excessive nasal resonance. Conversely, for other persons it may be difficult or impossible to add any nasal resonance. In either case, medical intervention may be needed prior to, or in conjunction with, speech therapy.

Articulation

When we watch a skilled piano player's fingers we see an impressive display of coordination, but those who have witnessed X-ray motion pictures of the tongue in action, or who have watched it directly through a plastic window in the cheek of a cancer patient, have observed the ultimate in motor coordination. The precision of the tongue contacts, the constant shift of contours, and the rapidity of sequential movements are almost unbelievable. The articulation of speech sounds, the consonants, vowels, and **diphthongs** that are the basic **phonemic** elements of our language, demands incredibly intricate coordinations of the tongue, lips, **mandible,** and velum. And the movements of these structures must occur in synchrony with those of the respiratory and phonatory systems. It is a minor miracle that most of us have acquired normal articulation skills so uneventfully and that we employ them so automatically.

Certain sounds require the rounding of the lips; some require lip retraction; others demand their firm closure; still others need the upper teeth to be in contact with the lower lip. The mandible must be lowered to help create a larger mouth cavity for some vowels than for others. While adjustments of these types are occurring, the velum and pharyngeal walls also must perform precisely timed movements. Our tongues, perhaps the most remarkably agile of the articulatory structures, continuously must

Velum.
Soft palate.

Diphthong.
Phoneme produced by the blending of two vowel sounds into a single speech sound.

Phoneme.
A "family" of speech sounds that may differ slightly from one another (allophones) with no effect on meaning; the smallest contrastive sound unit in a language.

Mandible.
Lower jaw.

assume different shapes and postures as our speech carries us forward through various combinations of vowels, diphthongs, and consonants.

Before continuing our discussion of speech articulation, however, we should introduce the use of phonetic symbols—tools that greatly facilitate the study of spoken language.

A Phonetic Alphabet.   It is nearly impossible to use the regular orthographic *abc's* of English spelling to represent speech sounds. As you well know, a letter of our written alphabet may represent more than one sound, or *phoneme,* in our spoken language (and, of course, a given phoneme is represented in more than one way in written language). If a non–English-speaking visitor were to ask what sound is represented by the letter *u,* how should you answer? Most likely, you'll have a hard time answering, at least if you pause first to consider how *u* actually does sound in such words as *flu, put, but,* and *upon.* If she had asked what letter is used to represent the vowel sound in the spoken word *do,* your answer would have to take into account words such as *sue, through, flew,* and *boot.* And, speaking of *through,* just imagine how confused your guest will be when she works her way from the correct pronunciation of this word while trying to pronounce *rough, thought,* or *although.*

As noted by MacKay (1987, p. 46), the famous playwright George Bernard Shaw once observed that the word *fish* could just as well be written "ghoti" if we just used the "gh" of *enough,* the "o" of *women,* and the "ti" of *nation.*

In order to minimize these complications and confusions, we will be using the International Phonetic Alphabet (IPA) when we refer to a particular phoneme. Each written symbol of the IPA represents *one,* and *only one,* phoneme, and the IPA also includes diacritical marks that can be used to show features of a misarticulated sound. Anyone preparing to become a speech-language pathologist will take coursework in descriptive phonetics in order to become able to recognize, report, and analyze abnormal articulation; but, even if you are not leaning in the direction of this profession, you will find it very useful to become acquainted with the IPA. And for purposes of this book, our use of the IPA should help to ensure that you understand more exactly how the correct and incorrect articulations of our illustrated therapy clients actually *sound.*

Table 2.1 shows the IPA symbol for each phoneme of our language, though not all possible dialectal variations have been included (and you will find minor variations among certain of its symbols from one source to another). Many IPA symbols correspond pretty directly to familiar alphabetic letters, others you may not have seen before. Alongside each IPA symbol are some key words to help you recognize the referents of unfamiliar symbols. Each key word then is written in phonetic symbols. Whenever we use symbols of the IPA in this book they will be set off from other text by diagonal slash marks, or virgules (/).[2]

TABLE 2.1 The phonetic alphabet

	Key Words			Key Words	
Phonetic Symbol	English	Phonetic	Phonetic Symbol	English	Phonetic
Consonants					
b	*b*ack, *c*ab	bæk, kæb	p	*p*ig, sa*p*	pig, sæp
d	*d*ig, re*d*	dɪg, rɛd	r	*r*at, poo*r*	ræt, pur
f	*f*eel, lea*f*	fil, lif	s	*s*o, mi*ss*	so, mɪs
g	*g*o, e*gg*	go, ɛg	t	*t*o, wi*t*	tu, wɪt
ʤ	*j*ust, e*dg*e	ʤʌst, ɛʤ	ʃ	*sh*e, wi*sh*	ʃi, wɪʃ
h	*h*e be*h*aves	hi, bɪhevz	ʧ	*ch*in, it*ch*	ʧɪn, ɪʧ
k	*k*eep, tra*ck*	kip, træk	θ	*th*ink tru*th*	θɪŋk truθ
l	*l*ow, ba*ll*	lo, bɔl	ð	*th*en, ba*the*	ðɛn, beð
ļ	simp*le*, fab*le*	simpļ, febļ	v	*v*est, li*ve*	vɛst, lɪv
m	*m*y, ai*m*	maɪ, em	w	*w*e, s*w*im	wi, swim
m̩	kingdo*m*, mad*am*	kɪŋdm̩, mædm̩	hw	*wh*ere, *wh*en	hwɛr, hwɛn
n	*n*ot, a*n*y	nɑt, ɛnɪ	j	*y*ell, *y*oung	jɛl, jʌŋ
n̩	ac*ti*on, mis*si*on	æk ʃn̩, mɪn̩	ʒ	mea*s*ure, ver*s*ion	mɛʒɚ, vɝʒn̩
ŋ	si*ng*, u*n*cle	sɪŋ, ʌŋkļ	z	*z*ebra, o*z*one	zibrə, ozon
ʔ	oh oh!	ʔo ʔo			
Vowels					
a*	f*a*r, s*a*d	far, sad	ɒ*	la*w*, wr*o*ng	lɒ, rɒŋ
ɑ	f*a*ther, m*o*p	fɑðɚ, mɑp	ɝ	*ear*ly, b*ir*d	ɝlɪ, bɝd
e	gr*ea*t, *a*che	gret, ek	ɜ*	*ear*ly b*ir*d	ɜlɪ bɜd
æ	s*a*d, s*a*ck	sæd, sæk	ɚ	p*er*haps, nev*er*	pɚhæps, nɛvɚ
i	intr*i*gue, m*e*	intrig, mi	u	t*o*, y*ou*	tu, ju
ɛ	h*ea*d, r*e*st	hɛd, rɛst	ʊ	p*u*dding, c*oo*k	pʊdɪŋ, kʊk
ɪ	h*i*s, *i*tch	hɪz, ɪʧ	ʌ	m*o*ther, dr*u*g	mʌðɚ, drʌg
o	*o*wn, b*o*ne	on, bon	ə	*a*bove, s*u*ppose	əbʌv, səpoz
ɔ	*a*ll, d*o*g	ɔl, dɔg			
Diphthongs					
aɪ	m*y*, *eye*	maɪ, aɪ	ɔɪ	t*oy*, b*oi*l	tɔɪ, bɔɪl
au	c*ow*, ab*ou*t	kau, əbaut			

(continued)

TABLE 2.1   CONTINUED

Key Words			Key Words		
Phonetic Symbol	English	Phonetic	Phonetic Symbol	English	Phonetic

			Centering Diphthongs		
ɛr	*wear*, *fair*	wɛr, fɛr	ɪr	*beer, weird*	bɪr, wɪrd
ɑr	*barn*, *far*	bɑrn, fɑr	aɪr	*wire, tire*	waɪr, taɪr
ʊr	*lure*, m*oor*	lʊr, mʊr	aʊr	*hour, flower*	aʊr, flaʊr
ɔr	sh*ore*, b*orn*	ʃɔr, bɔrn			

Some Additional IPA Signs and Symbols

:	sign to prolong the preceding sound: [ʌnːɛsəsɛrɪ]	ǀ	comma; pause
ʰ	sign to release consonant breathily: [tʰek]	ʍ	a *hw* made as a single sound
ˈ	primary stress mark: [ˈsæləd]	ɹ	a trilled *r*
ˌ	secondary stress mark: [ˈsælə, mændɚ]	ˆ	lateral [ŝ]
ʔ	the glottal stop	ω	rounded [r̫]
.	syllabic consonant sign: [sɪmpl̩]	~	nasalized [ã]

*Sounds commonly used in the East and South.

Vowels.   Vowels are produced in a relatively open vocal tract and all require laryngeal tone (voicing). The contours of our tongues vary with each vowel, for there are front, middle, and back vowels, each vowel family having several members distinguished by the height of the tongue constriction and the amount and rounding of the lip opening. Thus the /u/ vowel as in *flute* /flut/, for example, is the highest back vowel and has the narrowest lip rounding while the *ee* /i/ is the highest front vowel. Notice, too, how your jaw opens and closes again when you utter the vowels /i/, /a/, and then /u/. The central vowels such as /ʌ/ or /ə/ are produced with the tongue lying in an almost neutral, or nearly relaxed, position on the floor of the mouth cavity. The position of the primary vowels is shown schematically in Figure 2-5 by superimposing an enlarged vowel quadrilateral on a side view of the oral cavity. Keep in mind, though, that there is considerable variation from individual to individual in the production of both vowels and consonants.

Diphthongs.   A diphthong (/dɪfθɔŋ/), in the simplest sense, is a phoneme that involves the combination of two different vowel sounds.

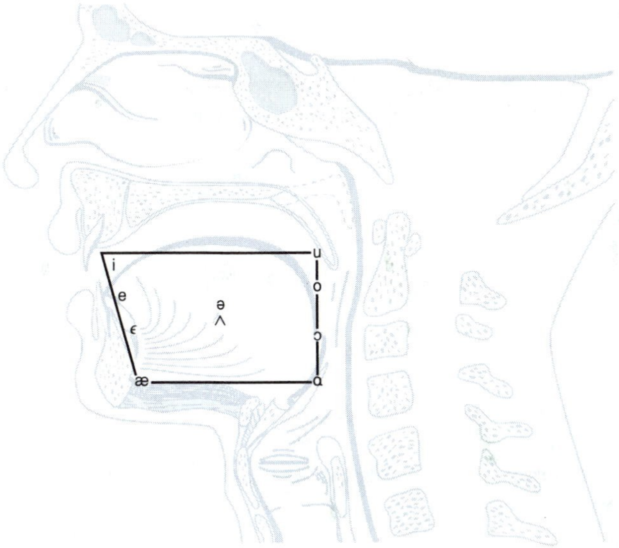

FIGURE 2-5 The primary vowel positions shown in enlarged schematic relationship to their respective tongue placements within the oral cavity

As we see in Table 2.1, for example, the second phoneme in the word *cow* is a diphthong that begins as the vowel /a/ and ends as the vowel /ʊ/. As you say this diphthong aloud you will indeed feel the changing postures of your tongue and lips as you move from one vowel into the next. Some of our vowels tend routinely to be diphthongized if they are at all prolonged or emphasized in a word. Some versions of the IPA will show /eɪ/ and /oʊ/ diphthongs, for example. Prolong your utterance of an /e/ or /o/ to feel for yourself the shifting positions. We have chosen to simplify our approach at this point, however, using just /e/ or /o/, even when they may happen to be diphthongized.

Consonants.   Children generally learn all these different postures, contours, and coordinations for uttering vowels with very little difficulty, and they learn them very early, but deaf children may never get some of them right in a lifetime. Because they require greater precision in placement of the tongue and proper direction of the airstream, learning to produce consonant sounds acceptably is a bit more difficult. Although there are a great number of possible hisses, clicks, and explosions which could be used for speech, most children learn the correct *place* and *manner* of articulation and *voicing* characteristics needed for uttering the consonants of their language. Let's use this classification system (see Table 2.2) to examine how consonant sounds are produced. In Table 2.2, two phonemes sometimes appear side by side in the same column without a comma between them. In these instances, the first phoneme is voiceless and the second is voiced; the two *cognate* phonemes otherwise are virtually identical.

Place of articulation refers to the anatomical *site* where the breath stream is interrupted or constricted to produce a speech sound. There are seven valve sites along the vocal tract:

Bilabial. Sounds (/p/, /b/, and /m/) are made with lips pressed together.

Labiodental. Only two sounds, /f/ and /v/, are produced by placing the upper teeth on the lower lip and blowing air through the narrow slit. One of our clients made a perfectly acceptable acoustic /f/ by using his lower **incisor** teeth and upper lip. Watch yourself in a mirror while you duplicate his error and you will see why he was referred for speech therapy.

Dental. The /θ/ as in *thin* /θɪn/ and the /ð/ as in *them* /ðɛm/ are made by forcing the airstream through a narrow slit between the tongue tip and the teeth.

Alveolar. By inspecting Table 2.2, you can see that there are more sounds made by moving the tongue tip upward and forward to make contact with the upper gum (or alveolar) ridge than at any other articulatory port.

Palatal. The /j/ as in *Yale* /jel/, /l/ and in *bell* /bɛl/, /ʃ/ as in *ship* /ʃɪp/, and /ʒ/ as in *rouge* /ruʒ/ are all produced by lifting the tongue tip to the hard palate.

Velar. Sounds (/ŋ/, /g/, and /k/) are made by lifting the back of the tongue up to the soft palate (velum).

Glottal. Only one legitimate English speech sound, the /h/, is made by simply blowing air between the vocal folds. Children

Incisor.
Any one of the four front teeth in the upper or lower jaws.

TABLE 2.2 Classification of the consonants

	Nasals	Glides	Liquids	Fricatives	Affricates	Plosives
Bilabials	m	w hw				p b
Labiodentals				f v		
Dentals				θ ð		
Alveolar	n		l, r	s z	tʃ dʒ	t d
Palatal		j		ʃ ʒ		
Velar	ŋ					k g
Glottal				h		

who cannot close their soft palates sufficiently to make velar sounds often substitute a glottal stop /ʔ/, a tiny coughlike sound produced by the sudden release of a pulse of voiced or unvoiced air from the vocal folds.

When we describe *how* a sound is made, the way in which the airstream is obstructed, and how the air is released from the vocal tract, we are referring to *manner of articulation.* Consonants can be grouped into six categories on the basis of how they are formed:

Nasal. The sounds /m/, /n/, and /ŋ/ are made by lowering the soft palate, blocking the oral airway, and directing sound through the nasal passages.

Glides. A few sounds can only be made on the wing—with the mouth in motion. These are called **glide** sounds because you must move you articulators from one position to another during their production. For example, to produce the /w/ as in *we* /wi/, you must form your tongue and lips for the vowel *oo* /u/ and then shift or glide into the vowel *ee* /i/, the distinctive sound of /w/ being made during the transition, during the shift.

Liquids. The English language has two liquid sounds, the /l/ and /r/, half consonant and half vowel, in which the voiced airstream flows around or over the elevated tongue.

Fricatives. These sounds are made by forcing air through a narrow vocal tract creating a hissing or turbulence against the teeth and gum ridge. The /s/ and /z/ sibilant **fricative** sounds, for example, are made by forcing air through a narrow groove on the upper surface of the tongue; for the *sh* /ʃ/ and *zh* /ʒ/ sibilants, a slightly wider groove must be employed.

Affricates. In the *ch* /tʃ/ of *choke* /tʃok/ and the *j* /dʒ/ of *joke* /dʒok/, a child must learn to link a plosive and a fricative sequentially. (Try saying *it* and *she* swiftly, and you'll be uttering "itchy" before you know it.) These consonant combinations are called **affricates,** and many children need help if they are to learn to combine their components.

Plosives. Make the sounds /p/, /b/, /t/, /d/, /k/, and /g/ several times and observe what they have in common. Try the /p/ and /b/ first since they are the most visible. Note that you close your lips tightly, build up air pressure behind the seal, and then suddenly release the air with a popping sound. Where are the articulatory seals for /t/ and /k/?

Voicing is the last dimension commonly used for classifying consonant sounds. This refers to whether a consonant is accompanied by laryngeal tone. Consonants that do have vocal fold activity are termed *voiced; voiceless* is the term applied to consonants that are not accompanied by vocal

Glide.
A class of speech sounds in which the characteristic feature is produced by shifting from one articulatory posture to another. Examples are the *y* in /j/ in *you,* and /w/ in *we.*

Fricative.
A speech sound produced by forcing the airstream through a constricted opening. The /f/ and /v/ sounds are fricatives. Sibilants are also fricatives.

Affricate.
A consonantal sound beginning as a stop (plosive) but expelled as a fricative. The *ch* in /tʃ/ and *j* /dʒ/ sounds in the words *chain* and *jump* are affricates.

fold vibration. Many consonants, for example, /s/ and /z/, occur in cognate pairs that differ solely by the variable of voicing.

The classification system we presented may seem confusing and a bit cumbersome to you at first, but assigning sounds to the categories of place, manner, and voicing provides a convenient way in which to understand how consonants are produced. More important for the speech clinician, by comparing a client's inventory of speech sounds with the expected repertoire delineated in Table 2.2, we can discern patterns underlying the client's errors.

So there you have the sounds of our English language, sounds that you have mastered in just a few years and that your own infants someday will have to master, too. Knowing that any prospective student of speech pathology will have to take courses in phonetics, we have presented just the bare bones of the information needed to work successfully with persons who cannot utter these sounds correctly. Indeed, anyone who tries to help a child with an articulatory problem should have at least this basic knowledge, but our major point is that we should not be surprised, given the complexity of our own speech, to find so many persons with defective articulation. Instead, we should be amazed to find so few, especially when we take into account the fact that phonemes typically are not uttered as isolated entities.

Syllables, Clusters, and Coarticulation. In actual speaking, phonemes are incorporated into syllables. Each syllable has as its nucleus a vowel or diphthong, and consonants are used to begin (release) or terminate (arrest) the syllable, although a diphthong or diphthongized vowel can stand alone as a syllable (as in *eye* or *oh*). The letters C for consonant and V for vowel are used to show the shape of a syllable. The word *me*, for example, is a **CV** syllable; *egg* is a VC syllable; *soap* has a **CVC** shape.

Consonants often occur in blends and clusters. The word *straw* has a cluster of three consonantal phonemes, /s/, /t/, and /r/, before its vowel, so this syllable is said to have a CCCV shape. Children may find the mastery of these consonant clusters difficult and so they simplify them, saying *taw*, or saying *poon* for spoon. Certain cluster simplifications, however, may be the products of normal **dialectal** variations, especially when they occur at the end of a syllable.

When phonemes are incorporated into syllables, their production is influenced by the sounds that precede or follow them. For example, the /r/ in the word *rope* is made with the lips already rounded. This is because the /o/ vowel that follows the /r/ is articulated with lip rounding. We find no such preliminary rounding occurring in the word *red*. Try saying aloud the words *geese* and *goose*, paying some attention to what your tongue is doing. Why do you suppose the /g/ is not produced with identical placement in these two words?

CV.
A syllable containing the consonant-vowel sequence as in *see* or *toe* or *ka*.

CVC.
A syllable containing the consonant-vowel-consonant sequence, as in the first syllable of the word *containing*.

Dialect.
Regional, social, or cultural variation of a language.

Finally, we should note that phonemes that precede or follow a nasal consonant usually are themselves somewhat nasalized. This type of **coarticulation** is called *assimilation nasality.*

Not producing a sound alone

Regulation

Respiration, phonation, resonation, and articulation—all these diverse processes that combine to produce speech are regulated by the nervous system. "Orchestrated" might be a better word, for there are at least one hundred muscles that must work together with precise timing. Airflow and voicing must be programmed to match the speech sound requirements, words and word meanings must be retrieved from storage and formulated into acceptable units, and then the whole activity must be monitored *as it occurs* to determine if the form and content of the message fulfill the speaker's communicative intent (see Figure 2-6). And yet the central and peripheral nervous systems work so swiftly and smoothly that they make the act of talking look simple.

Unlike all other components of the speech chain, that are temporarily borrowed from their basic biological duties, the central nervous

Coarticulation.
Influence of adjacent phonemes on the articulation of a speech sound (also see *assimilation*).

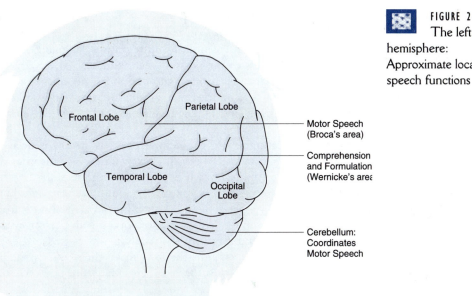

FIGURE 2-6
The left cerebral hemisphere: Approximate location of speech functions

Parietal Lobe

Frontal Lobe

Motor Speech (Broca's area)

Comprehension and Formulation (Wernicke's area)

Temporal Lobe

Occipital Lobe

Cerebellum: Coordinates Motor Speech

system has specialized segments that fulfill the sole purpose of receiving, organizing, and formulating messages. We now review the major functions of the nervous system in relation to the production of speech. Remember that the system is extremely complex and that much still remains to be discovered about how the 14 billion neurons regulate oral language.

The cortex or thin bark of the hemispheres of the brain has an amazing capacity to *store information*. As one of our colleagues demonstrates dramatically through hypnosis, events experienced by a person as a child can be recalled in vivid detail. Individuals thus hypnotically regressed in age to five or six years can name who sat next to them in school and list the presents they received at a birthday party. This is an example of *long-term memory* and it is obviously very important for formulating messages. But we also possess a very brief or *short-term memory*, which is essential for tracking incoming messages, remembering and sequencing items dictated to us, and monitoring what we ourselves have said. Persons with aphasia show losses in both long-term and short-term memory. One former client could not recall the make of his car, the street on which he lived, or even his wife's first name. Interestingly, he could recognize all three words when they were presented to him as a multiple-choice task. Another person with aphasia with whom we worked had extreme difficulty reading or listening because of an impairment in short-term memory; by the time she got to the end of a sentence, she had already forgotten the first few words she had said.

The central nervous system is also the *motor command center*; it is the site for originating, planning, and carrying out the transmission of messages. The command center for integrating language is the left hemisphere, regardless of the person's handedness.[3] Orders are relayed to specific muscle groups through the peripheral nervous system. It is easy to understand that injuries or malfunctionings of this system may be reflected in speech and language problems. Let us give just a few illustrations.

When the maturation of the central nervous system is delayed the child will be slow to talk. Later in this text we discuss a disorder due to brain damage called apraxia in which the client cannot *voluntarily* lift the end of his tongue to produce a /t/ or /l/ sound even though he might be able to move its tip perfectly in licking a bit of peanut butter from the same contact in the mouth. We have also worked with persons with only half a functional tongue in whom the paralysis was caused by peripheral nerve damage and we've taught them to make their sounds adequately anyway. Again, certain voice disorders occur when one of the vocal folds is similarly paralyzed. In aphasia we deal with the result of brain injury, and in the speech of certain people with cerebral palsy we find the coordination difficulties produced by inadequate integration of the motor impulses controlled by the **cerebrum** and **cerebellum**. These few illustra-

Cerebrum.
Refers to the general structure of the brain.

Cerebellum.
Structure of the brain that regulates and coordinates complex motor activities.

tions present only a tiny sample of the problems in speech pathology that are due to neuropathology. Those who specialize in this field will need to explore this area intensively.

Finally, the nervous system is responsible for *processing information;* detection of, attending to, and patterning of incoming messages are only a few functions of this component. The structure of the ear has a primary responsibility for information processing and its importance to speech is obvious.

Deaf babies will **babble** for a time, but because they cannot hear that babbling or the speech of others, their speech and language are bound to be impaired. In a later chapter we present basic information about hearing and its disorders. Here we wish merely to remind all those who may deal with persons with communicative problems that hearing impairment and auditory perceptual problems may be responsible for deviant speech, or for inadequate language, or for learning disabilities.

> We were once asked by a teacher of the emotionally disturbed to observe the speech of one of his pupils. "Frank gives me more trouble than all the others combined," he said. "He's always negative; won't follow directions; will not cooperate with the other children in any of our projects. All he does is raise hell. His speech isn't bad, for I can usually understand him and the other children do not even seem to notice his mispronunciations. Perhaps he's just oversensitive about the way he talks." We found that Frank's speech had the kinds of errors characteristic of a conductive hearing loss. Referral to an otologist resulted in the removal of heavy wax deposits in both ear canals and once the boy could hear again, his behavior changed so dramatically he was able to return to a regular classroom.

LANGUAGE

Students who enter the field of speech pathology soon find themselves confronting the nature of language itself, a fascinating but also very complex topic. The Book of Genesis in the Old Testament tells how the ancient Babylonians began to erect the Tower of Babel with its top in the Heavens as a challenge to God. Whereupon "He confused the language" of the workers so they no longer understood each other and the result was that the tower was never finished. Those of us who have tried to teach children whose language is "confused" or stroke patients with aphasia to read or write or speak again can easily appreciate the havoc so wrought.

There are literally thousands of languages being spoken at this moment on our planet and only a handful of us can understand more than one of them. These languages differ widely one from another. The Hottentot click language and the Chinese tonal language or that polyglot

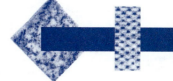

Babbling.
A continuous, free experimenting with speech sounds.

monstrosity called English would seem to have very little in common, yet they do.

All languages share five characteristics:

1. The use of symbols
2. A limited (finite) set of different sounds or phonemes
3. A vocabulary or **lexicon** of meaningful combinations of these phonemes into units called **morphemes**
4. A set of rules for linking these units together
5. A set of rules for using language in a social context

Every child must acquire this fivefold repertoire and do so at the same time he is learning hundreds of other new coordinations, exploring the territory of his new world, and testing the limits of his freedom. It is probably good that the student who feels overloaded by the unreasonable demands of his professors has forgotten the incredible amount he had to learn before he was four years old.

Symbols

Language is comprised of a system of arbitrary symbols. A symbol is a surrogate; it is something that stands for an object, an event, some feature of reality. The word "cow," for example, stands for a creature with four legs and hooves that gives milk. But the word "cow" is purely arbitrary—it could just as well be "woc" or any other combination of letters or sounds. We simply find it convenient to use this particular utterance, "cow," as a shorthand way of identifying a Holstein, a Jersey, or Old Bossy. It sure is easier to utter or write the word "cow" than it is to run out in the pasture and lead in a large lactating quadruped every time we want to refer to that particular domesticated mammal. Our point is this: Words are simply metaphors, mental analogs of reality. Apparently, the human nervous system is uniquely equipped biologically to process reality, not directly on a concrete level, but through the use of symbols. In short, we bind experience by translating sensory events into symbols; order and meaning are created by the act of symbolization.

But it is important to remember that a word is not the thing or event. The name is not in or on the cow somewhere; we will not find a label saying "cow" on Old Bossy's ear or tail. All of us have trouble at times remembering that words do not *create* reality, they merely stand for it. But how do *you* respond when someone calls you a chicken, a cretin, or an s.o.b.? We once observed a mental patient write the word "hamburger" on a piece of paper and then eat it with relish (pardon the pun). Signs, however, do have a closer, more direct relationship to behavior.

A sign is a direct representation of an object or event, and it has a single, fixed meaning regardless of the context. A red traffic signal means stop! A wailing siren portends an ambulance or police vehicle. Puddles on

Lexicon.
The stock of terms in a vocabulary.

Morpheme.
Smallest meaningful combination of phonemes; may be a word, a prefix, a suffix.

saying = symbol
the act = s

a forest trail and water dripping from the trees are *signs* of rain; but when you turn to your hiking companion and say, "It's raining," you are using a *symbol*. Furthermore, signs differ from symbols in having a physical resemblance to the thing they represent. The 🚺 sign on a door allows you to find the women's restroom much faster than the symbol *damas* in a Costa Rican airport.

Phonology

In our presentation of the speech mechanism, we described the speech sounds or phonemes of our English language that comprise its **phonology.** As we noted, they fall into natural groupings according to how they are produced and where. Of course, you probably knew all this phonology long ago, or rather your lungs, larynx, velum, tongue, and lips did, and long before you could even read.

As we now know, the term for a distinctive speech sound is *phoneme,* and the concept is important in speech pathology. You perhaps may be surprised to learn that the phoneme /s/ is not really a single sound but a family of sounds. However, if you listen carefully to the *s* sounds in the words *see* and *Sue* you will notice that the latter /s/ seems lower in pitch than the former. They are not the same sound but they are similar enough to be perceived as being identical. Moreover, there are no two words in English that have different meanings just because the two /s/'s differ in pitch. The difference between these two /s/ sounds makes no difference in meaning. To give another example, the /t/ in the word *take* is **aspirated;** it is released with audible airflow. On the other hand, in the word *stake* we do not hear that tiny rush of aspiration on the /t/ yet both /t/'s belong to the same sound family, to the phoneme /t/. Variant members of a phonemic family are called **allophones.**

And what has an allophone to do with speech pathology? Let us give just one example. A child with a **lateral** lisp produces a very low pitched slushy **sibilant** for the standard /s/ phoneme and usually he is completely unaware of his error. Why? Because he perceives his defective sibilant as one of the *permissible* allophones or variants of the phoneme /s/. If he says *soup* using this laterally emitted allophone it still means *soup* to him and nothing else. His trouble lies in the fact that this particular variant is not permissible; it lies outside the boundaries of the phonemic family of /s/. This difference, of course, is what we must teach him. In other words, many articulation errors are not substitutions of one phoneme for another, but rather, they are the impermissible allophones we call *distortion errors.* They are hard to eliminate because to the child they make no differences in meaning. When such a child is corrected, he often says, "But I did say soup," using his slushy /s/. In the development of speech, then, the child must not only learn to produce all the standard phonemes of our language but also to recognize which allophones of those phonemes are

Phonology.
The linguistic rule system dealing with speech sounds and their characteristics.

Aspirate.
Breathy; the use of excessive initial airflow preceding phonation as in the *aspirate* attack.

Allophone.
One of the variant forms of a phoneme.

Lateral.
A sound such as the /l/ in which the airflow courses around the side of the uplifted tongue. One variety of a lateral lisp is so produced.

Sibilant.
A class of fricative consonant sounds characterized by high-pitched noise. Examples are /s/ and /z/.

Distortion.
The misarticulation of a standard sound in which the latter is replaced by a sound not normally used in the language. A lateral lisp is a distortion.

acceptable and which are not. He must learn, too, that in rapid connected speech, sounds are not produced one at a time like beads on a string; there is considerable overlapping and the movement patterns for two or more phonemes may take place simultaneously.

But how does the child acquire the more than forty phonemes he needs to speak English? The basic process seems to be one of discrimination and experimentation. Through matching his own production with the models provided by other speakers, he comes to recognize that each of these forty phonemes consists of its own unique bundle of **distinctive features.** Any sound that does not have all of the set of distinctive features possessed by a particular standard phoneme is perceived as being a different phoneme or as an unacceptable distortion. The /s/ in *Sue* and the /z/ in *zoo* have several features in common since their manner and place of articulation are identical, but they are different phonemes because the /z/ is voiced and the /s/ is not. Voicing, then, is one of the distinctive features of the /z/ in our language. The child gradually comes to recognize or has to be taught that all the distinctive features belonging to a specific phoneme must be present if that sound is to be spoken correctly.

Morphology

It takes more than a collection of phonemes to make a language. Only when those phonemes are combined into meaningful units does one have the vocabulary needed to communicate. Although there is great latitude, certain combinations of phonemes are not permissible. In English, for example, a word cannot start with /ŋ/ or /ʒ/. The following array of phonemes, *syzygy,* seems highly improbable for a legitimate word—but is it?

The linguist's term for the *smallest* meaningful unit of a language is *morpheme. Baby* is a morpheme but the word *baby's* consists of two morphemes, the first refers to the infant while the second, the *'s,* adds a second meaning, that of possessiveness. (The term morpheme, then, is not just a synonym for "word.") The phrase, "The baby's bottle," consists of only three words, but there are four morphemes in it. When a morpheme can exist by itself and still be meaningful (as baby or bottle can) it is called a *free morpheme.* Prefixes, suffixes, and other such "adders" of meaning are called *bound morphemes.* They cannot exist alone. The word *girls* has both types, the first meaningful unit referring to a young female and the second, the /s/, referring to plurality. Further complicating the learning task, some words change phonemically to form plurals *(mouse-mice, woman-women)* or tense *(sing-sang, run-ran),* for example.

Why is this information important? For a number of good reasons, of which we cite but one. If a person says "I see two boat" she may not have a disorder of articulation that results in omitting the /s/, even though your own first impulse may be to think in terms of articulation. The child may instead have a language disorder because she has not learned the use

Distinctive features.
Acoustic and articulatory properties of phonemes.

of the bound morpheme /s/ to indicate that she saw more than one boat. It also is possible that the person is evidencing no disorder at all but, rather, a language or dialectal difference. Even among speakers of English, as we know, all do not use the same variety of the language. We may be hearing the report of a child, or it might just as easily be an adult, whose linguistic rules differ from those of Standard American English (see, for example, Iglesias and Anderson, 1993).

In any event, by the time normal babies are one year old, regardless of their language or dialect environments, they have a production vocabulary of perhaps two to ten words and a recognition vocabulary of many more. From that time until well into adolescence we add to our vocabularies at amazingly rapid rates, and our vocabularies generally continue to grow for as long as we live. At every stage, our recognition vocabulary is far greater than the expressive vocabulary that we use to communicate, in part because of our fundamental understanding of the phonologic and morphologic rules that govern our language.

Syntax

To speak a language more than phonemes and morphemes are needed. The speaker must also know how to combine these into phrases and sentences. In speech pathology we often meet children who have difficulty doing this. Perhaps they still speak in "one-word sentences" at the age of four. Or perhaps they arrange the many words they do have in improper sequences. Also, some of your future clients may have failed to learn the grammatical rules they must follow in sending their messages and so they will need language training. Let us see how Tommy learned his language over the period between fourteen months and four years of age.

> The list is not complete for there were also other transitional forms used, yet they illustrate how one child mastered his **syntax.** At fourteen months the boy was using several one-word sentences with intonations and gestures to indicate his meaning. Most of them were declaratives or commands. Among them were "Daddy," "Tommy," and "lake" (Tommy loved to splash in it and go to it as often as he could). Here are some sequential samples of his speech. Note how his mastery of the language evolved.
>
> "Lake! Lake! Tommy lake!" (One-word sentence; two-word sentence.)
>
> "Pity (pretty) lake" (while splashing in it). (Noun phrase.)
>
> "Tommy lake! Daddy lake!" (An imperative. He demanded to go.)
>
> "Tommy go lake and Daddy go lake!" (Note conjunction linking the two **kernel sentences**.)
>
> "Tommy and Daddy go lake now!" (A better way, though shorter).
>
> "Tommy and Daddy go car and go to lake now!" (Note the first use of preposition.)

Syntax.
The grammatical structure of a language.

Kernel sentences.
The early primitive sentence forms from which other transformations later develop.

"Tommy go in lake now and go in, Daddy too!"

"Tommy and Daddy go in the car and go to lake." (Note the "the.")

"Me and Daddy go to the lake in car, now!" (Note personal pronoun and use of prepositional phrases.)

"Daddy, Tommy want to go to lake in the car now." (Two rules are still not applied.)

"Daddy no go lake now? Tommy wanna go in car and go to lake too." (Note length of utterance.)

"You going lake, Daddy? I wanna go."

"Why you no take me the lake, Daddy? I want to go to the lake."

"Mommy, why won't Daddy take me to the lake?" I want to go fimmin (swimming)."

Some of the children with whom you'll work may not develop the same ways of expressing meanings that Tommy discovered. A few may never get past the early noun-phrase or verb phrase level. Some may never learn the rules that govern personal pronoun usage or negatives or questioning. Some develop odd, inappropriate rules of their own. Still others may be bound by the linguistic rules of a dialect such as, for example, Black English (Terrell and Terrell, 1993). The student of speech pathology needs to know something about syntax. So does any teacher who must help a child with language.

The person with **dysphasia** often has difficulties with syntax, as well as with word finding. Trying to say "I now have to go to the bathroom" she might struggle and gesture and begin and hesitate before uttering "I . . . uh . . . bath . . . no . . . uh . . . go . . . now." The rules for ordering the words of her message have escaped her and are lost momentarily; without having these rules available she is helpless.

Any attempt to describe the syntax of our language in any detail would be inappropriate since this is an introductory text. Nevertheless, we can outline some of the standard English rules for joining words together that must be mastered. First, we must be able to understand and produce noun phrases and verb phrases and then to link them together. "The boy" is a noun phrase consisting of the *determiner* "the" and the noun "boy." "Can hit" is a verb phrase, with "hit" as the verb and "can" as its auxiliary. The sentence "The boy can hit the ball" adds another noun phrase. The diagram of this typical sentence (see Figure 2-7) may be thought of as the skeleton model for thousands of the sentences each of us will generate every year. Hidden in the linking of these words are eight rules, one of them being that a determiner must precede the noun (*the* must precede *boy*) and another that an auxiliary must precede the verb. "Boy the hit can ball the" breaks these rules and produces something that isn't standard English. A baby then must master something be-

Dysphasia.
The general term for aphasic problems.

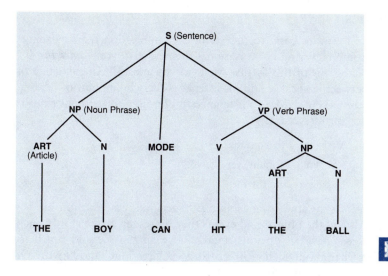

FIGURE 2-7 Tree diagram of a sentence

sides these words: not only how they must be combined but also how they shouldn't be linked together.

Of course, the illustration we have provided falls far short of portraying the whole picture of language structure. We do not speak only in such simple declarative sentences. Although thousands of sentences can be formulated in which different words can be placed in the slots of our diagram to say many different things, we need more complicated patterns to express other meanings. Expansion, coordination, and subordination require much more elaborate diagrams.

For example, the child, in learning a language, must also master some transformational rules. "The ball is being hit by the boy" is an example of the application of a passive transformation. "Can the boy hit the ball?" is a rearrangement of the words and phrases so that they pose a question. (As any parent of a two-year-old child knows well, these interrogative transformations are mastered early). These two examples of transformations show that there must be different rules governing the order of the words of a declarative or interrogatory utterance, as well as an active or passive one. The language learner will have to know these rules even if he cannot verbalize them. Again, all we provide here is the briefest of glimpses of the nature of the transformations in syntax. Not only the position of the words is changed; new words may have to be inserted or embedded in the new sentence structure. Modifying phrases or qualifying clauses that have their own rules may be necessary to express the altered meaning. Those who work with children who show language delay must be able to analyze their speech linguistically.

Semantics

What could be more basic to the act of communication than meaning? Consider some recurring conversational themes: "Do you *understand?*" "I can't make *sense* of this." 'Just what do you mean?" An exchange of meaning between a speaker and his listener is the whole point of talking. Parents correct their children's utterances more often for content (meaning) than for form (syntax):

Child: Alaska are a warm state.

Parent: No, "cold," Johnny, very "cold."

Child: Alaska are a cold state.

Semantics is the study of meaning; and meaning is the relationship between words and the objects and events they represent. Some words, such as "pine tree," have an obvious referent—we all can see and touch its trunk. But what about such abstract words as "freedom" and "love"? Or short connector words, for example, "to," "of," or "the" that derive meaning only from context. In dictionaries we find the *denotative* meanings of words: "Water" is a clear liquid composed of molecules of one part hydrogen and two parts oxygen. But if an individual has had a near-drowning experience, the morpheme "water" takes on a very personal or *connotative* meaning.

But language is a dynamic tool, and meanings are not found solely in dictionaries or even in the words themselves—meaning is derived from how people respond to or use morphemes. To illustrate we present now a portion of a diagnostic report on a language-delayed child. The speech clinician is describing how Myron uses four categories of meaning in his oral language:

Myron was observed during a "free play" session with two other children about his same age. The children were playing with small toy cars, trucks, and a garage. Myron used several categories of meaning in the session:

Nomination (naming or specifying objects) Example: "That car."

Possession (indicating ownership) Example: He took a blue car away from Stephen and said, "My car!"

Recurrence (indicating repetition) Example: "More crashes."

Nonexistence (noting when object not present) Example: "No fire truck (looking about)."

Before concluding our brief discussion of semantics, we must note that the very same word may have quite different meanings even to different speakers of the same language, depending upon such factors as age, socioeconomic status, or cultural background. The adjective *bad*, for example, seems to have meant just the opposite among teenagers and young adults not too long ago; *pig* does not always refer to a farm animal; and the word *head* certainly has different meaning to the sailor than to the landlubber. Communication among individuals can and does break down easily when differences such as these are unrecognized or ignored.

Pragmatics

The utterance of certain words that are combined in a grammatical sequence may constitute speech, but it does not necessarily constitute communication. Any sending of purposeful messages back and forth between speaker and listener requires the observation of rules of appropriate communicative interaction. The term **pragmatics** refers to skills involved in the social use of language.

The child is encouraged to say "Please pass the beans," rather than "Gimme the beans." But pragmatics is far more than the learning of good manners. It also involves knowing how to phrase a request, how to ask a question, how to start a conversation, or keep it going.

The words we use and the manner in which we speak depend to a great extent on our purpose and the constraints of the social situation. Talking is a sociopsychological event and there are distinct rules that govern how we use language within different social contexts. We offer congratulations at weddings and condolences at funerals, and in elevators we remain quiet. Students talk differently in the dormitory than they do when conversing with their grandparents over Sunday dinner. We overheard the following very rapid exchange between two collegians late one afternoon—can you decipher it?

First student:	D'ja-eat?
Second student:	Naw, d'jew?
First student:	Naw, s'twirly.

The term **code switching** is often used with reference to the change of speaking style as people interact with different listeners. We may use quite different styles when speaking with an authority figure than when the listener is our closest friend; the style that we tend to use with males may not be the same one we use with females. But code switching also can refer to dialects or even to languages. For example, you might switch to Spanish (or at least try to) while visiting in Mexico, or to French while touring Quebec. An example of code switching that probably is more familiar is seen in the person who speaks **Black English** but who sometimes chooses to use standard English in particular situations.

Pragmatic concepts have found their way into diagnosis and treatment with children who have language disorders, and we shall return to this important aspect of communication in a later chapter.

Pragmatics.
How communication is used in a social context.

Code switching.
Conscious shifting from one language or dialect to another, depending on speaking situation.

Black English.
Dialects of Standard American English often used by persons of African descent; also called Black English Vernacular (BEV).

Prosody

Each language has its unique melody and rhythm patterns, in addition to its other unique features, and to speak their own language children must learn when and how to pause, how to pace an utterance, how to use pitch inflections, and how to stress and emphasize certain syllables. Consider the differences in the way we say the following sentences.

"Are you going to the store?"

"I'm going to the store."

"Go to the store!"

Each one of these has a different inflection pattern, depending on whether it is a question, a statement, or a command. Try reading the following sentence aloud four times, each time giving emphasis to a different word (the capitalized word).

"Did you see him TAKE my book?"

"Did YOU see him take my book?"

"Did you see HIM take my book?"

"Did you see him take my BOOK?"

You'll no doubt agree that each question has a different thrust, which calls for a contrasting type of answer from the listener. Can you come up with at least one other way to ask the question that would require yet a different sort of answer?

We also can change the meaning of an utterance by altering its juncture characteristics. By putting in a pause after the first and third words of this sentence we probably can effect a very significant change in our listener's reaction. First, just read it aloud as a simple declarative sentence: "Woman without her man would be a beast." Now introduce the suggested prosodic changes and it becomes: "Woman! Without her, man would be a beast." The beast has changed sex!

Prosodic patterning is learned very early in our lives and is exceptionally resistant to change. In the babbling of infants we can sometimes recognize the intonations of questions or commands; and, even though they may have limited vocabularies and may keep the flow of "speech" going by using jargon, children exhibit the same tonal patterns as adult speakers of their language. Stroke patients with aphasia often retain the **prosody** of their utterances even when they have lost the words they need to express themselves. At times we have helped them by tapping the rhythm of the words they want to say. And you may have noticed, as have we, that non-native speakers of English who have acquired an excellent command of our phonology, vocabulary, and grammar often still sound "foreign" to our ear. They tend to use the prosody of their native language, and we know immediately that they come from another land. Perhaps this

Prosody.
Linguistic stress patterns as reflected in pause, inflection, juncture, melody or cadence of speech.

prosodic persistence also explains, at least in part, the difficulty you may have experienced when you tried code switching to Spanish.

SPEECH ACOUSTICS

Do Not Read Beyond this point

"It's not easy, but this is a really interesting topic. It puts so many things together for me. It's like . . . oh, Yes!! Now I can understand how tongue positions are able to change a sound so much even when the position changes ever so little." Such was the unsolicited commentary of one student following her recent immersion in speech acoustics.

We noted early in this chapter that our understanding of communication disorders derives in part from knowledge about normal speech processes. For this and other reasons, it is important to examine speech as a series of dynamic acoustic events. *Acoustic* refers simply to sound or hearing; and by *acoustics* we mean the scientific study of sound generation, propagation, and perception.

Our particular interest is in speech (and the hearing of speech), of course; but, because speech is a very complicated type of sound, we must limit ourselves here to an abbreviated overview of speech acoustics. Your future coursework will explore this topic in much greater depth, if you continue to study either audiology or speech-language pathology; but, for now, if you wish more detailed information, you may find Denes and Pinson (1993) to be a very readable and useful resource.

Speech acoustics necessarily incorporates information about sounds in general, and you may have become acquainted with the basics of sound in a physics class or in a class that reviewed the ear and hearing, but it's also possible that some readers may be encountering information of this type for the first time. In either case, you may not yet be certain that the study of sound or of speech acoustics has much, if any, relevance to your study of communication disorders.

Consider again, then, that at the level of physical events our utterances are nothing more (and also nothing less) than complex sound waves that happen to be generated by our speech mechanisms. However, these particular acoustic signals are intriguingly potent. Somehow they are able to represent all manner of messages and subtle meaning when they reach the brain of a listener. Under some circumstances it is not even necessary that the entire intact signal reach the listener's ear in order for the speaker's message to be understood. Moreover, these sound waves carry information enabling you to recognize the identity of speakers with whom you are acquainted, and they can provide clues to the emotional state of the speaker. Exactly how all of this (and more) can occur is not entirely clear, although scientists have studied such matters intensively for decades.

Acoustic.
Pertaining to sound.

With the help of sophisticated computers we have learned how to artificially produce simple speech signals that are understandable to ordinary listeners. These synthesized speech samples do not always sound very natural, though, and they seldom would be mistaken for actual human speech. Computers also can be programmed to recognize simple speech signals, especially if only one specified individual produces the speech. However, if that individual happens one day to have laryngitis or perhaps a stuffy nose, the computer may well be stumped. If some other person does the speaking, a computer quite likely will make errors, and if that different person is of the opposite sex, or perhaps speaks with a slightly different intonation pattern, the computer again may prove unreliable in deciphering the signal.

Amazingly, the most refined speech synthesizers and the most advanced speech recognition programs are unable to do some of the things that children, by and large, do *well* and *easily* long before they enter kindergarten.[4] On the other hand, as we know, some people do *not* process these acoustic events well or easily (or at all). Difficulties in producing, receiving, or interpreting speech signals are central to the communication disorders of the people we seek to serve.

It stands to reason, then, that as more becomes known about speech acoustics we generally will be better able to serve our clients. Evidence that this is true already is at hand, as we shall see in later chapters, especially in areas such as hearing amplification and **augmentative communication.** Of even greater importance, our understandings of speech acoustics eventually may help enable us to facilitate the normal development of communication skills and to prevent or minimize the occurrence or severity of certain disorders.

The Nature of Sound

Augmentative and Alternative Communication (AAC). The use of non-speech techniques and devices (e.g., picture boards, symbol systems, computerized speech) as a substitute or supplement for speech communication.

Sounds occur when objects are set into vibration or oscillation, if the vibratory motion repeats itself from about 20 to around 20,000 times per second (the range of frequencies to which our ears normally respond). Vibratory rates slower than 20 Hertz (Hz) are not perceived as sound. Rates more rapid than 20,000 Hz are not audible to the human ear (even though they may be heard by your dog) and are referred to as *ultrasonic* acoustic frequencies.

Just about anything that can be set into vibration (for example, a violin string, the reed in a clarinet, the neck of an inflated balloon, a loudspeaker diaphragm, a slammed door, a tuning fork) can be a source of sound. And our vocal folds are a major sound source, as we know, during the utterance of speech sounds, although other parts of our speech mechanism also produce sound by impeding or stopping the flow of air.

Vibrations become sound by creating regular or irregular disturbances in the air (or in other substances with which we are not concerned here).

We can illustrate this by observing the prong of a tuning fork (Figure 2-8) as it impacts on the air surrounding it. When at rest and undisturbed, the surrounding air normally would be said to be at ordinary atmospheric pressure.

In our simplified figure we have used a single line of dots, to the right the tuning fork, to represent the countless air particles (molecules) that actually would surround the tuning fork. Simplifying even a bit more, we can see that as the prong moves "outward" from its resting position it pushes against nearby air particles and forces them to be closer together, or **compressed,** compared to their resting state. The air pressure immediately adjacent to the prong is now greater than atmospheric pressure.

Compression. The phase during a vibratory cycle when molecules are pressed more closely together, creating a region of high pressure.

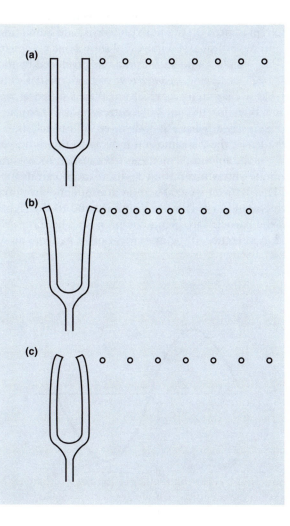

FIGURE 2-8 Air particles (a) at rest, (b) in compression, and (c) in rarefaction, as the prongs of a tuning fork move through a cycle of vibration

Then, when it has reached its maximum "outward" position, the prong springs back "inward." This motion pulls those very same compressed air particles apart from one another. Soon the particles are separated even more from one another (**rarefaction**) than we found them in their resting state. The air pressure here is now less than atmospheric pressure.

Again, lest you be misled by our simplification of this process, we remind you that the tuning fork is completely surrounded by air. We've been disturbing a multitude of air particles in every direction, not just some few and nearby particles that were convenient to depict. In any event, air disturbances continue as the prong returns toward its rest position and then immediately begins a second cycle of vibration, causing another cycle of alternating compression and rarefaction to begin in the adjacent air; then, a third cycle; then a fourth; a fifth; and so on (at least 20 times or more within one second, if sound is to be generated).

Sound is often shown graphically by picturing its **waveform,** a display in which time units are represented on the horizontal axis, and amplitude or intensity is shown on the vertical axis. Figure 2-9 shows one complete cycle of the waveform of a simple sound such as the one produced by the tuning fork that we've been observing. A *pure tone* of this type has only one frequency, and it has a characteristic waveform that is called a *sine wave*. The horizontal line bisecting the sine wave corresponds to zero amplitude. Let's look more closely at what a sound waveform can tell us.

Beginning from the left at the zero line and moving to the right, we can follow along visually as the amplitude increases from instant to instant. At the zero line our vibrator was in its resting position and no air disturbance was occurring. The particles were at rest, at atmospheric pressure. During the time in which our curve is moving upward and to the right, in a *positive* direction, the particles are being compressed. The term *displacement* is often used in reference to the movement of air particles away

Rarefaction.
The phase during a vibratory cycle when molecules are spread more distantly from one another, creating a region of low pressure.

Waveform.
Graphic representation of sound pressure variations or vibratory amplitudes over time.

FIGURE 2-9   The waveform of a pure tone, such as that produced by a tuning fork, is a *sine wave*

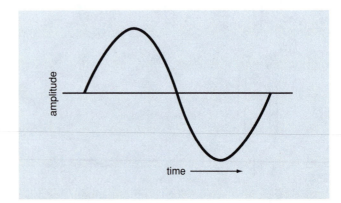

from their normal rest state. So the particles are in a maximum state of compression, or positive displacement, and the pressure is greater than atmospheric pressure, when our wave reaches its maximum positive amplitude. Then, as the curve begins to descend, compression and pressure begin to decrease. The zero (atmospheric pressure) line soon is crossed, pressure continues to decrease, and rarefaction quickly reaches a maximum, where our waveform is at its maximum *negative* amplitude (and particles have reached their maximum negative displacement). The wave now begins its return toward the zero line, and momentarily the next cycle will be underway. Our tuning fork will vibrate, and the waveform display could continue, at a regular and unchanging rate (although amplitude, or displacement, will gradually decrease as the vibrations gradually subside) until vibration has come to a halt. Remember that each of these vibrations is occurring in just a brief fraction of a second. If we were using a 2000 Hz tuning fork, for example, it would complete 2000 complete cycles in just one second.

When we say that *pitch* is the perceptual correlate of *frequency,* we simply mean that the pitch of a sound depends upon the rate at which the source is vibrating. Faster rates are perceived as higher in pitch than slower rates. In the case of our tuning fork, as we've seen, the sound is produced by simple periodic motion and is called a pure tone. Its acoustic energy is concentrated at a just one frequency, usually called the *fundamental frequency,* corresponding to the rate at which the prongs are vibrating.

Most of us are not accustomed to thinking in Hertz—except, perhaps, when we rent a car (if we may be forgiven a moment of irreverence toward science)—so it might help here to relate frequency to a scale that may be more familiar to the beginning student. In more advanced studies you may learn that pitch is sometimes measured by psychoacousticians in units called *mels.* For our purposes, we'll stick to more familiar territory, namely the Equal Tempered Musical Scale (ETS). It can be useful to know that the frequency of 440 Hz corresponds to A4 (the A above middle-C) on the ETS. It's this note to which orchestra instruments tune before the concert. Middle-C (C4), which happens to be at the middle of a piano keyboard, has a fundamental frequency of approximately 260 Hz. Women's speaking voices, by and large, tend to be produced with average fundamental frequencies in the range of 190 to 220 Hz; men's, in the range of 100 to 125 Hz.

We don't spend much time listening to tuning forks, and very few of the sounds we hear are pure tones. Most sound sources, unlike a tuning fork, vibrate in very complex patterns, even when they vibrate in a regularly repetitive fashion; hence, most periodic sounds have acoustic energy at many different frequencies. It is important to remember that even the most complex sound, *if its waveform is repetitively replicated* (i.e., *periodic*), actually is made up of simple periodic sounds that occur simultaneously. (*Noise,* to which we shall attend in a moment, is another story.) We need to be aware that the combination of two or more sine waves of different frequencies always produces a complex periodic waveform.

Pure tones of the same frequency, if combined in particular ways, can "reinforce" one another to produce a simple periodic tone of the same frequency, but with an amplitude greater than either tone taken separately. And, combined in yet another way, two pure tones of the same frequency can "cancel" each other, resulting in no sound at all. All of these possible results of "mixing" sounds together play a role, as we shall shortly see, in our production especially of vowel sounds.

The sounds generated by vibration of our vocal folds, as you will recall, are complex periodic tones comprised of a *fundamental frequency*, together with *harmonics* at frequencies that are whole-number multiples of the fundamental. Figure 2-10 shows the waveform of a human voice (albeit, after the laryngeal tone has been resonated in the vocal tract) during an utterance of the vowel /ɑ/. Its regularity (periodicity) is quite easy to see, in that the same waveform pattern is repeated again and again. The presence of additional components beyond the fundamental frequency can be confirmed by noting how much this waveform differs in shape from the simple waveform of our tuning fork. We cannot tell *which* harmonic frequencies are represented merely by looking at the waveform, we can only know that other frequencies are present. The fundamental frequency, in any event, continues to govern our perception of pitch in *complex periodic* tones.

The amount of time (usually expressed in milliseconds) consumed by one complete cycle of vibration is known as the ***period*** of the tone. For example, the period of a 100 Hz tone is 1/100, or ten one-thousandths (.010) of a second; in other words, its period is ten milliseconds. When we know the frequency, we always can calculate the period by means of a simple process of division: *1/frequency*. Another way to say this is to say *period is the reciprocal of frequency*.

In Figure 2-10, as it happens, we know that the period was 10.7 milliseconds. What was the fundamental frequency of this voiced sound? You're correct if you answered "about 93 Hz," and your mathematical approach was right if you divided *one* (second) by *.0107*. To calculate the

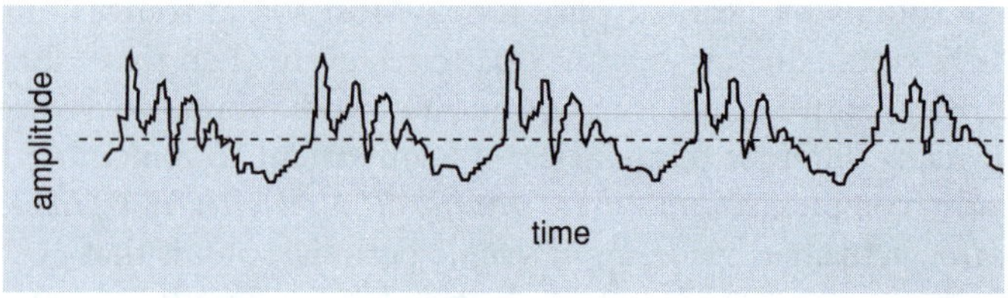

Period.
In acoustics, the duration of one vibratory cycle.

FIGURE 2-10   Complex periodic tone: Waveform recorded during utterance of the vowel /ɑ/

frequency, when we know the period, we always perform this same division operation. *Frequency is the reciprocal of period.*

Not all sources vibrate in a regular repetitive fashion. Some have irregular vibratory patterns, and they have no period. We hear these *a*periodic complex sounds as *noise,* which really has no discernible fundamental frequency. This does not mean, however, that noises may not have characteristic sounds which are unique to particular sources. You might well recognize the noise outside your window as coming from a neighbor's lawnmower. Indeed, many of our consonant sounds are basically noises, but we are able to distinguish among them on the basis of how their predominant acoustic energies are distributed. For example, the /s/ tends to have a greater concentration of its energy in very high frequencies than do /θ/ or /ʃ/.

A second attribute of sound, *loudness,* is the perceptual correlate of the *intensity* of compression and rarefaction of the air particles surrounding our source. In a sense, we can think of this in terms of the distance (from its resting position) that the prong of our tuning fork travels before it reverses and begins to travel in the opposite direction. When we strike the tuning fork forcefully, each vibratory cycle will carry the prongs further from their resting state than if we strike the fork lightly, and we will perceive greater loudness. The resultant waveform will show greater excursions above and below the zero line (greater amplitude, or displacement) for a loud sound than for a quiet sound. Knowing what you now know, look at Figure 2-11. Assuming that the same amount of time is represented in each display, which of these pure tones would be perceived as having the higher pitch? We hope you've answered "b"—because more vibratory cycles have occurred per unit of time in (b) than

FIGURE 2-11 Waveforms: Frequency and amplitude differences

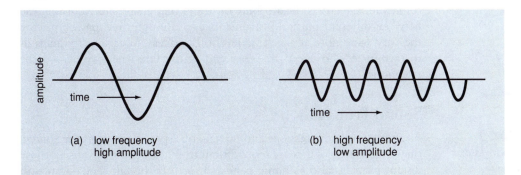

in (a). Your answer should be the same if we had asked which tone has the briefer period. And, of course, you'd know that waveform (a) represents the louder of the two tones, since its amplitude is greater than the amplitude of (b).

Intensity or loudness actually correlates in the world of physics to the amount of energy or power in the sound wave, and the human ear is capable of detecting an enormous range of sound powers, from about .000,000,001 watt up to 50,000,000 watts. It would be inconvenient, to say the very least, if numbers of these magnitudes were used to provide an index of loudness. Instead, a logarithmic scale of **decibels** (one-tenth of a Bel, after Alexander Graham Bell) is used to measure intensity. The "zero dB" sound pressure reference level is about the softest sound that the average ear might normally detect in a quiet listening environment.

When we say that the "average whisper" has a sound level of 30 dB (see Figure 2-12), we are saying that its intensity is 30 dB (or 3 Bels) greater than the reference intensity. This means that the whisper is 10^3 (or 1,000) times more intense than the reference intensity. The intensity of the "average busy street," at 60 dB, would be about 1,000,000 (10^6) times greater than the reference level; but the street would be only ten ($10^6 - 10^5 = 10^1$) times more intense than "moderate restaurant clatter," at 50 dB. To explore further details of this ratio scale would go far beyond our present purposes, but Figure 2-12 may help you to appreciate the range of loudness ratios are measured relatively easily by using this scale.

Quality or *timbre* (/tæombɚ/) is the third feature we need to consider. The quality of a sound is related to the manner in which acoustic energy is distributed among the various frequencies that are present. The number and relative intensities of any harmonics in a periodic sound source are important determinants of quality. Also important is the manner in which the original sound is modified by any associated resonator(s). Just as the laryngeal tone does not sound like "voice" until it is resonated, the plucked string of a guitar does not sound very musical until it has been resonated. Quality is the attribute of sound that enables us to distinguish between different musical instruments even though they may be playing the very same note at the same level of loudness. Vocal quality helps us to recognize who is on the other end of the line when we answer the telephone.

Sound Propagation

Decibel (dB).
A unit of loudness or sound intensity.

As alternating compressions and rarefactions spread out from the source, they affect particles that are more distant from the source by causing those distant particles also to bump back and forth (although they bump with decreasing force as distance increases). It is important to understand that,

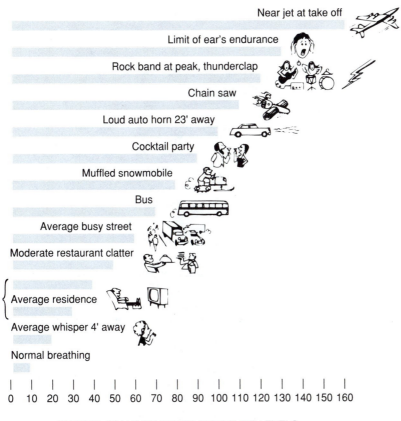

Near jet at take off

Limit of ear's endurance

Rock band at peak, thunderclap

Chain saw

Loud auto horn 23' away

Cocktail party

Muffled snowmobile

Bus

Average busy street

Moderate restaurant clatter

Average residence

Average whisper 4' away

Normal breathing

| | | | | | | | | | | | | | | | |
0 10 20 30 40 50 60 70 80 90 100 110 120 130 140 150 160

DECIBEL SCALE OF SOUND PRESSURE LEVELS

FIGURE 2-12
Comparative loudness of familiar sounds and noises

except for this oscillating back and forth, forth and back motion, the air particles do not actually travel anywhere. They do not race away from the source, for example, to some eventual destination (such as our ears). Rather, they simply displace adjacent particles that, in turn, displace yet other particles.

These successive positive and negative displacements result in wavelike patterns of air pressure variation that *do* travel across space through the air. The pressure variations spread out in a spherical pattern, something akin to the circular pattern suggested by Figure 2-13, but in three dimensions. As their distance from the source increases, the actual amount of displacement also decreases. If we are far enough from the tuning fork, the disturbances will have become so tiny that we'll not be aware of any sound at all. If we're close enough to the source, though, our eardrums will be set into vibration by these minuscule oscillations of air pressure. When the ear drums vibrate, the **ossicles** will transmit the vibrations to the **cochlea,** and, lo, we're about

Ossicles.
The three smallest bones in the body—the malleus, incus, and stapes; the ossicles convey vibrations of the eardrum to the oval window of the cochlea.

Cochlea.
The spiral-shaped structure of the inner ear containing the end organs of the auditory nerve.

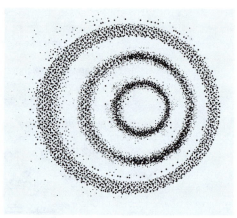

FIGURE 2-13   Alternating waves of compression and rarefaction spread in all directions from a vibrating sound source

to hear a sound. You'll find more information about this part of the process in Chapter 13.

How rapidly will these waves of air pressure travel away from the source and toward our ears? Right! They will move at the speed of sound! At sea level, sound waves travel at about 770 miles per hour, or about 1,130 feet per second. Light waves, by the way, travel with incredibly greater speed (about 186,000 miles per second), reaching our eyes almost instantaneously from any reasonably nearby source. When we hear a clap of thunder five seconds after we've seen the bolt of lightning, for example, we know—because of the difference between the speed of sound and the speed of light—that the lightning was about a mile (5 × 1,130 feet) away from us. And it makes no difference how loud the sound is. Very quiet sounds travel through space at exactly the same speed as very loud sounds.

It also makes no difference what the pitch of the sound is. Very low frequency sounds and very high frequency sounds move at exactly the same speed. Since this is true, then the distance in space between compressions occurring at a high frequency will have to be shorter than the distance between compressions occurring at a lower frequency. In other words, the number of compressions occupying any given distance in space will be greater for a high frequency sound than for a low frequency sound. And the greater the number of compressions within a given space, the shorter will be the distance between successive compressions.

This leads us to consider another important feature of sound that requires our attention. The **wavelength** of a sound is defined as the distance in space between successive compressions (or between successive rarefactions) as these disturbances travel through space. The concept of wavelength is easily confused with wave*form*, but you should try to keep these two notions quite separate as you seek to further your understanding of

Wavelength.
The distance in space between successive compressions (or successive rarefactions) in a sound wave.

acoustics. A waveform, per se, is of little relevance to us when we are dealing with the transmission, or propagation, of sound. But wave*length* is all-important, especially when we consider what happens to sound as it moves through the vocal tract.

You can compute the wavelength of any sound rather simply, if you know its fundamental frequency. Just divide that frequency into the speed of sound, and you'll have its wavelength (often symbolized by the small Greek lambda, λ). The wavelength of a 100 Hz sound wave, for example, is 11.3 feet. A 200 Hz sound will have a wavelength just one-half that long, 5.65 feet. What, then, would be the wavelength of a 2,000 Hz sound? Your answer should be 0.565 feet, or 6.78 inches. We will call upon you understanding of wavelength as we look briefly now at speech spectra and **formants.**

Speech Spectra, Formants, and Perception

By the *spectrum* of a sound we mean the manner in which sound energy is distributed among the various frequencies that the sound contains. This information can be presented graphically in either a "line spectrum" or a "continuous spectrum" (which is essentially a smoothed curve version of the line spectrum). In a spectral display, frequency is represented on the horizontal axis, while amplitude or intensity is represented on the vertical axis. The spectrum shows us the exact distribution of sound energy at one quick instant in time (therefore, it cannot tell us how the distribution changes over time).

Figure 2-14 shows the line spectra of three sounds. A pure tone, as we know, has all of its energy at just one frequency, and in (a) we see a graphic representation of such a tone. In this example we can see that all of the energy is focused at 2,000 Hz. The second, (b), shows the approximate distribution of energy we might discover in the spectrum of a trumpet that is sounding the ETS note D4 (about 300 Hz). We see energy in that fundamental frequency and in a series of harmonics (600 Hz, 900 Hz, 1200 Hz, and so on, up through 3,000 Hz, though this would not truly be the upper limit if we analyzed an actual trumpet tone). Harmonics, by the way, are also known as "*overtones,*" especially in the world of music. Finally, 2-14(c) shows a random distribution of sound energy—illustrative of one type of spectrum which might be associated with an aperiodic complex sound (noise).

We turn now to the sound of the *glottal source,* a term commonly used in reference to the sound produced at the level of the vocal folds—the sound we actually never hear until after it has been resonated in the cavities of the vocal tract. Figure 2-15(a) displays a line spectrum of the glottal source. At this particular instant in time the vocal folds are vibrating at a rate of 100 Hz; so we see, furthest to the left, a vertical line representing the intensity of that fundamental. Looking to the right from the funda-

Formant.

Frequency range in which the acoustic energy of a speech signal is concentrated by vocal tract resonance.

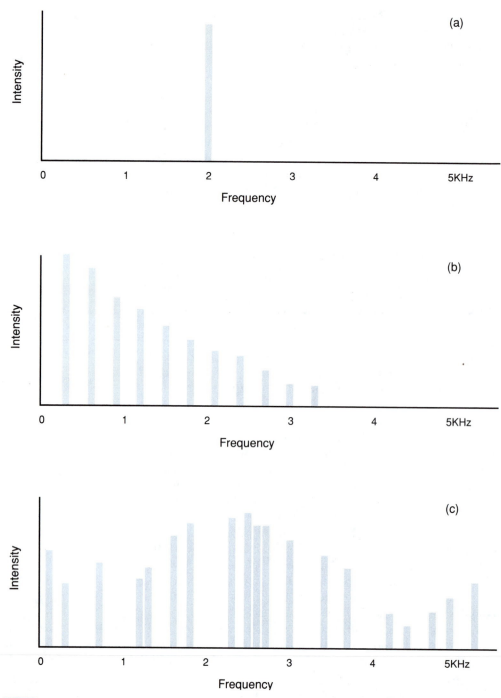

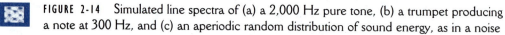

FIGURE 2-14 Simulated line spectra of (a) a 2,000 Hz pure tone, (b) a trumpet producing a note at 300 Hz, and (c) an aperiodic random distribution of sound energy, as in a noise

mental we see a harmonic at 200 Hz. Additional harmonics are seen also at 300 Hz, 400 Hz, 500 Hz, 600 Hz, . . . 5,000 Hz. If our display were expanded horizontally, we possibly might see harmonics as high in frequency as 8,000 Hz or even a little higher, depending on the individual larynx involved; but only energy in the range below 5,000 Hz generally is regarded as important to the study of speech production and perception.

Note that the preponderance of intensity of the glottal source is in the lower frequencies. To the right, moving from low toward higher frequencies, the intensity declines at a rate of about 6 dB per octave. We would see basically this same spectrum for any normal larynx, and the general shape of the spectrum would not change much, regardless of the pitch or intensity of the voice. We would, though, see harmonics more widely spaced if the fundamental frequency were greater, or more narrowly spaced if the fundamental were lower in frequency.

In Figure 2-15(b) we have simply drawn a continuous smooth curve that connects the point of maximum intensity at one frequency to the point of maximum intensity at the next higher frequency. Now, if we were to delete the vertical lines in (b), leaving just our superimposed curve, we would be displaying what is known as a "continuous spectrum" or "spectrum envelope" of the glottal source. A continuous spectrum still tells us a great deal about the nature of a sound (even though it does not show the exact location of harmonics) and about how the sound likely will be interpreted by a human listener.

For speech perception purposes, the ear does not need to attend to discrete individual harmonics. Rather, it attends to concentrations of sound energy within certain regions or ranges of frequency. When we analyze the spectra of vowels and diphthongs and of some consonants, these ranges or regions of energy concentration are known as *formants*. The glottal source itself has no formants; and, as we've previously noted, the audible sound at the level of the glottis is more like a rather nondescript buzz than like a voice. By the time that sound emerges from the mouth, it has undergone considerable change. It sounds like a voice, and it even may sound like a recognizable phoneme. As you would expect, the spectrum of this "output" signal also looks quite different from the glottal source spectrum.

You earlier saw the waveform of a vowel /ɑ/ utterance in Figure 2-10, and now in Figure 2-16(a) we have displayed the continuous spectrum of that same utterance. The peaks in the spectrum are the locations of five formants of the /ɑ/. For analysis and discussion purposes, formants are numbered in sequence, beginning with F1, the formant with the lowest frequency location. F2 then is the next higher formant, F3, the next higher, and so on (through F5 in our /ɑ/ example).

Information about the frequency locations of F1 and F2 generally has been thought to be sufficient information to enable our ear (and brain) to recognize vowels accurately. The third formant, F3, sometimes may assist us with this identification task and may help to make the vowel seem more natural sounding. Any additional higher frequency formants are regarded

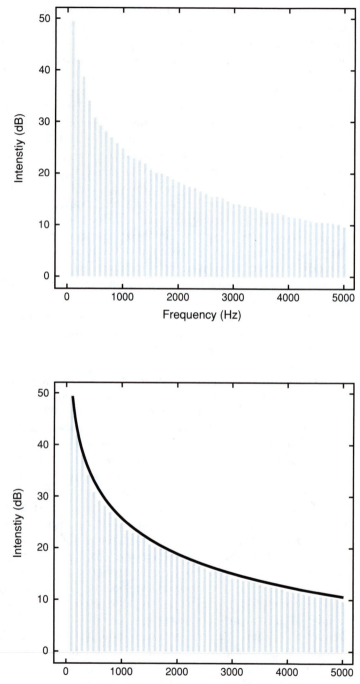

FIGURE 2-15   Line spectrum (a) and continuous spectrum (b) of the human glottal sound source with vocal folds vibrating at 100 Hz

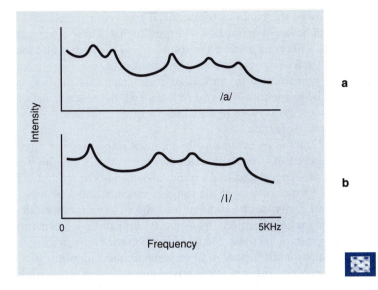

/a/

a

/I/

b

Intensity

0   Frequency   5KHz

FIGURE 2-16   Continuous spectra of two vowels /ɑ/ (a), and /ɪ/ (b)

as contributing to our perception of quality or timbre of the voice rather than to phoneme identification.

The continuous spectrum of an /ɪ/ utterance is shown in Figure 2-16(b), and you quickly will note that only four formants appear. The critical difference, however, is that the frequency locations of F1 and F2 differ considerably from those of the /ɑ/. Each vowel of our language has typical or characteristic F1, F2, and F3 frequency locations. These locations for adult males (with large vocal tracts) will differ somewhat from the locations for adult females (with somewhat smaller vocal tracts) and for children (with even smaller vocal tracts), but the general patterning of formant locations remains constant from speaker to speaker.

Our /ɑ/ was spoken by an adult male, and his first three formant locations are at about 770 Hz, 1230 Hz, and 2620 Hz, respectively. The /ɪ/ was spoken by an adult female, and her first three formants for /ɪ/ are found to be at approximately 530 Hz, 2160 Hz, and 2965 Hz. These frequency locations, in both cases, correspond very closely to the locations reported by Hillenbrand, Getty, Clark, and Wheeler (1995) in what undoubtedly is the most thoroughly detailed study of average vowel formant frequencies yet reported in our literature.

It is far beyond the scope of our text to examine in detail the manner in which formant frequency locations arise, but we would point out that formants reflect the resonation (selective emphasis and suppression) of the frequencies that are present in the original glottal source spectrum. Once our vocal folds begin to vibrate, the sound waves begin to travel toward the listener. En route, however, the glottal sound will be reflected and bounced about within the confines of our vocal tract. And the effects of this resonation will be heard in our final "output" signal. These effects are comparable to the effects of passing the sound signal through a filtering process (which is something you do with the amplifier of your own stereo system each time you adjust it to emphasize or de-emphasize the bass or treble "tone" of the music to which you're listening). Because resonation has similar results, the process we're describing is often called the "*source-filter theory of vowel production.*"

But the vocal tract is an exceptionally complex **resonance** (or filtering) system, comprised of irregularly shaped cavities. Moreover, the size and shape of the pharyngeal and oral cavities are quickly changed, easily and continuously, by movements of the tongue, jaw, lips, and pharyngeal walls; and the nasal cavity can be coupled into the system in varying degrees, or it can be excluded entirely from the system, all by adjustments of the velum and pharyngeal walls. Depending upon the configuration of the vocal tract at a particular instant in time, some frequencies of the glottal source will combine with reflected waves and be reinforced, while others will combine and be suppressed or nearly cancelled.

These varying degrees of reinforcement and cancellation are determined basically by two factors. One factor relates to the wavelengths of the various harmonics of the glottal source spectrum. A second factor relates to the dimensions of the vocal tract. Whenever a sound wave travels through a resonating tube, the resonance effect, if any, depends upon how the length of the tube relates to the wavelength of the sound. Some wavelengths will be reflected back strongly, others weakly, and some not at all. The resultant interactions between a reflected wave and the original wave then will determine whether the original sound wave is strengthened, weakened, or relatively unaffected.

Each harmonic in the glottal spectrum has its own wavelength, however, and we know that the vocal tract is not a *simple* resonating tube. The vocal tract is not even a *single* tube, as we also know, considering that the tongue may act to divide the tract into a pharyngeal cavity and an oral cavity and that the nasal cavity may or may not be included. It should not surprise us, then, that the output signal of the vocal tract will contain a complex patterning of frequency regions that are relatively strong and others that are relatively weak or even nonexistent.

In essence, we might say that formants will show up in the output spectrum at those frequency regions where the greatest reinforcement has occurred. The "valleys" between formants, on the other hand, represent frequency regions in which suppression (or at least little or no reinforcement) has occurred.

Another display that provides information about formant locations is called a **spectrogram.** In the spectrogram, the horizontal axis represents frequency, and the vertical axis represents time. Darkness and lightness in the pattern shown by a spectrogram are related to the relative intensities

Resonance.
Phenomenon whereby acoustic energy present at various frequencies in the complex laryngeal tone is selectively emphasized or suppressed by the vocal tract.

Spectrogram.
Graphic display of the frequency components of a complex sound where time is shown on the horizontal axis, frequency on the vertical axis, and intensity is shown by relative darkness of the graph.

of sound within different frequency ranges. A formant region shows up more darkly than do frequency regions where sound is less intense.

A spectrogram enables us to visualize spectral changes over time. We are not limited, as we were in the line spectrum and continuous spectrum displays, to examining just one brief slice of time. Figure 2-17 is a spectrogram which shows three consecutive utterances: first (on the left), the vowel /a/; in the middle, the diphthong /aɪ/; and on the right, the vowel /ɪ/.

We have included this particular spectrogram in order to show you the change of formant frequency locations that occurs during production of a diphthong (the combination of two vowels into a single phoneme). As our resonating cavities move from their configuration for the first vowel element toward the configuration required for the second vowel, these adjustments are reflected in movements of formants. The change in frequency location of a formant is known as a *formant transition*. Note in our diphthong, near the white arrowhead mark, how the frequencies of F1 and F2 are beginning to move from their /a/ locations toward the F1 and F2 frequency locations of the /ɪ/.

Formant transitions play an important role in our perception of consonants, too. Hearing such transitions helps us to know, for example, what tongue posture preceded (and/or will follow) a vowel sound in an utterance. This subtle information about the extents and durations of formant transitions somehow registers in our minds; and, from that information, we have learned to draw inferences about probable associated articulatory adjustments. Even when the sound energy of an adjacent phoneme is diminished or absent, we are able to perceive the "missing phoneme" with amazing accuracy. No doubt this greatly facilitates our recognition of

FIGURE 2-17   Spectrograms of the diphthong /aɪ/ and of its component vowels, /a/ and /ɪ/

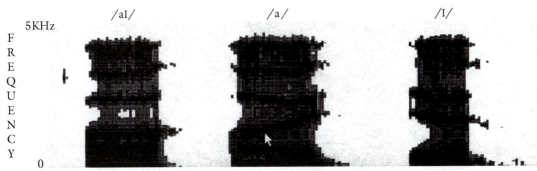

phonemes that may have extremely brief durations in ongoing speech or which, especially in the case of voiceless consonants, may be very difficult to recognize merely from their somewhat ambiguous spectral features. Other factors, such as our knowledge of linguistic probabilities, obviously also come to our assistance in the perception of speech; but, nevertheless, the fact that we typically understand the spoken word so effortlessly seems at least a minor and still mysterious miracle.

One day, as our knowledge base continues to be expanded and further refined, there is little doubt that the results of research in these areas will have contributed even more substantially to our understanding of speech, language, and hearing disorders. Already, as you will learn in later chapters, significant benefits are being realized by many of our clients. Individuals who are physically incapable of producing speech are able to take advantage of systems that synthesize quite intelligible speech. And the effective utilization of implanted cochlear bypasses in persons who are deaf or profoundly hearing impaired is far more successful than it could be without accurate information about the acoustic nature of speech signals.

It is clear that even our incomplete understandings have been quite useful to clinicians and clients and are not simply of interest to laboratory scientists. Furthermore, we are likely to see an accelerated development of additional clinical applications as communication scientists continue to fill in missing parts of the speech perception puzzle. You will be better prepared to work effectively, today and in the future, if you possess at least an elementary understanding of some basic aspects of speech production, linguistics, speech acoustics, and speech perception. In this chapter we've provided just a first glimpse into each, hoping to whet your appetite.

STUDY QUESTIONS

1. Explain the differences in the meanings of "language," "speech," and "communication."
2. Why is speech said to be an *overlaid* function of the respiratory, laryngeal, and oral/nasal structures?
3. Describe the basic elements of phonation. What structures and processes are involved, and how do they work together to produce voice?
4. What factors account for the differences that we typically hear between the adult male and the adult female voices?
5. Transcribe the following words, using symbols of the International Phonetic Alphabet: *aphasia, chew, diphthong, either, formant, larynx, pharynx, shoe, teeth, to, too, two*
6. At what seven sites along the vocal tract do we "valve" the airstream in order to produce consonant sounds? Give an example of one consonant for each place.

7. In what ways may adjacent phonemes affect one another when they are combined in the utterance of a syllable or word?

8. Avoiding the use of technical jargon, explain what is meant by the term "morpheme."

9. How is sound produced, and how does sound travel through the air from one location to another?

10. What acoustic features differentiate one vowel sound from another, and how do we produce these differences even while our basic voice signal remains unchanged at the laryngeal level?

ENDNOTES

[1]We should note, however, that some scholars believe the process of evolution may have favored the survival and refinement of structural features in the throat and mouth that facilitate speech production.

[2]/ðə mæstɚ-ɪ əv fonɛtɪks ɪznt æz hɑrd æz ju maɪt θɪŋk for mɛnɪ ɪf nɑt most əv ðɛm ɑr sɪmɪlɚ tu ðə lɛtɚz əv aʊr ɔrdɪnɛrɪ æl fəbɛt ‖ jul sun rɛkəgnaɪz ðɛm/

[3]In almost every individual the left hemisphere is the dominant hemisphere for processing and planning speech and language events. It is responsible for "logical" thinking and problem solving. The left hemisphere generally is larger and has a more extensive blood supply than the right. Among other functions, the right side of the brain is responsible for understanding nonspeech sounds and spatial relationships. The right side also is the hemisphere usually responsible for creative and artistic activity and for recognizing a familiar face.

[4]Even infants as young as six months are known to be able to discriminate auditorily among different vowel utterances (and to be able to do so even when the vowels are spoken by different individuals).

REFERENCES

Denes, P., and Pinson, E. (1973). *The speech chain.* New York: Doubleday.

Denes, P., and Pinson, E. (1993). *The speech chain: The physics and biology of spoken language,* 2d ed. New York: W. H. Freeman and Co.

Hillenbrand, J., Getty, L., Clark, M., and Wheeler, K. (1995). Acoustic characteristics of American English vowels. *Journal of the Acoustical Society of America,* 97, 3099–3111.

Iglesias, A., and Anderson, N. (1993). Dialectal variations. In J. Bernthal and N. Bankson, *Articulation and phonological disorders,* 3d ed. Englewood Cliffs, NJ: Prentice Hall, Inc.

MacKay, I. (1987). *Phonetics: The science of speech production,* 2d ed. Austin, TX: Pro-Ed.

Terrell, S., and Terrell, F. (1993). African-American cultures. In D. Battle, *Communication disorders in multicultural populations.* Stoneham, MA: Butterworth-Heinemann.

Development of Speech and Language

> *... you and I belong to a species with a remarkable ability: we can shape events in each other's brains with exquisite precision. ... That ability is language. Simply by making noises with our mouths, we can reliably cause precise new combinations of ideas to arise in each other's minds. The ability comes so naturally that we are apt to forget what a miracle it is.* (Pinker, 1994, p. 15)

Before reading this chapter you should have a baby immediately. If this is impossible, then read it for that wonderful future prospect. You also should read Pinker's book, *The Language Instinct: How the Mind Creates Language* (1994), for a comprehensive and unusually lucid discussion of this intriguing topic.

Most parents never really appreciate the marvelous process that occurs when their infants learn to talk. They take great joy in seeing the child change from being a creeper to become *homo erectus,* but few of them have the knowledge to understand the much greater miracle when *homo erectus* becomes *homo sapiens* by acquiring language and speech.

No one knows when or why the very first word was spoken. It was probably little more than a sigh, perhaps an expletive or a groan accompanying some heavy lifting or hauling. Nevertheless, with that primitive harbinger of oral language, our ancestors started an immense journey in the use of symbols. No other creature has been able to duplicate the long pilgrimage. When a child utters his own first word, he rediscovers a well-marked pathway to the magic of speech.

Since many of the disorders of communication have their onset early in life and reflect delays in maturation or acquisition of basic skills or competencies, we should understand something about how speech and language develop normally in the child. We begin our account from the moment of birth, trace the course of development through the stage of reflexive cooing and crying sounds, then through the period of babbling, and finally, into the acquisition of full-fledged language.

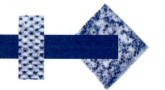

PREREQUISITES FOR SPEECH DEVELOPMENT

No doubt you have heard the anecdote about the naïve American tourist in Paris who was astonished to observe that even the small children there could speak French. Anyone who has tried to *learn* a second language, particularly after age twelve or thereabout, knows that it is far more demanding than *acquiring* one's own native tongue. Babies just seem to develop speech naturally as they mature, and most parents are not even aware of how the process unfolds. But not all children begin talking at the appropriate time, and, to determine where the normal sequence of development went awry, the speech pathologist must review the prerequisites for the acquisition of speech (see Emerick and Haynes, 1986, p. 91).

Does the Child Have a Normal Vocal Tract?   Although we have seen children who learned to talk despite anatomical abnormalities, the acquisition of speech is obviously fostered by having an intact vocal tract.

Does the Child Show Normal Neuromotor Maturation?   Speech is a very rapid, complex motor act and requires very finely tuned neurological regulation.

Longitudinal studies of children show a parallel course of development between key motor skills and the acquisition of speech. Consider the following examples:

Age	Motor Skill	Speech
6 months	Sits alone	Prespeech: babbling
12 months	Stands; takes first step	First words
18 to 22 months	Walks alone	Two-word phrases

Delay in acquisition of motor skills is often associated with slow speech development.

Does the Child Have a Normal Auditory System?   Speech is acquired primarily through the ear, and children who have a hearing loss, auditory localization, or discrimination problems will often show delay in the development of speech and language.[1]

Does the Child Have Adequate Physical and Emotional Health to Support and Foster the Growth of Oral Language?   Physical and emotional illnesses drain energy, restrict and distort relationships with family members, and hinder normal sensorimotor exploration and growth of independence.

Does the Child Show Normal Intellectual Capacity and Cognitive Development?   To acquire oral language, a child must have the mental capacity for using symbols. To use symbols appropriately, the child must, among other **cognitive** functions, be able to attend, recognize, make associations and generalizations, and store items in memory. Facility with language is an outgrowth of a child's expanding ability to reason; mental development is the necessary base for performing symbolic operations. In other words, a child can talk only as well as he can think.

An example will help to clarify the point we are making. Around age nine to twelve months, a child acquires the notion that objects have per-

Cognition. Higher mental functions, thoughts, interpretations, ideas.

manence; he becomes aware that an item, such as a favorite toy, exists even when he cannot see it. Before a child discovers he can use words to label objects and events, and thus call them forth, he must develop the concept of object permanence.

Does the Child Have a Nurturing and Stimulating Environment?   At least three environmental factors are crucial in fostering speech development: (1) an emotionally positive relationship (bonding) with a caregiver who provides reinforcement for the child's communicative overtures; (2) at least one speech model (person) who uses simple but well-formed language patterns; and (3) opportunities for exploration and a variety of day-to-day experiences that stimulate the urge to communicate.[2]

When parents have their first child they often wonder how well the child is doing in acquiring the ability to talk. They ask for tables of maturation so they can compare their child with others. The guidelines parents seek are available, but unfortunately they provide only general information, usually expressed in terms of what should be expected of the "average" child. Each baby is unique, however, progressing unevenly and rarely fitting neatly into arbitrary age norms. Nevertheless, most children do seem to pass systematically through various stages of speech development, and we provide Table 3.1 to illustrate the process.

We wish to emphasize that these stages merely highlight only the major characteristics of a progressive learning process. No child suddenly shifts from one stage to another. Always there is overlap. Even when she begins to say her first words she may still be doing some babbling and vocal play.

Though most children of different nationalities must learn different languages, the early development of their speech is similar from nation to nation. DeBoysson-Bardies, Sagart, and Bacri (1981) found that the babbling of French babies could not be distinguished from those who had English parents. A similar result for Spanish and English infants was shown by Oller and Eilers (1982) and for Swedish babies by Roug, Landberg, and Lundberg (1989). Very early babbling apparently follows the same universal pattern around the world, only later to be altered in ways that begin to reflect the speech characteristics of the particular language community to which the infant is exposed (Levitt and Utman, 1992).

Now let us examine the development of speech and language in more detail.

Many linguists, doubtless because their field is focused on language rather than on speech, have shown only minor interest in the output of the baby's mouth prior to the emergence of the first meaningful words. The linguists point out that the sounds of crying, comfort, and babbling are not phonemic, which, of course, is true. These early utterances are sounds (*phones*), not phonemes, and often they lack any precise identity because their boundaries are difficult to determine and their variability is

❖ TABLE 3.1	Development of speech and language

Age	Speech and Language
1–3 months.	Little sign of speech comprehension. Much crying. May cry differently in expressing pain, hunger, or need for attention. Produces cooing and comfort sounds. Does show response to sounds and moving objects.
3–6 months.	Seems to pay attention to the speech of others and to react to it. Less crying and more cooing and the beginning of babbling. Responds to parental speech and behavior by vocalization and imitation.
6–9 months.	Marked increase in babbling and word play. Vocal play shows inflections. Comprehends certain words such as "Eat" or "Up." Uses signs and some syllables to express wants.
9–12 months.	Comprehends a few words and even phrases: "No." "Daddy come." "All gone." "Go car." Crude imitation of parent's speech. Practices syllable strings.
12–15 months.	Appearance of first words, usually monosyllables or repeated syllables: "Mama," "Byebye," "No." Much jargon and self talk. Can point to objects, toys, animals. Understands simple directions and the word "NO." Has a speaking vocabulary of six to eight words. Understands short phrases.
15–20 months.	Seems to understand most of what is said, if said simply. Regularly uses words and short phrases to express desires. Imitates environmental noises. Much self talk when alone. Begins to combine several words into primitive sentences: "Eat all done." "More milk."
20–30 months.	Comprehends most adults if they speak slowly and simply. Knows names of all familiar objects and activities. Speaks in phrases and sentences. Has a vocabulary of about 100 words.

great. Moreover, although the baby may repeatedly utter a few clearly defined sounds in babbling, some of them drop out and seem to have to be relearned once words begin to be used in true language. However, some contemporary experts (Golinkhoff, 1983; Blake and Fink, 1987; Reich, 1986) insist that there is continuity from prelinguistic to linguistic vocalizations. Stoel-Gammon and Dunn report that "results of studies covering the transition from babbling to speech reveal that the phonological patterns of babbling are quite similar to those of early meaningful speech in terms of syllable types and phonetic repertoires" (1985, p. 21).

At any rate, during the period of prelanguage, the child does build the foundation for the true speech that is still to come. In the very early reflexive sounds of crying and comfort-cooing, we certainly find babies practicing the basic synergies of respiration and phonation. In their babbling we see them exploring articulation.

Reflexive Utterances

During the first three months of life a child has a very limited repertoire of vocal behavior. The two main types of nonpurposeful reflexive utterances the very young baby will produce are the crying and comfort sounds.

Crying Sounds.   Even the father of a baby will recognize the difference between them, although he may not be able to distinguish between the wail due to hunger or the howl caused by an open safety pin. For the first month parents should expect more crying than whimpering, and more whimpering than comfort sounds. The ratio, it is hoped, will change as the diapers go by. If the parents listen carefully to the crying, they'll probably be able to detect vowel-like sounds resembling the /æ/, /ɛ/, and /aɪ/ of our language, but they will be nasalized. And if the parent's imagination is good enough, he may hear a few sounds that crudely resemble the consonants /g/ or /k/, but since these sounds are reflexive they should not be viewed as the true ancestors of the phonemes that the baby will eventually master.

When the baby is about two months old, parents can identify several distinct types of crying—signifying rage, hunger, pain—all having a distinct cadence and pitch level. Furthermore, high-risk babies—those who have jaundice, respiratory problems, and other infant ailments—can be recognized because they produce distinctive crying patterns (Zeskind and Lester, 1981; Petrovich-Bartell, Cowan, and Morse, 1982). If the crying sounds make any contribution at all to the mastery of speech (which you may doubt at midnight), that contribution lies in the practicing of essential motor coordinations and the establishment of the necessary feedback loops between the larynx and the mouth and ear. In addition, crying, particularly when it becomes differentiated, establishes a primitive communication link between child and parent.

Comfort Sounds.   These reflexive utterances are difficult to describe in words. Gurgles and sighs, grunts, and little wisps of sound, you will probably lump them together under the category of "cooing." They mainly appear during or just after feeding, or diaper changing, or some other form of relief from distress. Again, if you listen carefully, the front vowels and back consonants will seem to predominate, but they are not as nasalized as in crying.

Over and over again in taking the case histories of children with very severe articulation disorders or speech delay we have found parents telling us that these children cried much more than their other babies. If we were to hazard a guess as to the significance of these reports, it would be that the feedback loops between the ear and the vocalizing mechanism became loaded with the static of pain or unpleasantness. In contrast, when the ear of the baby hears the sound of her own voice in the context of pleasurable sensations, that baby may be more likely to experiment with her utterances and so achieve better speech sooner. Anyway, of one thing we're sure. You'll enjoy those comfort sounds more than the crying. Crying may build parental character, but the comfort sounds engender love. You'll need both.

Even when very young, babies will be far more sophisticated at receiving than in sending messages. At about two months of age, they will show early signs of social awareness—tracking an adult's movements with their eyes and smiling. Babies show a particular fascination with facial expressions and are able to mimic facial gestures of adults when they are as young as three weeks old (Figure 3-1). Newborn infants also respond selectively to the speech of adults. Not only do they coordinate their body movements with the melody of speech, but they also can easily discriminate speech from nonspeech signals. At an early age they can even detect differences among vowels and the very small changes between voiced and nonvoiced plosive sounds. Infants just one

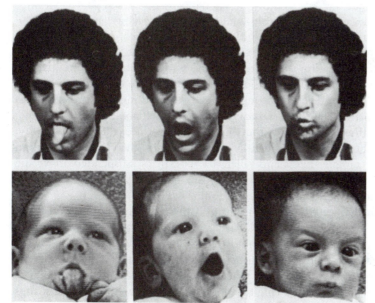

FIGURE 3-1 Infants can mimic facial expressions (from A. Meltzoff and M. Moore, "Imitation of facial and manual gestures by neonates." *Science* 198: 75–78, 1977).

and two days old have been shown to be able to hear the difference between **canonical** and **noncanonical syllables** (Moon, Bever, and Fifer, 1992). Evidently, babies are born with a special capability for recognizing and processing speech, so be careful what you say during the 2 A.M. feeding!

Babbling

Emerging from the stage of reflexive vocalizations is the appearance of babbling, a universal phenomenon found in all human infants. It is characterized by the chaining and linking of sounds together on one exhalation. We hear syllables of all types, the CV (consonant vowel as in "ba"), which is most common, with the VC (vowel followed by a consonant, as in "ab") and the VCV ("aba") being found less frequently. These strings of syllables have no more semantic meaning than did the comfort sounds, although their component sounds are perhaps more similar to our standard phonemes. The baby just seems to be playing with his tongue, lips, and larynx in much the same fashion as he plays with his fingers or toes. A good share of this **vocal play** is carried on when the child is alone, and it disappears when someone attracts his attention. One of the senior author's children played with her babbling each morning after awakening, usually beginning with a whispered "eenuh" and repeating it with increasing effort until she spoke the syllable aloud, whereupon she would laugh and chortle as she said it over and over. The moment she heard a noise in the parent's bedroom this babbling would cease and crying would begin.

Parents who joyfully rush in and ruin this speech rehearsal are failing to appreciate its significance in the learning of speech. The child must simultaneously feel and hear the sound repeatedly if it is ever to emerge as an identity. Imitation is essentially a device to perpetuate a stimulus, and babbling is self imitation of the purest variety. When the babbling period is interrupted or delayed through illness, the appearance of true speech is often similarly retarded. Deaf babies may begin to babble at a normal time, but since they cannot hear the sounds they produce, they probably lose interest and hence have much less true vocal play than the hearing child (see, for example, Eilers and Oller, 1994). Mirrors suspended above the cribs of deaf babies have increased the babbling through visual self-stimulation (Stoel-Gammon and Otomo, 1986).

And what are the contributions of babbling to the acquisition of true speech? As we have mentioned earlier, many linguists would say they are few. Certainly the babbling sounds are not phonemic, but in babbling we often hear the repetition of intonation and stress patterns so similar to the patterning of adult sentences that many parents swear that their baby is talking to himself or is trying to tell them something. Some of the strings of syllables have the intonational patterns of command; others, of decla-

Canonical.
Canonical syllables have a vowel nucleus and consonant margins (CVC).

Vocal play.
In the development of speech, the stage during which the child experiments with sounds and syllables.

ration or questioning; most are just randomly varied in pitch and stress. During this babbling period we find sounds from many languages other than English (even the tongue clicks of Hottentots) occurring in the free speech flow.

Socialized Babbling.   In about the fifth or sixth month, when the infant can sit up, fixate an object with its eyes, grab an object to put into its mouth, or hoist its hind end up to crawl, some of the babbling appears to have an instrumental function. It *seems* to be used to get attention, to support rejection, to express a demand. She babbles more in a social context. Sometimes she even seems to listen and certainly is aware of the speech of others.

A bit later the child begins to use vocalization for getting attention, supporting rejection, and expressing demands. Frequently he will look at an object and cry at the same time. He voices his eagerness and protest. He is using his primitive speech both to express himself and to modify the behavior of others. This stage is also marked by the appearance of syllable repetition, or the doubling of sounds, in vocal play. He singles out a certain double syllable such as *da-da* and frequently practices it to the exclusion of all other combinations. Sometimes a single combination will be practiced for several weeks at a time, although it is more usual to find the child changing to something new every few days and reviewing some former vocal achievements at odd intervals. True dissyllables (*ba-da*) come relatively late in the first year, and the infant rejects them when the parent attempts to use them as stimulation.

At this time the child will often "answer back." Make a noise and he makes a noise. The two noises are usually dissimilar, but it is obvious that he is responding. In his vocal play, most of the vowels are still the ones made in the front or middle of the mouth, but a few *oo* and *oh* sounds (which are back vowels) can be detected. There are also more consonants to be heard, the /d/, /t/, /n/, and /l/ having appeared; but it's still hard to separate them out of the flow of unsorted utterance unless you have long, sharp ears. Some private babbling continues throughout these months, but now the child seems to take more pleasure in public practice. He's listening to himself but also listening to you. He is talking to himself but also sometimes to you. This is *socialized vocalization*.[3]

Inflected Vocal Play

Although some squeals and changes in pitch and loudness have previously occurred in the babbling, it is not until about the eighth month that inflection or intonational changes become prominent. It is then that the vocal play takes on the tonal characteristics of adult speech. We now find the baby using inflections that sound like questions, commands, surprise, ponderous statements of fact, all in a delightful gibberish that has no meaning. We hear not only the inflections and sounds of English but those of the Oriental languages as well. No baby can be sure that he will end up speaking English. So he practices a bit of Chinese now and then. We have tried hard to imitate some of these sounds and inflections and have failed. The baby can often duplicate whole strings of these strange beads of sounds.

The private babbling and social vocal play continue strongly during this period from eight months to a year. The repertoire of sounds increases. There is a marked gain in back vowels and front consonants. Crying time diminishes, even though few fathers would believe it. They begin to get interested in their sons and daughters about this stage, however. The infant is becoming human. He'll bang a cup; he'll smile back at the old man. He'll reach out to be picked up. He begins to understand what "No!" means. But most important of all, he begins to *sound* as though he is talking.

We have previously spoken of various stages of development, but it should be made very clear that, although most children go through these stages in the order given, the activity in any one stage does not cease as soon as the characteristics of the next stage appear. Grunts and wails, babbling, socialized vocalization, and inflection practice all begin at about the times stated, but they continue throughout the entire period of speech development.

It is during this period that the baby begins to use more of the back vowels /u, ʊ, o, ɔ/ in his babbling. It is interesting that when we work with adult articulation cases, we prefer syllables such as *see* and *ray* and *lee* to those involving the back vowels like *soo* and *low*. Front vowels seem to be more easily mastered.

The baby, through vocal gymnastics, gradually masters the coordinations necessary to meaningful speech. But it must be emphasized that when he is repeating *da-da* and *ma-ma* at this stage, he is not designating his parents. His arm movements have much more meaning than do those of his mouth. It is during these months that the ratio of babbling to crying greatly increases. Comprehension of parental gestures shows marked growth. The child now responds to the parent's stimulation, not automatically, but with more discrimination. His imitation is more hesitant, but it also seems more purposive. It begins to resemble the parent's utterance. If the father interrupts the child's chain of *papapapapapapapapapa* by saying *papa*, the child is less likely than before to say *wah* or *gu* and more likely to whisper *puh* or repeat the two-syllable *puhpuh*. During this period, simple musical tones, songs, or lullabies are especially good stimulation. The parent should observe the child's inflections and rhythms and attempt to duplicate them. This is the material that should be used for stimulation at this period. In this socialized babbling or vocal play of the baby we find the basic pattern of communication, of sending and receiving, although it is only sounds, not meaningful messages, that are being batted back and forth.

By the eighth month pitch inflections are very prominent and the prosodic features or melody of his gibberish make the give-and-take of a "conversation" with the baby a delightful experience. Social reinforcers such as a parental smile or gesture or touch or spoken word increase the frequency of his vocal behaviors. You will imitate him more than he will you, but you'll note that his repertoire of sounds is growing rapidly, with a marked gain in back vowels and front consonants. It is about time for him to say his first meaningful word.

THE FIRST WORDS

When you have that first baby someone is sure to present you with a "Baby Book" in which you are to record a host of its accomplishments. One of them will surely be a section of "First Words." We have examined many such books without much profit from their perusal. (One mother claimed that her child's first word was "Kalamazoo" spoken at the age of seven months while babbling. It was probably just a sneeze.) The linguistic literature and our own observations of our own children and grandchildren have been more illuminating than these baby books.

For a host of reasons, including parental pride and faulty as well as wishful memories, reliable reporting of a child's "first word" can be an elusive matter even for the trained linguist. While actual words "co-occur in the period of transition . . . with a variety of non-word vocalizations, little attention has been given to the formidable problem of identifying these earliest words" (Vihman and McCune, 1994). It is not surprising, then, that the criteria for recognizing those first words show wide differences from parent to parent and that the average age reported for first words varies from about nine to eighteen months for normal children. When the criterion for the emergence of true verbal utterance is increased from the very first word to a vocabulary of ten words, the average age is about fifteen months. A few children begin to speak much later, and when they do, they may speak in multiple-word sentences, thereby showing again that comprehension precedes performance (Barrett, 1985).

Words are acquired (comprehended) before they are used, and long before the first one pops out, the child has shown by his behavior that he understands the gestures, intonations, and meanings of some of the parent's speech. Since parents at this time tend to speak to their children in single words or short phrases and sentences when really trying to communicate with them (rather than adoring them, which produces a host of multiword nonsense), it is not surprising that the first meaningful utterances of babies are single words.

The first words spoken by the child are usually single syllable (CV) words or two-syllable reduplicate words (CVCV) such as /dɑ/ or /mɑmɑ/. Here is one explanation.

"In order to suck, the child makes a lip closure around a nipple and presses the nipple up against the **alveolar ridge** with the tongue. The basic movements to and away from these constrictions involve the CV-like syllables as the child alternately presses the lips together and then opens the mouth" (Hoffman, Schuckers, and Daniloff, 1989).

As you might expect, salient objects, events, and persons from a child's daily experience are singled out for his very first words. The senior author's son's first word was "aga," meaning "all gone" in the contexts of no more milk in his cup or the turning off of a light.

The first words are sentence words, and you will soon hear the same utterance spoken at one time with the intonation and stress of a declarative statement, or at another as a command, or even as a question. Often an appropriate gesture will accompany the utterance. Even though only one morpheme is used, the tone of the voice and the gesture show the other parts of the implicit sentence. When one of our daughters heard the sound of the car in the garage, she said, "Dadda?" with an upward inflection and looked toward the door through which he usually entered. Then when he came in, she held up her arms to be picked up and imperiously demanded, "Dadda! Dadda!" with the appropriate inflection and stress of command. These were sentences even though only single words were spoken.

As you probably have observed, children often "misuse" these new words: a word may be limited (*underextension*) to a very narrow range of reference ("dog" is reserved for only *one* particular canine); or a word may be expanded (*overextension*) to cover a large range of referents (*all* creatures with four legs are "dogs").

How are the first words acquired? This question looks innocently simple, but it has troubled many students of language and still has no universally accepted answer. Since you may have to teach a nonverbal child to talk someday, your own or somebody else's, you should be interested in the various explanations.

Assume for a moment that it were possible to bring up an infant in some remote spot where he would receive basic care but never be talked to or even hear other people conversing. What language would he speak? Would his first words be uttered in Hebrew—the original universal language according to King James—as some theologians believed? On the basis of our clinical experience with several experience-deprived children, as well as familiarity with the literature, a child so isolated from human discourse would have no intelligible speech. Experts agree that normal speech and language development requires the dual contributions of good native endowment and a reasonably stimulating environment.

Children do, after all, acquire only the language that is spoken to them. But why do children in disparate cultures learn to speak about the

Alveolar ridges.
The ridges on the jawbones beneath the gums. An alveolar sound is one in which the tongue makes contact with the upper-gum ridge.

same time, follow the same developmental sequence, and use linguistic forms that are remarkably similar?

How Children Learn Their Morphology

1st word

How children learn their first words (morphemes) is still something of a mystery despite many investigations. Those first words are free morphemes, words that stand alone. The morphemic modifiers such as plurals and past tense (bound morphemes) come later.

Nelson (1993) lists six theories that seek to explain how babies learn their first words. We will summarize four of them—two relating to learning theory, and two relating to native endowment. Each seems to make some sense, but none has gained complete acceptance.

Learning Theory

For many decades, speech pathologists relied on learning theory as their primary source of information about language acquisition. In this frame of reference, language is seen as a behavior acquired by the right amount of motivation, environmental stimulation, and parental reinforcement. A baby must be endowed with the normal sensory and motor equipment, of course, but he is basically a blank tablet for the script of experience. The core element in all learning theory explanations is the necessity to associate verbal behavior with rewarding conditions. We now present brief reviews of two prominent learning theories of speech and language development: **operant conditioning** and the autism theory.

Operant Conditioning.

Advocates of operant conditioning believe that whenever a parent smiles, cuddles, or responds favorably to a child's vocalization, that vocalization or something like it will tend to increase in frequency. If that vocalization has some similarity to the intonation or phonemic patterns of adult language, it will get more reinforcement immediately, and then with each closer approximation the parent will tend to show more approval. Children echo or imitate the word of the mother, saying something like *milk* when she says it, and lo, there is the bottle and the mother's smile. When the word is emitted and then rewarded, the probability that it will be uttered again in future but similar situations is thereby increased. The development of syntax is explained by some theorists in terms of the chaining of operants, each word of a phrase or sentence carrying a cue that evokes the next one or next group of words. This simplistic account does not do justice to the operant learning explanation, but it describes its major features.

> **Operant conditioning.** The differential reinforcement of desired responses through the systematic control of their contingencies.

The Autism Theory.

Experiments in teaching birds to talk led a famous American psychologist to formulate what is known as the autism theory of speech acquisition (Mowrer, 1950). Mowrer found that his birds would reproduce human words only if these words were spoken by the trainer while the birds were being fondled or fed. After this had happened often enough, the word itself could apparently produce pleasurable feelings in the bird. Since myna birds and parakeets produce a lot of variable sounds, it is almost inevitable that a few of these sounds might resemble the human word that produced such pleasant feelings, Thus when the bird hears itself making these similar sounds, it feels again the pleasantness of fondling and being fed. So it repeats them, and the closer the bird's chirp-word comes to resemble the human word, the more pleasant the bird feels. By properly rewarding these progressive approximations, we can facilitate the process. However, finally the bird will find that "Polly-wants-a-cracker" is pleasant enough to be self-rewarding. The word "autism" refers to the self-rewarding aspect of the process. At any rate, these phrases seem to sound almost as good to the bird as a piece of suet tastes.

When this theory is applied to the child's learning of his first words, it seems to make a lot of sense. Certainly, the mother says "Mama" or "baby" a thousand times while feeding, bathing, or fondling the child. Also it is certain that the baby will find *mama mama* or *bubbababeeba* sometime in his babbling and vocal play. If these utterances flood him with pleasant feelings, he will repeat them more often than syllables such as "gugg," which have no special pleasant memories attached to them. It is also true that the closer the child comes to the standard words, the more reward he will get from the mother. There still remains the problem of giving meaning to utterance, and this is explained in terms of the context. "Mama" is used when the mama is present; "baby" is used when he sees himself in the mirror or plays with his body.

Native Endowment Theory

Linguists have asked persistent questions about speech and language development that the learning theories could not answer: Why do languages all over the world have such remarkably similar characteristics? Why does language acquisition commence at the same time and proceed in the same orderly fashion in all cultures? How can children *learn* language forms when parents reward speech attempts indiscriminately rather than grammatically correct utterances? There are two closely related points of view regarding language development as a preprogrammed human trait: the *nativistic theory* and *cognitive determinism*.

Nativistic Theory.

This explanation states that the child has an inborn capacity for language learning that is mobilized when he discovers that the parent's noises have meaning and a structure that somehow fit those innate patterns. Just as Helen Keller, deaf and blind, suddenly discovered that water had a name when the word was traced upon her hand by her teacher, so little children discover that things and experiences and people have words (names) for them, that there are different classes of words, and that words can be arranged sequentially according to certain basic rules to represent other meanings. Even as the child organizes his visual perceptions to recognize the bottle from which he drinks his milk, so he is programmed to organize his auditory perceptions of language. Born in all human beings is a basic competence or propensity for language learning and the parent's speech merely triggers that latent capacity (Chomsky, 1968).

The development of language, in this view, is an outgrowth of general maturation and, as we pointed out in a prior section of this chapter, the phases of language acquisition are synchronized with maturation of key motor skills. Adherents of this theory insist that other theories cannot account for the child's surprisingly rapid acquisition of the complexities of language or for his ability to generate novel phrases and sentences (and even new words such as "bringed" for "brought") that he has never heard before. Finally, proponents of this viewpoint maintain that there is a "readiness window" or "critical age period" during which proper environmental stimulation triggers language acquisition. If this critical period is bypassed because of severe illness or environmental deprivation, that portion of the brain devoted to language and related cognitive abilities may functionally atrophy.

Cognitive Determinism.   It is entirely possible to teach a child a few words by intensive operant conditioning. But to then suggest that he has achieved the use of language is like claiming that an adult is a playwright because he has memorized a few lines of Shakespeare. True language use has a cardinal feature: the expression of meaning. And to express meaning, a speaker, whether a child in the one-word stage or a garrulous adult, must have his mental clutch engaged before he can make sense with his mouth. This notion is the centerpiece of the cognitive determinism theory of language acquisition.

There is little doubt that the ability to use language rests upon a foundation of higher mental (cognitive) functions. Advocates of the cognitive determinism viewpoint assert that language development depends upon (is determined by) intellectual growth. Before a child can use her first word in a meaningful way, she must have acquired the mental sophistication to realize that a hidden object still exists. She must, in other words, be able to substitute mental imagery for, let's say, a teddy bear that has been placed playfully behind a sofa. The next step, then, is for the child to substitute the label "bear" for the missing toy. To put it differently, an uttered word is an outward and audible expression of an understanding.

In the cognitive theory of language acquisition, a child's gradually refined awareness of relationships, his development of concepts about the world, precede and are prerequisites for verbal expressions of meaning.

The environment serves to release and do some minor shaping of language development. Once a child begins to use words, however, his cognitive growth is facilitated.

The wrangling of scholars about how babies learn their first words does not help much. Perhaps all their theories are partly true. More helpful may be an account of how one of the senior author's children managed the feat.

> Cathy, by the age of one year, had gone through all the stages of speech development that we have sketched and at ten months it was clear that she comprehended many single words and even short phrases such as "No," "Go bye-bye," "ball," "eat," and "Mama" and "Daddy." When we spoke to her, she answered back but in jargon and gibberish. She still did some babbling and vocal play when alone but that was all.

> We had stimulated her a lot with simple speech and had encouraged her to imitate us in many ways. Whenever she was engaged in a repetitive activity such as banging her cup or clapping her hands or babbling, we would interrupt it by doing the same things ourselves and often she would return to the activity. Finally she would even thrust out her tongue when I did or wave bye-bye back at me when I left her. Nevertheless, there were no meaningful words.

> I was determined that her first word would be "Daddy" or something like it, and my wife was equally determined that it would be "Mama," and so we tried hard to make this happen by strongly reinforcing any time she said "da" or "ma" in her babbling or vocal play because these syllables occurred frequently.

> But her first word was neither. It was "pitty" /pɪtɪ/ for *pretty* and it was her name for a flower. I presume she had heard us say it but not nearly as often as we had other words. It was meaningful. She would point to a flower, any flower, and say "pitty" over and over again, then gurgle with triumph and delight. She never used it for any other object. He second word was "dah" /dɑ/ for *dog* and within two weeks she had mastered nine other words, all of which were names for objects or for activities. Within six more weeks she was speaking in phrases and short sentences. I still can't explain how she acquired that first word.

Conclusions

Even though we presented only a very brief review of the major theories of how children acquire speech and language, it still may seem confusing and unnecessarily complicated to you. Since we do not wish to end this section on such a note, let us present five general conclusions to use as stepping stones for finding your own path through the theoretical thickets:

> Although the precise contribution of each is not yet known, *both nature and nurture are involved in the process of language development*. While a child does seem to be biologically programmed for acquiring symbols

and the rules of early syntax, environmental stimulation may be very important for learning speech sounds and subtle nuances of more complex sentence structure. The variables of *sex* (females have a slight edge in rate of development), *order of birth* (firstborn and only children develop faster), and *socioeconomic status* (middle- and upper-class children seem to acquire language faster than do lower-class children) influence to some extent the rate of speech and language development.

While the rate at which they move through the stages of speech and language development may vary from individual to individual, the sequence is similar for all children. A child will not use inflected vocal play and then back up to begin babbling. Deviations in the sequence of development may signal a problem and should be thoroughly investigated.

At each stage of development, a child's manner of communication is an integrated whole, not an incomplete version of the form adults use. His performance is best described as a special type of language, "childese," if you will, complete with its own "rules."

The acquisition of language is all of one piece. All components, syntax, phonology, semantics, are acquired simultaneously; a child does not learn sentence structure and then phonology, for example. But the core of language development is the expression of meaning. The ability to express meaning depends on cognitive development.

The way in which a person conceptualizes the process of language development will determine what he does to foster development in a normal child or help a language-impaired child. Theory, whether explicitly formulated by a speech pathologist or simply a parental intuition, dictates the form of therapy.

Although we have observed our own children and grandchildren learn to speak, and have helped scores of troubled youngsters overcome the barriers of silence, we still look upon the process of language acquisition as a major miracle.

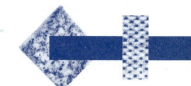

SYNTAX: LEARNING TO TALK IN SENTENCES

At about eighteen months of age, when they have acquired a vocabulary of about fifty words, many children begin to join words together, and this is probably the most important discovery the child will ever make—even were she to become the first person to walk on Mars. Indeed, it is probably the most important one the human species has achieved, for it enabled this two-legged race of mammals to exploit the immense potentials of symbolization. Were we restricted to one-word utterances, we would be woefully handicapped.

The development of syntax is amazingly swift: An eighteen-month-old child surges from telegraphic two-word utterances to complex sentences in a little more than a year and a half. There are several early signs that the child is getting ready for this great leap forward. One of our former students made these observations about her daughter just before the child began to put words together.

> Martha is seventeen months old and, like the books predict, she seems to be preparing for putting words together. (1) Her comprehension of speech has improved and she now will follow simple one- and two-step directions. (2) There are little nuances of prosody she uses to express different meanings with her one-word statements. (3) Her vocabulary has grown and peaked now at about forty-five words. (4) Her use of words is more "sophisticated" now. Rarely does she show overextension; cats, dogs, and horses now have separate names; every man in the supermarket is not "Daddy!" (5) Conceptually, too, she uses words in a more sophisticated way. She recognizes that the label "chair" can mean her father's Lazyboy, a rocker, or even her highchair. And, finally, (6) Martha is using symbolic play. She is much more imaginative now, pretending that a block is a cookie and an oatmeal box is a miniature oven.

How, then, does the child learn to join words together and to do so correctly? Some theorists have suggested that they come to recognize that there are two different kinds of words, *open-class* words and *pivot* words. Open-class words are similar to those the child has already been using in his one-word utterances. They are content words; they refer to things or activities; they are labels and can stand alone. *Milk, cup, car, Jimmy, shoe, drink, go* are all samples of open-class words. Pivot words are handles. By themselves they cannot constitute a sentence. They can modify ("*more* milk") or locate ("*that* cup") and do other things, but they need another word (an open-class word) before they make sense. Some linguists believe that when a child learns to join the two kinds of words together the first primitive sentences are formed.

Other linguists, however, reject the pivot grammar approach, mainly because it ignores the semantic or meaningful aspect of language. Instead, they claim that the child begins to join words together when he recognizes the need for modifiers, for ways of expressing subject-predicate, action-object, possessor-possessed, and other relationships. They feel that the pivot grammar explanation of how a child learns to combine words is too simplistic, preferring an explanation that shows how the four basic kinds of one-word utterances (declarative, imperative, negative, and interrogative) are expanded in the interest of meaningfulness. Table 3.2 (taken from Wood, 1976) provides an illustration of this point of view.

Advocates of this view assert that by focusing upon the meanings a child seems to convey (and how he uses utterances to make things happen in his environment) rather than on sentence structure, it is possible to

TABLE 3.2 Development of sentence structure

Sentence Type	Sequential Stages in Sentence Formulations		
Declarative	"Big boat"	"That big boat."	"That's a big boat."
Negative	"No play."	"I no play."	"I won't play."
Interrogative	"See toy?"	"Mom, see toy?"	"Did you see the toy?" *age question*
Imperative	"No touch!"	"You no touch!"	"Don't touch it."

B. Wood, *Children and Communication*. Englewood Cliffs, NJ: Prentice Hall, 1976, p. 137.

gain a better insight into how he organizes and conceptualizes his world. Neither explanation is completely satisfactory.

How then do children learn their syntax (the joining of words together to express their meanings)? Again, there are different theories with which we shall not burden you because none has achieved complete acceptance.

It does seem clear, however, that a certain progression occurs. First the child learns to use two-word *noun phrases*, such as "big ball" and "baby bottle" in which the first word modifies, locates, designates, or describes the noun.

Next, the child begins to use two-word *verb phrases*, saying "me go" and "kitty eat" with the verb following the noun to form the essential subject-predicate shape of a primitive sentence. Soon after this achievement, the verb may precede, as in "bang cup" or "eat banana." Then follows the child's use of prepositional phrases and clauses to modify the meanings expressed in the simple phrases he has used before. Many different types of clauses become embedded in the child's utterances. Instead of saying "go" or "go bye bye," he now may add to it by saying "go bye bye in car now."

Thereafter, the acquisition of various language structures is astoundingly swift. He discovers conjunctions such as "and"; he learns the rules for plurals and tense and dozens of other features and rules. To the knowledgeable observer, the process can only be described as miraculous. In all the rest of his life he will never learn so much in such a short time. Rather than dwelling further on details in an introductory text, we describe now how the senior author's grandson learned to speak.

For the first six months of his second year we heard only one-word utterances, but they were accompanied by intonations and gestures that supplemented their meaningfulness. Thus "bye-bye" might be uttered as a question or as a command or merely as a comment on the fact that he was already in the car. He also had two negatives, "uh-uh" and occasionally "No!" "Ah-gah" (for "all gone") seemed to be a single sentencelike word and was used interrogatively, imperatively, and declaratively depending on the situation. Jimmy had achieved a vocabulary of about thirty-two words at eighteen months. Most of these, such as *milk, cup, car, plane, shoe,* were open-class words, but the boy also had some modifiers that could be termed members of the pivot class, such words as *here, more, big,* and *that.* At any rate, by one year and ten months he had learned to combine these into two-word utterances that again were used with the appropriate intonations of command, questioning, commenting, and so forth. Many of these were novel combinations that certainly he had never heard before such as "bye-bye bed." He would say "more milk," which certainly had been modeled for him, but he also said "more shoe" when he wanted the other one put on, and this too could not have been learned by any sort of imitation.

Within a month Jimmy showed clearly that he had discovered how noun phrases and verb phrases could be constructed: "my cup," "that shoe," "that car," "big milk." In naming pictures he would use the article "a" or the demonstrative "that" before each of them. No longer would he merely say "cow" or "house." It was always "a cow" or "that house." If we forgot to put in the prefatory word, he would become enraged and say, "No, no! 'a' cow," and correct us. He wasn't going to have his newly learned rule violated. If we said "big cow," that was all right, but no more single words for him! Something similar also occurred with verbs, although this came later. Verb phrases consist of the combination of an antecedent verb with a noun or noun phrase. jimmy's first one was "bang cup," but within a week he was saying not only "pay pono" (play piano) and "wah miuk" (want milk) but also "weed a booh" (read a book) and, showing us that he could do so, "frow duh bih bah" (throw the big ball), thus combining the verb with a noun phrase.

For almost two months, Jimmy stayed at this level of speaking in noun phrases and verb phrases, making many gains in vocabulary and practicing many different applications of the rules he had discovered. The noun phrases were then expanded: "Daddy big shoe." Verbs were followed by noun phrases as well as single nouns. He would say such things as "Jimmy want big ball" and even "Doggie eat Jimmy toast," thus indicating some sense of the possessive. Some of these verb phrases soon showed expansion by linking adverbs or prepositional phrases with the verb: "Fall down," "Go now in big car." It was fascinating to see him experimenting with these noun and verb phrase combinations. That he was not merely repeating phrases that he had heard his parents use, but actually and deliberately linking the words together is shown by some of these utterances: "Here bye-bye" (I've got to go now), "Go Mummy bed," and "No that button." These were not imitations of parental speech. They were the result of his attempts to construct a grammar, to relate words appropriately and meaningfully.

Then one day we heard more true sentences. "Jimmy want coat." "Jimmy go car." "Big ball fall down." He had found a new way of combining. Noun phrases could be joined to verb phrases. Subjects could have predicates. He didn't know these terms, but he had the idea. Whee! When he said one of these new combinations, he would run around in circles, shriek with pleasure, and collapse on the floor in ecstasy.

For some time Jimmy seemed to be practicing these simple sentence combinations. Then we heard him restructuring them and adding the appropriate intonations of pitch and stress. "Jimmy want cookie!" (command); "Where Daddy go?" (interrogative); "Jimmy no go bed" (negation); "Jimmy big boy" (declarative). Soon he was no longer having to add two simple sentences together as in "Jimmy go car and Mummy go car" but was saying, "Jimmy and Mummy go in car now." Shortly thereafter, he was using more of what is called *embedding,* attaching a clause or phrase to the basic subject-predicate pattern. Instead of saying "Daddy go car?" he said, "I think Daddy go car?"

Next the boy showed a growing mastery in the use of prepositional phrases ("Jimmy go to store" instead of "Jimmy go store"); then possessives, plurals, past tenses, passive voice, and other constructions appeared until by age four he was speaking very much like an adult.

The grammatical morphemes emerge in a definite sequence (see Table 3.3). When you have that baby of yours, watch for these aspects of language growth. You will be amazed to see the unfolding of the potential he possesses for becoming human. Besides, your enjoyment of his lan-

TABLE 3.3 Brown's (1973) fourteen grammatical morphemes in developmental order

Present progressive	-ing
Preposition	in
Preposition	on
Regular plural	-s, -z, -es
Past irregular	ran, came
Possessive	-s, -z
Uncontractible copula	is, am, are
Articles	a, the
Past regular	-ed
Third-person regular	-s, -z
Third-person irregular	does, goes
Uncontractible auxiliary	is, am, are
Contractible copula	is, am, are
Contractible auxiliary	is, am, are

guage development may help you bear all the other responsibilities with which his birth has bedeviled you.

You will notice that we have not provided chronological ages for the steps in sentence development. This is because the rate of acquisition varies quite a bit, and it is impossible to predict very precisely when Jimmy or any other child will achieve the various levels of sentence formulation we just described. Age is a poor basis on which to predict syntactic achievement. A better index of linguistic maturity is the average or *mean length of a child's spontaneous utterances* (**MLU**).[4] Brown (1973) found that as a child's MLU increases, he begins to incorporate more and more complex syntactic features. Employing mean length of utterance as a way of grouping children, Brown identified five stages in the development of syntax. Although the children differed somewhat in the chronological age at which they reached the stages, within each stage they all used the same set of rules for forming sentences. The major features of the five stages are summarized in Table 3.4.

Mean length of utterance (MLU). A measure of average utterance length used in studying language development.

Later Syntax. By the time a child is ready to enter kindergarten, he will have acquired almost the entire repertoire of adult grammar. Only a few refinements remain to be learned, and these tasks are accomplished by

---

TABLE 3.4   Stages in the development of syntax*

Stage	MLU	Major Features	Examples
I	1.0–2.0	Telegraphic utterances showing simple semantic rules: agent + action, action + object.	"Doggie run." "Drink juice."
II	2.0–2.5	Acquisition of noun and verb inflections: *in, on,* plural *s, -ing;* articles begin, overgeneralizing.	"Dolly drinking juice." "Read the book." "Look at the 'meese'" (child plural for moose).
III	2.5–3.0	Simple sentences using noun and verb phrases; simple transformations: questions, negations.	"I want some juice." "Is doggie sleeping?"
IV	3.0–3.75	Embedded one sentence in another; use of clauses	"The waterfall is singing to me." "Mary's book is in the camper."
V	3.75–4.50	Complex sentences; use of "so," "because," "but."	"When are we going to the cabin?" "I came in because it's raining."

*Based on the work of R. W. Brown, *A First Language: The Early Stages* (Cambridge, MA: Harvard University Press, 1973).

about ten or twelve years of age. Some of the later-learned aspects of syntax include:

Comprehension and use of the passive voice. Upon hearing the sentence, "The cow was kicked by the horse," children under five or six years of age insist that the cow did the kicking.

Exceptions to general rules. The plurals of "goose" and "mouse" are of course "geese" and "mice." One eight-year-old child excitingly reported that he saw two "meese" (mooses) in Canada. What's the plural of mongoose?

Complex transformations. It requires considerable linguistic sophistication to restate a sentence such as "It's nice to live in Baraga," several different ways: "Baraga is a nice place to live." "Living in Baraga is nice."

More complete accounts of later syntactical development may be found in Lund and Duchen (1993) and Nelson (1993).

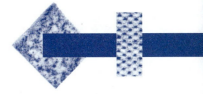

PHONOLOGICAL DEVELOPMENT

Thus far we have been tracing the way in which the child acquires the use of syntax, her grammar. Now let us see how she comes to master the sounds (phonemes) of her language. Although the process of mastering speech sounds takes a bit longer than with syntax, the same regular, predictable sequence is apparent. You will find comprehensive reviews of phoneme acquisition and mastery in the work of Bernthal and Bankson (1993) and Lund and Duchan (1993).

Occasionally we meet a proud mother who insists that her child pronounced sounds like an adult from the very first, but we have never observed such a paragon personally. Certain sounds appear before others in the child's early words, the /m/, /b/, /w/, /d/, /n/, and /t/ consonants being those most often used. Most of the vowels of these early words are produced fairly accurately from the first, although the /ɔ/ as in *ought,* the /ɛ/ as in *met,* and the /ʊ/ as in *cook* seem to cause some difficulty.

The mere presence of a standard phoneme in a word or two obviously is not the same as its mastery. Ordinarily, we feel that a child has really mastered a phoneme when he consistently uses it correctly in the initial, medial, or final positions of all the words which require it. We have little research on the age of the first appearance (acquisition) of phonemes. Instead, we have tables of mastery, such as those shown in Figure 3-2. Keep in mind when looking at this figure that there is a great deal of variability among children.

An inspection of Figure 3-2 reveals that the sounds first mastered are mainly the **labials,** nasals, **stop consonants,** and glides with the fricatives,

Labial.
Pertaining to the lips.

Stop consonant.
A sound characterized by a momentary blocking of airflow. Examples are the /k/, /d/, and /p/.

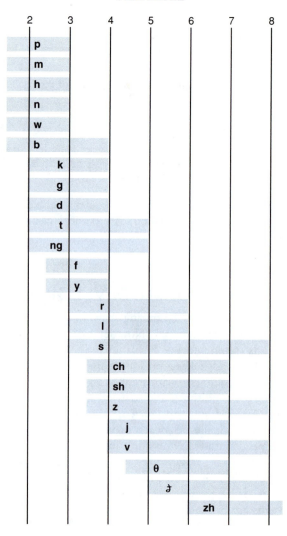

AGE LEVEL

2	3	4	5	6	7	8
p						
m						
h						
n						
w						
b						
k						
g						
d						
t						
ng						
f						
y						
r						
l						
s						
ch						
sh						
z						
j						
v						
θ						
ð						
zh						

FIGURE 3-2 Average age estimates and upper age limits of customary consonant production. The solid bar corresponding to each sound starts at the median age of customary acquisition; it stops at an age level at which 90% of all children customarily are producing the sound (from Sander, 1972).

affricates, and the /r/ appearing after the fourth year. We should also add that the consonant blends (such as /fl/, /str/, /gr/) often are in error even later. Various explanations have been offered for this sequence of development. One is that the earliest sounds to be acquired are those that involve the easiest coordinations. The /p/, /b/, and /m/, for example, are less complex motorically than are the fricatives, affricates, or the /r/ sounds, and they are also more visible. Another explanation is based on the distinctive feature concept, the belief being that the child masters the discriminations in the following order: voicing, nasality, stridency, continuancy, and place of articulation.

Mastering the standard phonemes of our language is not an easy task for the child. "Goggy" does not sound much different from "doggy" in the ears of a two- or three-year-old. One plosive seems similar to another; one fricative resembles several others, especially when the sounds are hidden in the flow of continuous parental speech. How then does the child ever master the discriminations he needs? In part, he learns what he needs to know through parental correction. ("Don't say 'thoup.' Say 'soup'; "That's 'soup,' not 'thoup'." This is a crude way of presenting contrasting pairs, the nonword and the real word.) And, of course, he never hears his parents using "rings" except in the context of fingers, whereas "wings" are what birds fly with. Unfortunately, not all the words in English have such contrasting pairs. If they did we suspect that we would have far fewer children with articulation errors. If the name for spinach were "tandy," no child would use that expression for "candy" more than once or twice.

In the mastery of a new phoneme, we often find the child going through a series of **approximations** before the standard sound is produced. "Choo-choo" for *train* may be uttered with the two vowels alone, as *oo-oo* /u u/, then change to /tutu/, then shift to /tsu tsu/, before many months later it appears as "choo-choo" /tʃutʃu/. The substitutions reflect the use of easier and earlier sounds for those that are acquired later, and they are usually similar in that they possess some, if not all, of the distinctive features of the correct phoneme. Thus, we have never heard a normal child substitute a back plosive such as /k/ for the /m/ sound when he tries to say *milk*. If the standard sound is voiced, the child's substitution tends to be voiced. If it is a glide, the error will rarely be a stop consonant. He may say "wummy" for "yummy" but he won't say "dummy" or "chummy." Why does a child say "tandy" for "candy" rather than "sandy," or "mandy," "randy," or "bandy"? The /t/ substitution used by the child has all the distinctive features possessed by the first sound of *candy* (/k/), all except one, the place of articulation. Both the /t/ and the /k/ are unvoiced, and stop plosives, and they are not nasal. They both involve the touching of the tongue to the roof of the mouth. It is the spot being touched that differs, the /t/ being in front and the /k/ in the back of the mouth. In terms of their distinctive features they differ in only one. Were a child to use an /m/, or /r/, or /b/ for the /k/ sound in *candy,* the substitution would be much more unlike the standard sound. That is, more than one distinctive feature would differ. The child may not be able to hit the target phoneme's bull's-eye at first, but he tries to come as close as he can; he does not fling out any old sound at random.

The mistakes children make in mastering the correct pronunciation of their sounds may be grouped into categories. Table 3.5 classifies the com-

Approximation. Behavior that comes closer to a standard or goal.

TABLE 3.5   Common phonological processes in the speech of normally developing children with examples from English

Process	Examples
Syllable Structure Processes	
Final-consonant deletion	boat [bo]; fish [fɪ]
Unstressed-syllable deletion	tomato ['medo]; elephant ['efənt]
Cluster reduction	snow [no]; brick [bɪk]
Reduplication	water ['wawa]; doggie ['dada]
Epenthesis	big [bɪgə]; blue [bə´lu]
Assimilation Processes	
Velar assimilation	sock [gak]; chicken ['gɪkɪn]
Labial assimilation	sheep [bip]; boat [bop]
Nasal assimilation	bunny ['mʌni]; down [naʊn]
Substitution Processes	
Stopping of fricative and affricates	very ['bɛri]; jaw [da]
Gliding of liquids	rose [woz]; look [jʊk]
Velar fronting	go [do]; cup [tʌp]
Depalatalization[1]	show [so]; chip [tʃɪp]
Voicing Processes	
Prevocalic voicing	pig [bɪg]; happy ['hæbi]
Final devoicing	big [bɪk]; nose [nos]

[1]This process is labelled "palatal fronting" by some researchers.
Used by permission from M. Yavas (ed.). (1991). *Phonological disorders in children*. New York: Routledge, Chapman and Hall, Inc.

mon errors. Read the phonetic representation of these errors so you can recognize them. (*Epenthesis* means that an extra and unneeded phoneme has been added to the word.)

When we look at the child's errors it seems obvious that she is simplifying the models of adult speech. She comes as close as she can to these models but they are for the time being beyond her ability, so instead of saying *dog* (dɔg) she will just omit the last sound, though she may prolong the vowel a bit as a substitution. Clusters of consonants—/skr/, /bl/, /fr/—are just too complicated so she will say /ku/ for *screw* and /bu/ for *blue*. She will omit a syllable if the word is too long and say /nænə/ instead of *banana*. Duplicate-syllable words are simpler and easier to say than those whose syllables differ so he will simplify the word *water* into /wɑwɑ/. According to Nelson (1993) these "simplification processes are observed in the speech productions of normally developing children but often persist among children with speech-language disorders beyond the ages when they usually disappear" (p. 38).

Finally, we should remember that progress in articulatory mastery is gradual. Even after the child has demonstrated that he is able to use the standard phoneme in some words, other words will still contain its usual error. Newly acquired phonemes seem very fragile. Under excitement, the child may return to the older forms and say "goggy" long after he has demonstrated that he can say "doggy." In certain phonetic contexts the new sound will tend to disappear. One child who had learned to say perfectly the word "fish" (instead of his earlier "fiss") could not say "Fish swim in water" for over a year because the /s/ in swim influenced the final sound of *fish* and turned it into another /s/ (assimilation). But eventually the child will master the phonemes he needs or have to have the help of a speech pathologist.

SEMANTICS: THE DEVELOPMENT OF MEANING

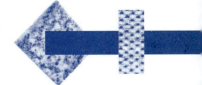

Although there is much we still do not know about how a child acquires the meanings of the words he hears and uses, it seems evident that in early years the developmental process involves both extension and contraction. One of the senior author's children's very first words was "pih" for *pig,* probably because she enjoyed the animal's feeding times on the farm. She would say the word and point to the pigs, big ones, little ones, alike. But, through extension of the meaning inherent in the words, she also called all other animals "pih" too: dogs, horses, cows, and even her father when he crawled on all fours under the fence. But then differentiation (contraction) appeared as she watched the cows being milked. She tried "pih-mik" (pig's milk?) a few times, then accepted our "moo-cow" by using her already acquired word for milk (mik) instead of our "moo" to produce "mik-kau." She never used "pih" for cow again, and very soon thereafter began eagerly to learn the names for other animals.

Children learn more than naming animals and objects (*referential* or structural meaning); they also acquire the ability to express relationships (*propositional* or functional meaning). Recently, we observed three children—all between two and three years old—as they played with a rabbit and an assortment of dolls, cars, and other toys. Here are some of the semantic categories recorded; note the wide range of meanings expressed despite their relatively simple sentence structure.

Semantic Relation	Example
notice-greeting	hi bunny
recurrence	more carrots
nonexistence	carrots all gone
possession	my truck
location	rabbit in box
agent-action	rabbit jump
agent-object	car hit
action-object	pet the bunny

We also know little of the internal dictionaries being developed by the child. There seems to be some evidence that the early entries may he filed not as words but as phrases, *cup* meaning *something to drink from* or *ball* as *throw ball*. With intellectual maturity and experience, these action phrases are gradually shaped into an increasingly complex system for segmenting and categorizing reality. There are interesting variations in language learning style from child to child. Some youngsters use their newly acquired verbal ability to label objects and events in their world. On the other end of the continuum are those children who tend to use words to regulate social interaction and to reveal their needs and desires. No doubt these styles reflect, to a great extent, the predominant type of communication parents use with their children. We do know that these internal dictionaries grow swiftly in volume. As noted by Pinker, "Around eighteen months, language takes off. Vocabulary growth jumps to the new-word-every-two-hours minimum rate that the child will maintain through adolescence" (1994, p. 267). Comprehension dictionaries are doubtless much more extensive. As is true for adults, children know many more words than they use in communicating.

Children also seem to learn the meanings of new words in a sequential fashion. First, they learn those that refer to objects, events, or actions; next, they seem to acquire the adjectives and adverbs that modify the words they've already acquired (e.g., "*big* dog," "go *fast*"); then they master a set of terms that describe spatial and then temporal relationships, as shown in Figure 3-3.

A final category of relational words, such as "here/there" and "this or that," that focus attention on a particular person or object by locating it in relation to the speaker are among the last learned.

We do not wish to imply that semantics is confined solely to vocabulary acquisition for, of course, it is the ways in which words are combined that enable us to communicate our meanings. Nevertheless, any child who lacks the words he needs is very handicapped, because he has to *have* them before he can string them together. We see this handicap vividly in

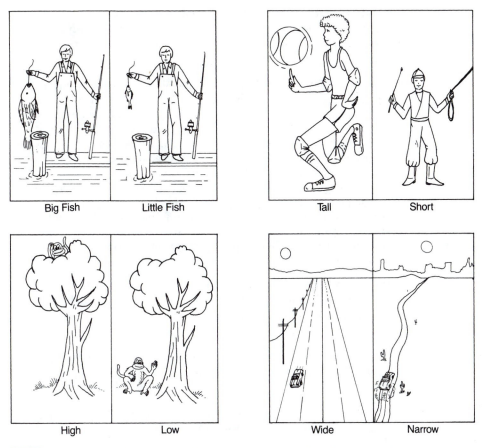

| Big Fish | Little Fish | Tall | Short |
| High | Low | Wide | Narrow |

 FIGURE 3-3   Developmental sequence of items related to size and space.

stroke patients with aphasia who often have tremendous difficulty in word finding. As one of our clients told us, "I have lost my voc . . . my vocab . . . my, oh dear, my alphabet." And then he cried with frustration, knowing well that "alphabet" was not the word he needed.

Most parents are eager enough to help the child to get his first twenty or thirty new words. Some parents are even too ambitious at first; they try to teach such words as "Dorothy" or "Samantha." But their teaching urge soon subsides. The child seems to be picking up a few words as she needs them. Why not let her continue to grow at her own pace? Our answer does not deny the function of maturation in vocabulary growth. We merely say that parents should give a little common-sense help at moments when a child needs a new word, a label for a new experience. When parents notice a child hesitating or correcting herself when faced with a new experience, they should become verbal dictionaries, providing *not only the needed new word, but a definition in terms of the child's own vocabulary.* For example,

> John was pointing to something on the shelf he wanted. "Johnny want . . . um . . . Johnny want pretty pretty ball . . . Johnny wanta pretty . . . um . . . ." The object was a round glass vase with a square opening on top. I immediately took it down and said, "No ball, Johnny. Vase! Vase!" I put my finger into the opening and let him imitate me. Then we got a flower and he put it in the opening after I had filled it partially with water. I said, "Vase is a flower cup. Flower cup, vase! See pretty vase! (I prolonged the *v* sound slightly.) Flower drink water in vase, in pretty vase. Johnny, say 'Vase'!" (He obeyed without hesitation or error). Each day that week, I asked him to put a new flower in the vase, and by the end of that time he was using the word with assurance. I've found one thing, though; you must speak rather slowly when teaching a new word. Use plenty of pauses and patience.

Besides this type of spontaneous vocabulary teaching, it is possible to play little games at home in which the child imitates an older child or parent as they "touch and say" different objects. Children invent these games for themselves.

> "March and Say" was a favorite game of twins whom we observed. One would pick up a toy telephone, run to the door of the playroom, and ask his mother, "What dat?" "Telephone," she would answer, and then both twins would hold the object and march around the room chanting "te-poun tepoun" until it ended in a fight for possession. Then the dominant twin would pick up another object, ask its name, and march and chant its name over and over.

In all these naming games, the child should always point to, feel, or sense the object referred to as vividly as possible. The mere sight or sound of the object is not enough for early vocabulary acquisition. It is also wise to avoid cognate terms. One of the senior author's children for years called the cap on a bottle a "hat" because of early confusion.

Scrapbooks are better than the ordinary run of children's books for vocabulary teaching because pictures of objects closer to the child's experience may be pasted in. The ordinary "Alphabet Book" is a monstrosity so far as the teaching of talking is concerned. Nursery rhymes are almost as bad. Let the child listen to "Goosey Goosey Gander, whither dost thou wander" if he enjoys the rhymes, but do not encourage him to say the rhymes. The teaching of talking should be confined to meaningful speech, not gibberish. The three-year-old child has enough of a burden without trying to make sense of nonsense. When using the pictures in the scrapbooks, it is wise to do more than ask the child to name them. When pointing to a ball, the parents should say, "What's that!" "Ball." "Doug throw ball. Bounce, bounce, bounce" (gestures). Build up associations in terms of the functions of the objects. Teach phrases as well as single words. "Cookie" can always be taught as "eat cookie." This policy may also help the child to remember to keep it out of his hair.

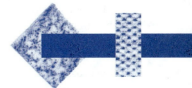

PROSODY AND PRAGMATICS

Our research on how children master their prosodic and pragmatic skills is very meager. With respect to prosody, the acquisition of adult inflections, such as those for asking questions, making statements or commanding, seem to be learned very early because they can clearly be heard in the babbling and vocal play of infants long before they are using words. Similarly, variations in the loudness of babbling segments can be heard. Prosody, the melody of speech, is probably learned by imitation of caregiver's utterances. One exception to the early onset of prosodic skills is that the melodic features of sarcasm appear later, usually in the later elementary grades.

As for pragmatics, again we have little information about how the child learns those skills. Although the pragmatic rule of turn-taking while conversing appears early, most of the other pragmatic rules are delayed until the child has become a fairly fluent speaker. Only then does he learn to speak differently to differing persons (to adults versus children); only then does he know whether his utterances are appropriate to the communicative situation. Only then does he learn when to talk and when to shut up.

So there you have an admittedly sketchy account of how your children learn to talk. We hope you will find that this information will enable you to enjoy watching them do so.

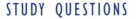

STUDY QUESTIONS

1. What types of speech and/or language behaviors tend to be characteristic of the average three-to-six-month-old infant?
2. Within about what age range, on the average, should you expect to hear a baby utter its first real words?
3. When might you expect first to observe signs of "social awareness" in the baby's behavior, and what are some of these signs?
4. Explain, as you would to the mother and father of a two-month-old baby, how babbling is different from reflexive vocalization and at about what age their baby probably will begin to babble.

5. For what reasons is it so difficult to be certain of the exact age at which an infant began to use actual words?

6. What is meant by the "autism" theory of speech acquisition, and how does it differ from "nativistic" theory?

7. What relationships appear to exist between a child's Mean Length of Utterance and the level of development of her syntax?

8. Among most children, in what general order is the correct articulation of phonemes demonstrated?

9. What are some of the common phonological processes that are observed to occur in the speech of normally developing children? Give at least one example of each.

10. Using Pinker's observation as the basis for your calculations, you would expect a child to add at least how many new words to his or her vocabulary between the ages of 18 months and five years?

ENDNOTES

[1] The importance of normal hearing to speech and language development has long been evident in many ways. For example, one recent study found that, while normal infants inevitably had canonical babbling before the age of 11 months, those with hearing impairments had none until after 11 months (Eilers and Oller, 1994).

[2] Adults often speak "motherese" when communicating with young children—using shorter sentences, raising the pitch of their voices, exaggerating speech melody patterns, and talking more simply (see, for example, Wanska and Bedrosian, 1985).

[3] Infants attempt to match the pitch of their vocalizations to that of their parents: They use a lower pitch when babbling to their fathers than to their mothers (Reich, 1986).

[4] MLU is determined by adding the number of morphemes spoken in a set of consecutive utterances and then dividing the sum by the total number of utterances. The utterance "my car" has two morphemes; "daddy's car" has three because the plural *s* alters the meaning of the message. Thus $(2 + 3)/2 = $ MLU 2.5.

REFERENCES

Barrett, M. (ed.) (1985). *Children's single-word speech*. New York: John Wiley and Sons.

Bernthal, J., and Bankson, N. (1993). *Articulation and phonological disorders* (3rd ed.). Englewood Cliffs, NJ: Prentice Hall.

Blake, J., and Fink, R. (1987). Sound-meaning correspondences in babbling. *Journal of Child Language*, 14, 229–253.

Brown, R. (1973). *A first language: The early stages*. Cambridge, MA: Harvard University Press.

Chomsky, N. (1968). *Language and mind*. New York: Harcourt Brace Jovanovich.

deBoysson-Bardies, B., Sagart, L., and Bacri, C. (1981). Phonetic analysis of late babbling: A case study of a French child. *Journal of Child Language*, 8, 511–524.

Eilers, R., and Oller, D. (1994). Infant vocalizations and the early diagnosis of severe hearing impairment. *Journal of Pediatrics,* 80(2).

Emerick, L., and Haynes, W. (1986). *Diagnosis and evaluation in speech pathology* (3rd ed.). Englewood Cliffs, NJ: Prentice Hall.

Golinkhoff, R. (Ed.). (1983). *The transition from prelinguistic to linguistic communication.* Hillsdale, NJ: Lawarence Erlbaum.

Hoffman, P., Schuckers, G., and Daniloff, R. (1985). *Children's phonetic disorders.* Boston: College Hill Press.

Lester, B., and Zachariah, C. (1985). *Infant crying: Theoretical and research perspectives.* New York: Plenum.

Levitt, A., and Utman, J. (1992). From babbling towards the sound systems of English and French: A longitudinal two-case study. *Journal of Child Language,* 19, 19–49.

Lund, N., and Duchan, J. (1993). *Assessing children's language in naturalistic contexts* (3rd ed.). Englewood Cliffs, NJ: Prentice Hall.

Meltzoff, A., and Moore, M. (1977). Imitation of facial and manual gestures by neonates. *Science,* 198, 75–78.

Moon, C., Bever, T., and Fifer, W. (1992). Canonical and non-canonical syllable discrimination by two-day-old infants. *Journal of Child Language,* 19, 1–17.

Mowrer, O. (1950). On the psychology of 'talking birds': A contribution to language and personality theory. In *Learning theory and personality dynamics.* New York: Ronald Press.

Nelson, N. (1993). *Childhood language disorders in context.* Englewood Cliffs, NJ: Prentice Hall.

Oller, D., and Eilers, R. (1982). Similarity of babbling in Spanish and English learning babies. *Journal of Child Language,* 9, 565–577.

Petrovich-Bartell, N., Cowan, N., and Morse, P. (1982). Mothers' perceptions of infant distress vocalizations. *Journal of Speech and Hearing Research,* 25, 371–376.

Pinker, S. (1994). *The language instinct: How the mind creates language.* New York: William Morrow and Co.

Reich, P. (1986). *Language development.* Englewood Cliffs, NJ: Prentice Hall.

Roug, L., Landberg, I., and Lundberg, L. (1989). Phonetic development in early infancy: A study of four Swedish children during the first eighteen months of life. *Journal of Child Language,* 16, 19–40.

Sander, E. (1972). When are speech sounds learned? *Journal of Speech and Hearing Disorders,* 37, 54–63.

Stoel-Gammon, C., and Dunn, C. (1985). *Normal and disordered phonology in children.* Baltimore: University Park Press.

Stoel-Gammon, C., and Otomo, K. (1986). Babbling development of hearing impaired and normally hearing subjects. *Journal of Speech and Hearing Disorders,* 51, 33–41.

Vihman, M., and McCune, L. (1994). When is a word a word? *Journal of Child Language,* 21, 517–542.

Wanska, S., and Bedrosian, J. (1985). Conversational structure and topic performance in mother-child interactions. *Journal of Speech and Hearing Research,* 28, 579–584.

Wood, B. (1981). *Children and communication* (2nd ed.). Englewood Cliffs, NJ: Prentice Hall.

Yavas, M. (ed.). (1991). *Phonological disorders in children.* New York, NY: Routledge, Chapman and Hall.

Zeskind, P., and Lester, B. (1981). Analysis of cry features in newborns with differential fetal growth. *Child Development,* 52, 207–212.

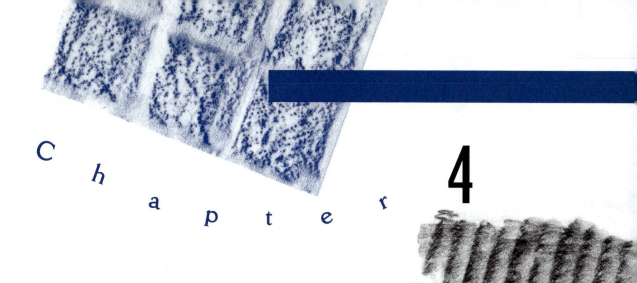

Chapter 4

Speech Disorders

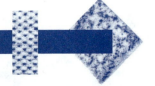

In the first chapter we provided a few glimpses of some speech disorders. In this one, we provide basic information that will help us identify all of the major ones.

DEFINITION

Our first diagnostic task, however, is to make sure that the person's speech is impaired. To accomplish this, we need a definition and the best one we have found is this. *Speech is impaired when it deviates so far from the speech of other people that it (1) calls attention to itself, (2) interferes with communication, or (3) provokes distress in the speaker or the listener.*

Let us consider each of the three parts of this definition in turn. The first part indicates that the speech is so different from that of other speakers that it is *conspicuous.* It varies too far from the prevailing and relevant norm. For example, a three-year-old child who says "wabbit" for "rabbit" would not be viewed as having a speech disorder because most three-year-olds make such mistakes, but an adult who said the word that way would be speaking in an abnormal way. A somewhat nasal voice in one geographic region might not be conspicuous; the same voice in another region could result in the speaker being urged to seek help from a speech clinician. All of us repeat and hesitate, but we are not all considered to be stuttering. Clearly, some speech differences fall into the range of normal variation and are not speech disorders.

Second, a person's speech tends to be diagnosed as impaired if it is *difficult to understand.* The main purpose of speaking is to send and receive messages and, when these messages are difficult to comprehend, we feel the speaker must have some kind of speech problem. We once heard and eighteen-year-old client of ours say " ''Poh ko an tebbuh yee adoh ow pojpadduh baw poh upah did kawinaw a nu naytuh." What was he saying? He was reciting the first part of the Gettysburg address. Speech must be intelligible; if it is not, then it is abnormal.

Part three of our definition stresses that when the speech behavior is unpleasant to either or both the speaker and listener, it tends to be diagnosed as being abnormal enough to require the services of a speech pathologist. You will read about clutterers who speak so fast and have so many slurred words or **fluency** breaks that their listeners just won't tolerate their efforts to communicate. Clutterers do not find their speech unpleasant but others do. Clergymen have come to us because their congregations complained about the harshness of their voices. Most of us find that listening to severe **stuttering** is both frustrating and unpleasant.

The person who stutters may be no less distressed than the listener, of course, nor is stuttering the only speech problem that can cause frustration and emotional stress in the speaker. As we shall see in Chapter 5,

Fluency.
Unhesitant speech.

Stuttering.
Disrupted speech, characterized by prolongations, hesitations, and blockages.

there are individuals whose communicative handicaps are due more to their emotional reactions than to the speaking disability itself.

In summary, our first task is to ascertain if the speech is conspicuous, unintelligible, or unpleasant enough to be diagnosed as impaired.

DISORDER CLASSIFICATION

It is not enough merely to decide that the person's speech is impaired. We must also determine the way(s) in which it is impaired. The speech-language pathologist immediately begins scanning to determine if the deviancy lies more in the person's *articulation, voice, fluency,* or *language.* This fourfold classification, it should be understood, refers to the outstanding aspect of the observed behavior. The person with aphasia, for example, may show articulation errors, broken rhythm, and difficulty producing voice; but the outstanding feature of aphasia is disability in handling symbolic meanings and language. Therefore, while describing and analyzing all problem areas, we would place aphasia under disorders of symbolization or language. Other individuals, such as the child with a cleft palate, also may have difficulty in more than one area—sometimes to the extent that one may not clearly be more outstanding than another.

FIGURE 4-1   The range of speech disorders

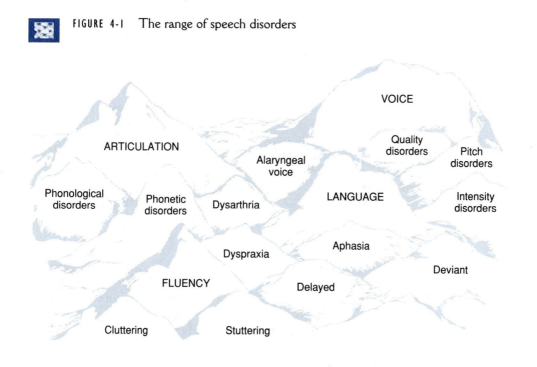

Each of these four aspects of human speech has its own criteria of normality, and each has a range of acceptable differences. The *s* sound in *Sue* is not the same sound as it is in the word *see;* it is lower in pitch, but this variation is within normal limits. But when that *s* is too slushy as in a person with a lateral lisp we would diagnose abnormality. *A difference to be a difference must make a difference.* If it calls attention to itself, interferes with the receiving of the message, or is unpleasant to the speaker or his listener, we then have a speech problem.

One of the common mistakes made by beginners in this field is the failure to scan all these four features of the speech of a person who obviously has some communicative abnormality.

> I learned another lesson today and I don't know why it took me so long. I have been working with a junior high school boy whose speech is full of distorted speech sounds due to the fact that he keeps his tongue flat in his mouth. Often he is unintelligible. Yet he could make every sound perfectly in isolation and often in single words if I said them first. Well, I began therapy by working to mobilize the lifting of the tongue tip and to disassociate it from any jaw movement and by stimulating him strongly with the sounds on which the distortions occurred. He was immediately successful in anything I asked him to do yet there was no transfer into real communication. Then just by chance I happened to overhear him talking to a girl in the hall and saw him have a severe stuttering block, so of course we discussed this at our next session. Come to find out, he doesn't have any articulation problem at all. He just uses this kind of speech as a way to keep from stuttering. Says he's only been using it for a few months and that though it helped at first because it was so novel and distracting, it was beginning to lose its effectiveness. After he told me this I realized that I had noticed many hesitations and gaps in his speech but had ignored them. The abnormal articulation had just been too conspicuous. Anyway, now we can begin to tackle the real problem.

Experienced speech pathologists do not make this mistake. Their diagnostic computers do not stop until they have scanned enough speech samples for deviancy not only in articulation but in voice, fluency, and language. They know the normal ranges of variation for each, and bells ring in their heads when they discover speaking behaviors that go beyond these boundaries.

Educators, counselors, health service providers, and other professionals who interact with individuals who may have communication disorders also must be alert to the necessity for recognizing the multiple aspects of speech that can show deviancy. The patient with Parkinson's disease who has difficulty with articulation often will be experiencing significant voicing problems as well. A child who is deaf, deafened, or severely hearing impaired will show not only articulatory errors, inappropriate vocal inflections, or a monotonous voice; he also often may have a language disability or the rhythm of his fluency will be broken by pauses in the wrong parts of a sentence. Similarly, the person with cerebral palsy may show deviancy in all four features. So may the child with mental retardation. The emotionally disturbed child may present the picture of a strange voice quality along with infantile kinds of articulatory errors. Although the speech of a child with a cleft palate is often conspicuously nasal, he will also tend to show speech sound errors, one of which may be the use of the **glottal stop** (similar to a tiny cough) for his *k* sounds. It is not enough merely to recognize that a person does not speak normally. We must know what features of the speech are abnormal.

Moreover, it is not enough merely to recognize that the deviancy exists in articulation, voice, fluency, or language. We must be able to analyze that deviancy so as to identify exactly what makes the speech conspicuous, hard to understand, or unpleasant. If a person has an articulation problem, we must know what sounds are produced incorrectly, for all of them are not defective. If the voice is abnormal, the speech pathologist will survey the pitch, loudness, and vocal quality aspects of that voice before zeroing in on the targets for therapy. It is not enough just to say that the person stutters, for there are literally thousands of different stuttering behaviors, though certain ones are demonstrated most frequently. If a person is aphasic (dysphasic is the more precise word), the language disability must be carefully analyzed if it is to be remedied.

In this chapter we present only the salient symptoms of the four major disorder categories. A more complete discussion of tile various disorders will be found in subsequent chapters.

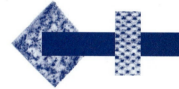

ARTICULATION DISORDERS

How does one learn to do diagnostic analyzing? The answer lies in training and experience. A speech clinician must acquire habits of careful listening and systematic observation. We begin your training by providing some brief word pictures of individuals with disorders of articulation.

When we first heard Lori's rapid unintelligible chatter, we suspected for a moment that she might be speaking a foreign language. At the end of a torrent of strange staccato syllables, all accompanied by seemingly appropriate gestures and vocal inflections, she looked at us expectantly for a response. When we just scrutinized her quizzically, she frowned slightly, sighed, and repeated her message in a slower but still incomprehensible manner. Showing the first-grader some pictures, we asked her to name them one at a time. Recording her responses, we then asked Lori to repeat words and short phrases and describe objects in the room. Later analysis showed that she produced all the vowel sounds correctly but substituted *t*, *d*, and *n* for all other consonants except the *h*. An interview with Lori's mother revealed that the youngster had been chronically ill

Glottal catch (or stop). A tiny cough-like sound produced by the sudden release of a pulse of voiced or unvoiced air from the vocal folds.

with respiratory ailments during her first three years. Also, she was overindulged by older siblings who had learned to interpret the child's defective speech. We enrolled Lori in the clinic, enlisted the aid of her parents and older sisters, and gave her intense daily speech therapy. By the end of the school year, she was using all speech sounds correctly—but still inconsistently—except *s*, *r*, and *l*.

When Craig came to the speech clinic, he was hurt and angry. A sophomore majoring in broadcasting, he had been dispatched posthaste to the clinic by the director of the university radio station. During his radio audition, Craig's **strident** *s* sound caromed the sensitive VU meter into overload. As far as we could discern, no one had confronted him about his sharp sibilants before his audition. This seemed astounding since we found it difficult not to wince when working with him in a small treatment room. A glib, fluent speaker, he had decided while still in junior high school to pursue a career in radio. Now he found his path blocked and he was bewildered and hostile. After utilizing the first few sessions for emotional ventilation **(catharsis),** we showed Craig how to make the *s* sound while anchoring his tongue tip below his lower teeth. When he combined this new articulatory placement with a more relaxed posture of his lower jaw, the strident *s* disappeared. Once he was able to make the new sound and compare it with his old sharp whistle, Craig's motivation zoomed. He practiced incessantly, and when he returned for a second audition at the end of the semester, he passed easily.

We do not wish to leave the impression that disorders of articulation present little difficulty to the clinician. Some of them have been our toughest cases. Somehow we remember our failures much more vividly than we do our successes. They haunt us. What did we do wrong or what did we fail to do? One of them was Joe.

Joe was in the fifth grade when we first worked with him. Only one of his sounds was defective—the vowel *r* sound as in *fur.* He was able to make the consonantal *r* perfectly, articulating it correctly whenever it occurred as the initial consonant of a syllable. He could say "run," "radio," or any other word beginning with *r* without error. Even the consonant blends, *pr*, *tr*, *gr*, and so on were uttered normally. But when the *r* occurred as a vowel as in *church*, he said "chutch." He said "theatuh," "mothuh," "guhl." When the *r* was part of a diphthong as in *ar*, *or*, *ir*, not only was the *r* distorted but the preceding vowel was often misarticulated. Instead of "far," he said "foah," and in these distorted diphthongs we heard sounds that we had never heard before. We worked hard with Joe and initially felt that the **prognosis** was good, that we could probably effect a transition from the consonantal to the vowel *r* with ease. We failed completely. He tried and we tried with all our might. We used every technique known to us. We vainly explored every possible reason for the persistence of the errors. We tried different clinicians. They failed. When Joe was a senior in high school we tried again with the same result. We still wonder what else we might have done.

Strident lisp.
Sibilants characterized by piercing, whistling sounds.

Catharsis.
The discharge of pent-up feelings.

Prognosis.
Prediction of progress or outcome.

As we have seen from our scrutiny of the preceding examples, the basic problem shown by a person with a disorder of articulation is that he has failed to master the speech sounds of his language. Each of these three persons could be characterized as having a phonological (articulatory) disorder rather than one of voice or of fluency or of symbolization. Although they differed one from the other in the pattern of their errors, they all showed one or more of the following types: (1) a substitution of one standard English phoneme for another (2) a distortion of a standard sound, (3) an **omission** of a sound that should be present. Some authorities include additions (the intrusion of an unwanted sound) as another type of articulatory disorder; in our experience, additions are generally the result of emphasis ("p*uh*lease close that door!") or idiosyncratic pronunciation ("I need some fil*u*m to take photographs of the ath*uh*letes by the el*u*m tree.").

Most young children during the course of their speech development show all these articulatory disorders at one time or another, but some children persist in their usage, having failed to perceive the contrasting features of the correct sound as compared with the defective one, or having been unable to achieve its correct production.

While we defer our discussion of the causes of articulation disorders until later (Chapter 6), there are two basic categories or types of impairments we should mention immediately: *phonetic* disorders and *phonological* disorders.

In the case of phonetic disorders, the individuals are unable to *produce* certain speech sounds correctly because of structural, motor, or sensory impairments; they have organic abnormalities that limit their speaking capabilities. In our present clinic caseload we have two clients with phonetic errors:

> Seven-year-old Cindy has a rare hereditary skin disorder that is **atrophying** her lips, tongue, and soft palate. Almost all speech sounds are difficult for her to produce, but she has particular difficulty with *s, l, r,* and *sh,* and *ch, k,* and *g.* Her clinician is attempting to teach the child to slow her rate of speech and use compensatory oral movements to articulate the defective sounds.

> By the time the physicians diagnosed his chronic and progressive muscular weakness as **myasthenia gravis,** Cliff Harris had to retire early from his position as high school English teacher and debate coach. He tires easily, talks in a soft nasal voice, and misarticulates most tongue-tip sounds. Mr. Harris is trying to learn to speak in short phrases, pause, and then continue. When he does this his speech is more intelligible.

Many children have phonological disorders of articulation (formerly termed *functional, dyslalic,* or *habit* errors). They misarticulate for no apparent organic reason. Although most of these youngsters can produce all the sounds of English speech, they seem to simplify the adult pattern or

Omission.
One of the four types of articulatory errors. The standard sound is replaced usually by a slight pause equal in duration to the sound omitted.

Atrophy.
A withering; a shrinking in size and decline in function of some bodily structure or organ.

Myasthenia gravis.
Chronic neuromuscular disorder characterized by progressive weakening of musculature without atrophy.

replace it with a contrived system of their own. They use phonemes differently. Interestingly, however, a careful analysis of their sound errors generally reveals an underlying system or set of rules by which they organize their repertoire of phonemes. Here is a portion of a student clinician's report on an eight-year-old child that illustrates a developmental disorder of articulation:

> Lance has inconsistent errors on *l, r, s, sh, f, v, th, k,* and *g*. He can produce each of the phonemes correctly by imitating the examiner's model. In spontaneous speech, however, he omits or substitutes other sounds for the phonemes listed in a seemingly random fashion. But he does appear to use a system for organizing his complement of speech sounds. His use of the *s* sound is typical of his misarticulation. When *s* begins a word, Lance substitutes the *t* sound ("toup" for "soup"); in words such as "basket," where *s* is in the **medial** position, he replaces it with the *th* ("bathkit"); for plurals, he omits the *s*. Interestingly, he substitutes *s* for *sh* when the latter sound occurs in the initial position.

Children with phonological disorders do not have "broken-down" patterns of sound production. On the contrary, they appear to have coherent strategies that guide their use of speech sounds; quite often these strategies evolve from the simplification techniques used by very young children who are learning to speak.

At this point we must remind ourselves that cultural and linguistic diversities abound in our nation. Standard American English is by no means the only dialect encountered by the speech-language clinician; and, although users of other dialects may *elect* to work on altering their speech patterns, the original pattern is not viewed as a disorder. The individual's background must be taken into account in the assessment of phonology.

> For example, if members of a child's speech community consist of individuals who are bilingual Spanish and English and the variety of English spoken in the child's community is Black English Vernacular (BEV), then the child will most likely speak . . . English which (is) influenced by BEV and Spanish. . . . Information on the characteristics of particular languages and dialects, together with information on normal phonological development can provide information for . . . differentiating children with dialectal differences from those with phonological disorders (Iglesias and Anderson, 1993, p. 147).

Even though we have described phonetic and phonological disorders as distinctly different types of articulation disorders, there can be a great deal of overlapping. A child born with a cleft palate may be unable to produce certain phonemes correctly because air leaks through his nose (**nasal emission**) when substantial oral air pressure is required. The same child may have other phonemic errors that are unrelated to the cleft. *The key feature of all articulatory disorders is the presence of defective and incorrect sounds.*

Medial.
The occurrence of a sound within a word but not initiating or ending it.

Nasal emission.
Airflow through the nose, especially during production of oral consonants.

Most people with articulation disorders have more than one error sound and are not always consistent in their substitutions, omissions, or distortions. This is not always the case, however. Thum lingual lithperth merely thubthitute a *th* for the *eth* thound. Othersh shkwirt the airshtream over the shide of the tongue and are shed to have a lateral lishp. Others thnort the thnound (nasal lisp). Many children have been known to buy an "ites tream toda" or an all-day "tucker."

People sometimes tend to regard articulatory errors as being cute and relatively unimportant. This view is unlikely to be shared by those who have such disorders, particularly if the problem is severe, as they seek to cope with even the simpler demands of modern life. We knew a woman who could not produce the *s, l,* and *r* sounds and yet who had to buy a railroad ticket to Robeline, Louisiana. She did it with a pencil and paper. A man with the same difficulty became a farmer's hired hand after he graduated from college rather than suffer the penalties of a more verbal existence. Many children are said to outgrow their defective consonant sounds. Actually, they overcame them through blundering methods of self-help, and far too many of them never manage the feat. One man, aged sixty-five, asked us bitterly when we thought he would outgrow his baby-talk.

Misarticulations can cause a great deal of difficulty in communicating. Mothers cannot understand their own children. Teachers and classmates fail to comprehend speech when it is too full of phonemic errors. Try to translate these familiar nursery rhymes:

Ha ta buh, Ha ta buh,
Wuhnuh peh, two uh peh,
Ha ta buh.

Tippo Tymuh meh a pyemuh,
Doh too peh,
Ted Tippo Tymuh to duh pyemuh
Yeh me tee oo weh.

("Hot Cross Buns" and "Simple Simon.")

Many children who are severely handicapped by unintelligible speech also find it very difficult to express their emotions except by screaming or acting out their conflicts. Most of us relieve ourselves of our emotional evils by using others as our verbal handkerchiefs or wastebaskets. We talk it out. But when a child runs to his mother crying "Wobbuh toh ma tie-tihtoh" and she cannot understand that Robert stole his tricycle, all he can do is fling himself into a tantrum. The same frustration results from his inability to use speech for self-exhibition. Often penalized or frustrated when he tries to talk, he soon finds it better to keep quiet, to use gestures, or to get attention in other ways. Some of the most handicapped people we have ever known were those who could not speak clearly enough to be understood.

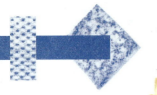

FLUENCY DISORDERS

While all of us hesitate and bobble at times, someone whose speech *habitually* shows abnormal interruptions in the form of hesitations, repetitions, or prolongations may be diagnosed as having a fluency disorder. About two million persons in this country suffer from disorders of fluency, primarily from the disorder called stuttering. Severe stuttering may be very conspicuous, and certainly it can be very distressing. When the flow of speech is excessively fractured, its meaning is hard to grasp. The contortions and struggling, the backing up and starting again, the prolongations of sounds, the compulsive repetition of syllables, and the difficulty in initiating utterances bother both the speaker and the listener alike.

Stuttering

It is difficult to find "typical" illustrations of this disorder since it is characterized by a high degree of variability. Nevertheless, some examples may be informative.

> By the time Colin's parents brought him to the speech clinic, the frequency of the child's speech interruptions exceeded the limits of normalcy for three-year-old children. The upsurge of disfluency began, according to his parents, three months before, on an extended family trip to attend a funeral and to settle a rancorous probate dispute. Prior to that time, Colin had been considered a normal, even a superior speaker. In fact, the child talked so well and was so skilled at echoing adult speech, his parents had often amused relatives and guests by having the child repeat polysyllabic words. Although the speech breaks seemed to come and go in waves, in the past few weeks Colin's disfluency had become more chronic. Our examination revealed that Colin was repeating whole words and syllables, and that these speech bobbles occurred more than fifty times in a thousand words. Most of the repetitions took place at the beginning of an utterance. For example, he uttered the word "I" (he was asking for a toy) with ten repetitions; the tempo of the iterations was irregular. We noted also that the child seemed to prepare himself to speak by uttering two or three "ums"; sometimes this **preparatory set** (utterance) was accompanied by several tiny inhaled gasps. Colin prolonged sounds. Once he said "mmm-mmme" and held on to the *m* for about 2 seconds. We detected a slight upward shift in pitch on one of his prolongations. We recommended that the child be accepted for therapy and that his parents receive counseling.

> Shawn was referred to the clinic by a public school speech clinician. Here is a portion of the clinician's report: "This nine-year-old child is having real troubles in her third-grade classroom. She has a severe fluency problem. Her stuttering is characterized by long silent blocks (as long as 10 seconds) and audible prolongations of sounds. During the longest of her

Preparatory set.
An anticipatory readiness to perform an act.

blocks, there is a **tremor** of the lower lip and chin. To terminate a **fixation,** she first clicks her tongue and then blurts out the word with a sudden surge of force. During the utterance she also blinks her eyes. She speaks and reads aloud very slowly—less than forty words per minute. When I talk with her, her most common response is 'I don't know.' When I do press her for a reply to my question, she lowers her head, fixes her eyes on the floor, and begins to cry. She is very quiet in the classroom, but her teacher says she does well on written work. Some of the children have teased and mocked her in the halls and during recess. She prefers to spend recess and lunch hour with the teacher. Shawn's mother reports that the child spends a great deal of time alone in her room talking with her dolls. Apparently she is fluent in this situation."

Barry, a high school senior, was one of the most severe stutterers we have seen. His speech was filled with rapid, explosive repetitions of sounds and syllables; the speech interruptions were accompanied by head jerks and a violent backward thrust of his upper body. He refused to give up a speech attempt. In a highly compulsive manner he would repeat a sound or syllable over and over until finally a fractured, grotesque version of the word emerged. For example, Barry attempted to say the word "Friday" in the following manner: the word was broken into four syllables, "fruh-high-un-day"; we counted forty-six repetitions of the first three syllables ("fruh-high-un), and it took him 27 seconds and three complete breath cycles to add to the last syllable. Almost immediately he plunged back into the word with a somewhat shorter but similar result. Barry's conversational speech was judged to be unintelligible. The only avoidance he seems to use is the phrase "Let's see," which he employs to start an utterance. He displayed open hostility toward the listener and on several occasions has been involved in fights at school and in his neighborhood.

In considering this disorder of fluency, let us observe its various aspects. Stuttering shows breaks in the usual time sequence of utterance. The usual flow is interrupted. There are conspicuous oscillations and fixations, repetitions, and prolongations of sounds and syllables. There are gaps of silence that call attention to themselves. If you ask a question, the answer may not be forthcoming at the proper time. Stuttered speech sometimes seems to have holes in it. Some sounds are held too long. Syllables seem to echo themselves repeatedly and compulsively. Odd contortions and struggles occur that interfere with communication and the person who stutters may show marked signs of fear or embarrassment. Stuttering fits our definition because this behavior deviates from the speech of other people in such a way that it attracts attention. All of us hesitate and repeat ourselves, but the person who stutters hesitates and repeats differently from us, and more often.

One of the interesting features of stuttering is that it seems to be a disorder more of communication than of speech. Most people who stutter can sing without difficulty. Most of them speak perfectly when alone. Usually, it is only when they are talking to a listener that the difficulty becomes ap-

Tremor.
The rapid tremulous vibration of a muscle group.

Fixation.
In stuttering, the prolongation of a speech posture.

parent. Stuttering varies with emotional stress and increases in situations invested with fear or shame. When very secure and relaxed, they often are very fluent. In extreme cases even the thinking processes seem to be affected—but only when they are thinking aloud, and again in the presence of a listener. The intermittent nature of the disorder is not only extremely unsettling for the speaker, it is also astonishing for family and friends.

Stuttering takes many forms; it presents many faces. *The only consistent behavior is the repetition and prolongation of syllables, sounds, or speech postures*. It changes as it develops, for stuttering usually grows and gets worse if untreated.

At the outset, generally around two and a half to four years of age, the child's speech is broken by an excessive amount of repetitions of syllables and sounds or, less frequently, by the prolongation of sound. He does not seem to be aware of his difficulty. He does not struggle or avoid speaking. He does not seem to be embarrassed at all. Indeed he seems almost totally unconscious of his repetitive utterance. He just bubbles along, trying his best to communicate. In many instances, it appears as if the child's need to talk exceeds his maturational capacity to coordinate thoughts and motor speech skills. An excerpt from a parent's letter may illustrate this early stuttering.

> I would appreciate some advice about my daughter. She is almost three years old and has always been precocious in speech. Four weeks ago she recovered from a severe attack of whooping cough, and it was immediately after that when she began to show some trouble with her speech. One morning she came downstairs and asked for orange juice, and it sounded like this: "Wh-wh-wh-where's my orange juice?" Since then, she has repeated often, and sometimes eight or nine times. It doesn't seem to bother her, but I'm worried about it as it gets a lot worse when she asks questions or when she is tired, and I'm afraid other children will start laughing at her. One of her playmates has already imitated her several times. No one else in our family has any trouble talking. What do you think we should do? Up to now we have just been ignoring it and hoping it will go away.

In some instances it does go away; apparently many children do seem to outgrow stuttering. Unfortunately, other youngsters, however, neither outgrow the problem nor does the stuttering remain so effortless. The child begins to react to his broken communication by surprise and then frustration. The former effortless repetitions and prolongations become irregular, faster, and more tense. As the child becomes aware of his stuttering and is frustrated by it he begins to struggle. Finally, he becomes afraid of certain speaking situations and of certain words and sounds. Once this occurs, stuttering tends to become self-penetrating, self-perpetuating, self-reinforcing. The more he fears, the more he stutters, and the more he stutters, the more he fears. He becomes caught in a vicious circle.

In the older person, stuttering occurs in many forms, since different individuals react to their speech interruptions in different ways. One German authority carefully described ninety-nine different varieties of stuttering (each christened with beautiful Greek and Latin verbiage), and we are sure that there must be many more. Individuals who stutter have been known to grunt or spit or pound themselves or protrude their tongues or speak on inhalation or waltz or jump or merely stare glassily when in the throes of what they call a "spasm" or a "block." Some of the imitations of stuttering heard in the movies and on radio may seem grotesque, yet the reality may be even more unusual.

Some develop an almost complete inability to make a direct speech attempt upon a feared word. They approach it, back away, say "a-a-a-a" or "um-um-um," go back to the beginning of the sentence and try again and again, until finally they give up communication altogether. Many become so adept at substituting synonyms for their difficult words, and disguising the interruptions that do occur, that they are able to pose as normal speakers. They have preached and taught school and become successful traveling salesmen without ever betraying their infirmity, but they are not happy individuals. The nervous strain and vigilance necessary to avoid and disguise their symptoms often create stresses so severe as to produce profound emotional breakdowns.

This general picture of stuttering gives you an overview of the disorder, but it does not show you how a speech pathologist would analyze the problem of a specific client. First she would ask the question, "What behaviors does this person show that are unlike those of a normal speaker?" She would be interested in the overt, visible, and audible manifestations of the problem such as repetitions, prolongations, tremors, inappropriate mouth postures, or abnormal foci of tension. She would note how the stutterer avoids or postpones the speech attempt. She would try to determine how the person seeks to release himself from the verbal oscillations and fixations that break up the flow of speech. Through interview and observation the speech clinician would probe the stutterer's inner world. What speaking situations are most feared? What words and sounds are viewed as difficult? How much frustration does he feel? How much shame and embarrassment? Is the disorder getting worse? How fluent can he be in certain situations? These and a host of other questions and scannings provide the diagnostic information needed to plan appropriate therapy.

Cluttering

Cluttering is a fluency disorder that is often confused with stuttering, but there are some major differences. People who clutter also have breaks in fluency, but they repeat words rather than syllables or sounds. They show few prolongations, few tremors, and rarely any of the tension and struggle that characterizes stuttering. Also they have no fears of words, sounds,

Cluttering.
A disorder of time or rhythm characterized by unorganized, hasty spurts of speech often accompanied by slurred articulation and breaks in fluency.

or speaking situations, and indeed have little awareness that their speech is disrupted. Most striking, however, is the very rapid rate of their utterances **(tachylalia).** They speak in torrents, their words stumbling over each other so that listeners just cannot understand much of what they are trying to say. Perhaps because of this excessive speed, speech sounds and entire syllables are often omitted or distorted, a feature that again affects intelligibility. Speech occurs in spurts rather than continuously, and sentence structure may be disorganized. Nevertheless, and curiously, individuals who clutter typically seem unaware of, and largely indifferent to, their speech. Very few refer themselves to the speech pathologist because of cluttering, but their teachers and employers certainly do and treatment is often difficult.

> Ralph was referred to us as a stutterer by his industrial education supervisor during his semester of student teaching. When we examined him, he revealed no fears or avoidances, exhibited only a few part-word repetitions, and had no fixations; he said he enjoyed talking, did a lot of it, and that he was asked frequently to repeat himself, "especially when I talk fast." Ralph's difficulty seemed to take place on the phrase or sentence level; his interruptions broke the integrity of a *thought* rather than a *word*. In addition, he frequently omitted syllables and transposed words and phrases: he said "plobably," "posed," and "pacific" for "probably," "supposed," and "specific." Ralph's speech was sprinkled with spoonerisms (he said "beta dase" for "data base") and malapropisms (he said he was under the "antiseptic" for two hours in a recent operation and that the students had made him so angry it got his "dandruff" up). His speech was swift and jumbled; it emerged in rapid torrents until he jammed up and then he surged on again in another staccato outburst. In spontaneous talking, his message was characterized by disorganized sentences and poor phrasing. He gave the impression of being in great haste. When we asked him to slow down and speak carefully, there was a dramatic improvement, but he soon forgot our admonishment and reverted to the hurried, disorganized style. Ralph was an impatient, impulsive young man, always on the go. His college coursework was characteristically done in a rush; he had difficulty reading and his handwriting was a scrawl.

Many clinicians suspect that cluttering may be one symptom of a central language disturbance or learning disability, citing the difficulties their clients often have with reading, writing, spelling, and other language-dependent skills. Cluttering also tends to run in families, suggesting a possible genetic basis for the disorder. Pointing to the occurrence of mixed laterality, brainwave irregularities, and deficits in auditory functioning, some authorities speculate that minimal but diffuse brain dysfunction may be involved.

Although our understanding of the cause of cluttering is limited, we can offer a rather comprehensive description of the disorder. The most salient feature is, of course, pell-mell, sputtered speech. We include here a comprehensive list of symptoms associated with the disorder. The items

Tachylalia.
Extremely rapid speech.

indicated with an asterisk are the essential features for a diagnosis of cluttering; the remaining symptoms may or may not be present.

*1. No seeming awareness of the excessive speed or garbled utterance; no fears or avoidance.
2. Speech characterized by
    *—rapid and irregular rate
    *—disorganized sentence structure
    *—articulatory imprecision or slurring
    *—repetitions of whole words and phrases
    —scoping (compressing two or more words into a holistic utterance, e.g., "she's expecting" becomes "shezezptn")
    —spoonerism (transposition of sounds of two words, e.g., "darn bore" for "barn door")
    —malapropism (incorrect use of words, e.g., "sales will rise for a while and then reach a *platitude*")
    —restricted vocabulary, redundant utterances, use of clichés
    —limited inflection, sometimes monotone voice
3. Reading problems (letter reversals, word emission)
4. Writing and spelling problems (both content and legibility)
5. Difficulty sustaining attention (some clients need to plan aloud, repeating instructions to themselves several times)
6. Difficulty imitating musical notes or simple melody patterns; some clients dislike or are indifferent to music
7. Personal characteristics: impulsive, careless, untidy, suggestible
8. Poor motor coordination
9. Case history revealing delayed speech and language development
10. Intelligence skewed toward arithmetical functions and skills requiring precision in nonverbal, concrete tasks

Since they are generally deficient in self-monitoring, persons who clutter are difficult to treat. They are surprised when others cannot understand them. They can speak perfectly when they speak slowly, but it is almost impossible for them to do so except for short periods.

The treatment of cluttering in school-age children requires the coordinated efforts of classroom teachers, learning disability specialists, and speech-language clinicians. Early intervention is important because some clutterers also become stutterers, although most do not.

VOICE DISORDERS

Except for instances in which the voice problem is sufficiently great to actually interfere with a speaker's intelligibility (or in which, for example, an individual's larynx has been surgically removed, or when an individual for

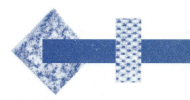

some other reason is not producing phonation at all), voice disorders are not necessarily easily identified or defined. The voice that "calls attention to itself" is not always perceived as a problem by either the speaker or the listener. On the other hand, a voice that is perceived by the typical listener as a relatively pleasant voice can be causing legitimate distress for its owner.

Diagnostic and treatment decisions relating to voice are even further confounded by many other considerations that we will begin to explore in Chapter 9. For now, we will simply note that the range of variation regarded as "normal" tends to be greater for vocal characteristics than for articulatory, fluency, or linguistic features of speech.

When speech pathologists become convinced that the speech impairment does involve voice (other than the voice loss associated with laryngectomy, which necessitates the utilization of some form of **alaryngeal speech**), they carefully scrutinize the client's voice for deviancy in *pitch, loudness,* or *quality.* They recognize that this simple three-dimensional analysis merely begins to scratch the surface and that a voice evaluation involves many other types of observations. We will need to know, for example, if the voice disorder *(dysphonia)* has some organic or neurologic cause and if medical or surgical treatment is warranted, or if the disorder seems instead to be a functional problem.

Nevertheless, one or more of these three basic features can show significant differences from the normal range of variation, and it is important to describe and define such differences as clearly as possible. Moreover, *pitch, loudness,* and *quality,* plus *alaryngeal speech,* afford us a useful framework for our first glance at voice disorders.

Deviations of Pitch

The normal range of pitch variations depends upon sex, age, and several other factors. The voices of men are generally lower in average pitch than are those of women. A deep-voiced male would have no voice disorder; the women who speaks with a bass voice is conspicuous. A six-year-old boy with a high-pitched treble voice would incur no penalty from society; a thirty-year-old man would find raised eyebrows if he began to speak in such tones. Under conditions of great excitement, many of us have voices that crack or show pitch breaks. But when an adult shows pitch breaks upward into the **falsetto** register when he orders a hamburger or says goodbye, we suspect the abnormal. There are times when it is appropriate to speak with a minimum of **inflection,** but a person who consistently talks on a monopitch will find his listener either irritated or asleep. In deciding whether a person has a pitch disorder we must always use the normal yardstick.

This discussion has anticipated our listing of the pitch disorders. They are as follows: *too-high pitch, too-low pitch, monotone* or **monopitch, pitch breaks,** *stereotyped inflections,* and **diplophonia.**

Alaryngeal speech.
Speech in which a sound source other than the larynx is used in place of normal voicing.

Falsetto.
The upper, high-pitched register of voice; produced with stretched, thinned vocal folds; also known as *loft register.*

Inflection.
Upward or downward change in pitch of the voice during a continuous phonation.

Monopitch.
Speaking in a very narrow pitch range, usually of one to four semitones.

Pitch break.
Sudden abnormal shift of pitch during speech.

Diplophonia.
Voice in which two separate tones are present simultaneously; associated with laryngeal pathology.

The following description was uttered by a 200-pound football player in his high, piping, shrill, child's voice:

> Yes, I was one of those boy sopranos and my music teacher loved me. I soloed in all the cantatas and programs and sang in the choir and glee clubs, and they never let my voice change. I socked a guy the other day who wisecracked about it, but I'm still a boy soprano at twenty-two. I'm getting so I'm afraid to open my mouth. Strangers start looking for a Charlie McCarthy somewhere. I got to get over it, and quick. Why, I can't even swear but some guy who's been saying the same words looks shocked.

The *falsetto* **register** used by this tortured young man involves more than simply a high pitch. Falsetto voice is produced with laryngeal adjustments that are different from the adjustments of the **modal register** in which we typically speak. In falsetto, our vocal folds are stretched long and thinly, and they vibrate in a fashion that differs markedly from the vibrations seen in modal register. When heard in the adult male, the high pitch of falsetto voice turns the heads of anyone within earshot. Some of our more troubled voice clients have been postadolescent males who told us that their voices never changed at puberty. Very rarely is there any physical cause, however, and therapy basically requires that we show them how to find the correct laryngeal adjustment for producing their true and mature voices. A high-pitched voice in the male, falsetto or otherwise, can definitely be a handicap—communicative, economic, and social.

An excessively low pitch in the male voice also can be problematic, particularly when it is used forcefully to convey the "voice of authority," although initially it may only damage the tissue of the larynx and contribute to the possible development of a **contact ulcer.**

Another interesting pitch issue that sometimes is seen in the clinic today is that of the transsexual person who is undergoing the process of gender reassignment. Pitch modification is only one of several aspects of speech that can help a former male sound more feminine (or vice versa), but it usually is a major concern for these individuals.

A woman's high-pitched voice (even, unfortunately, when it is an optimal pitch for her larynx) also is viewed too often as detrimental. A recent "how to succeed" article in a women's magazine irresponsibly advised its readers that the typical woman, to command respect, must "lower the pitch of her speaking voice by *one full octave.*" And we have had more than one female broadcaster request therapy to lower an already quite appropriate speaking pitch. Small wonder, then, that some women may abuse their voices while trying—either consciously or subconsciously—to alter their pitch levels toward a stereotypical, unrealistic vocal "standard."

At the other extreme, if the female voice has been forced to an excessively low pitch level, or if her pitch level is unusually low due to physical

Register.
Manner of adjustment of the larynx for voice production (e.g., falsetto register, modal or chest register).

Modal register.
The manner of laryngeal adjustment and vocal fold vibration used to produce voice in normal speech; sometimes referred to as chest register in singing.

Contact ulcer.
Small lesion on the posterior medial edge of the vocal fold; may be caused by reflux of stomach acids or abusive use of the voice.

conditions such as hormonal imbalance, she also may express concern. And we may agree that she has reason for concern.

When a woman's voice is pitched very low and carries a certain type of male inflection, it certainly calls attention to itself and causes maladjustment. The following sentence, spoken by a casual acquaintance and overheard by the girl to whom it referred, practically wrecked her entire feelings of security: "Every time I hear her talk I look around to see if it's the bearded lady of the circus."

The use of an excessively low pitch level in speaking, whether by a woman, man, or child, often is accompanied by frequent lapses into the *vocal fry* register of phonation. Vocal fry (sometimes called **"glottal fry"** or "dichrotic dysphonia" or "pulse register") is the very low-pitched, crackly, ratchet-like sound that can contribute to our perception of roughness, harshness, or hoarseness in a voice. Often it reflects simply a functional misuse or abuse of the voice, and it can help us identify habitual use of a pitch level that is too low for the *individual* even if it is not exceptionally low relative to group averages. But its presence also can be one sign of a potentially serious health condition such as **hypothyroidism.**

On every campus some professor possesses that enemy of education, a monotonous voice. A true monotone is comparatively rare, yet it dominates any conversation by its difference. To hear a person laugh on a single note is enough to stir the scalp. Questions asked in a true monotone seem curiously devoid of life. Fortunately, most cases of monotonous voice are not so extreme. Many of them could be described as the "poker voice"—even as a face without expression is termed a "poker face." Inflections are present, but they are reduced to a minimum.

By stereotyped inflections we refer to the voice that calls attention to itself through its pitch patterning. The sing-song voice, the voice that ends every phrase or sentence with the same rising or falling inflection, the "schoolma'am's voice" with its emphatic dogmatic inflections, are all types of variation that, *when extreme,* may be considered speech defects.

Pitch breaks may be upward and downward, usually the former. The adolescent boy, learning to use his adult voice, sometimes experiences them. Often they can be very traumatizing. To have your voice suddenly flip-flop upward into a falsetto or child's voice is to lose control of the self. When you want to speak you don't wish to yodel. Often individuals who fear this experience use a monopitch or too low or too high a pitch level to keep the flip-flopping from occurring. Pitch breaks can define the speaker as one who cannot control himself or who is very emotional. They often interfere with the person's ability to think on his feet, since he must forever be monitoring his voice. They may sound funny to others, but we have not found them so.

A curious pitch disorder, usually but not always organic, is found in *diplophonia.* The person uses two pitches at the same time, producing a voice that is very noticeable. We wish we could play for you a tape that

Glottal fry.
A low-pitched tickerlike continuous clicking sound produced by the vocal folds; also known as *vocal fry* and as *pulse register.*

Hypothyroidism.
Insufficient production of hormone by thyroid gland; can produce fatigue and other symptoms; may cause voice problems, especially in women.

would demonstrate it. One of our clients developed diplophonia as the result of having discovered that she could speak in a deep bass by adjusting her larynx in a certain way. She played with this deep voice, shocked her roommates in the shower or bedroom, and generally used it for kicks. Then she found that she could use both her normal voice and the deep voice at the same time, even being able to sing tunes in harmony with herself. About the time that she had decided to use it to go into show business, she found that she could no longer shift back and forth at will between the two voices but instead had the double voice, the diplophonia, all the time. Terrified, she came to us for help.

Loudness Deviations

Most of us, if we have abused our voices by excessive shouting or yelling, or have suffered from a severe cold or allergy, have experienced temporary dysphonia. For a time we cannot talk loudly or can speak only in a **breathy** whisper. In the latter case, we can be said to have had *aphonia,* the complete loss of voice. In either case, our voices usually have recovered relatively quickly, especially if we avoided placing heavy demands on an unhealthy larynx.

Loudness deviations come in other forms as well. The basic loudness level can be inadequate, as above, but a voice also can be too loud. The voice can be lacking in loudness variability, making it seem as monotonous as the voice that lacks appropriate pitch variability. Aphonia might occur during only some portion of an utterance (for example, as a breath phrase ends), but it also can occur rapidly and intermittently, virtually in spasms, even within the confines of a single syllable.

When a client is chronically dysphonic in these or other ways, the job of the speech pathologist can be quite challenging but also intriguing. The skilled clinician will try to identify the causes of the dysphonia through interviewing the client and try to sort out the predisposing from the precipitating causes, as well as identify the factors that may be maintaining the disorder. Is there a long history of vocal abuse, of regularly having to speak in an environment with high noise levels, of having to communicate too often with a family member who has become deafened? Does the client herself have any hearing impairments? Does the client have a long history of chronic laryngitis? Is she a college cheerleader? How many cigarettes does she smoke each day? Has there been a history of previous loss of voice and under what conditions? Speech pathology involves a lot of detective work, and these questions are only a few of those that are helpful in understanding the nature of the problem.

Associated behavior also interests us. How does this person with dysphonia attempt the production of voice? We may observe his thyroid cartilage, (his "Adam's apple"), to see if it assumes the position for swallowing at the moment he begins to phonate. We note any evidences

Breathiness.
Air wastage during phonation; voice quality heard when the vocal folds do not fully approximate during the vibratory cycle.

of excessive tension in the area of the throat. We look for the mistiming of the breath pulse or for other breathing irregularities. And, knowing that dysphonia may be one of the first signs of organic abnormalities, such as growths on the vocal cords, benign or cancerous, or the reflection of paralysis, the speech pathologist perhaps may save a life by insisting that his client be seen by a **laryngologist**.

Many dysphonias, however, do not have such an organic pathology. Our voices are the barometers or our emotional states. They reflect our feelings of anxiety, guilt, or hostility. When these acids begin to eat their human containers too often, voice disorders may ensue. Here is an illustration:

> For nine years since graduating from high school, Sgt. Maynard Gooch enjoyed a tranquil life in the U.S. Air Force. He had had it made, he told us in a strained whisper, as a clerk in the quartermaster's office. He relished the redundancy of the work and the secure certainty of military life. It all changed drastically when Sgt. Gooch was awarded another stripe for his sleeve and put in charge of twelve clerk-typist recruits. His new job was to train and supervise the men. Apprehensive about the responsibility at the outset, the client's fears were soon realized when the recruits showed no respect for him or the work; and they simply did not listen to Sgt. Gooch's patient pleading.
>
> Several days later, the client woke up and discovered his voice was gone. When we examined him, he seemed strangely unconcerned, even serene. "It's too bad," he whispered with a sad-sweet smile, "Now they will have to put me back on my old job." Instead of *being* a problem, the client's aphonia was a *solution* to a problem. It was easy to demonstrate that his vocal folds were not impaired: When we asked him to cough and clear his throat, he produced a normal baritone voice. Clearly, his sudden loss of voice had no physical basis, as reports from the Air Force medical officer and psychiatrist confirmed. The psychiatrist requested that we restore the client's phonation to facilitate individual and group psychotherapy. Using throat-clearing, sighing, and humming, combined with strong positive suggestion, we convinced Sgt. Gooch over several sessions that his larynx was again functioning normally. When we checked several weeks later, we learned that the client had made small gains in psychotherapy, that he experienced no relapse or transfer of symptoms, and that he was happily employed as a private secretary to the chaplain.

Speech pathologists, as well as physicians, may use certain adjectives before the term *aphonia* to indicate the presumed cause of the disorder. In our preceding illustration, Sgt. Gooch might be said to have the hysterical type of aphonia because of its evident neurotic nature. Someone whose loss of voice seemed to be due to vocal abuse and strain would have a **functional** *aphonia,* but not a hysterical one. On the other hand, when the loss of voice is due to paralysis or growths upon the vocal folds, it would be called an **organic** *aphonia* or *dysphonia,* depending upon whether the loss was complete or incomplete.

Laryngologist.
Physician specializing in diseases and pathology of the larynx; typically an *otorhinolaryngologist (ENT).*

Functional.
Refers to a disorder that has no organic cause; may or may not be "psychogenic."

Organic.
In the sense of causation, refers to an anatomic or physiologic etiology.

Although clearly more than a "loudness deviation," we mention here an unusual voice disorder that for many years bewildered physicians, psychologists, speech pathologists, and researchers, and that can severely disable the person who experiences it. Formerly known as **spastic dysphonia** (and, by some early observers, as "laryngeal stuttering"), it is more often called **spasmodic dysphonia** today. A person (somewhat more often female than male) with this problem may begin an utterance with a good voice, then the laryngeal and throat muscles tense so tightly that the voice comes out only spasmodically in small bursts of squeezed, strangled sound, with intermittent total blockages of airflow. Or, in a variation of this pattern, laryngeal muscles may slacken in spasms to the point that voicing is intermittently absent with only whispered airflow being present.

Like stuttering, spasmodic dysphonia can vary in severity with communicative stress. Persons with spasmodic dysphonia may briefly show normal voicing in, for example, the quick, automatic utterance of an expletive, and there may be little or no interruption of phonation when they sustain a vowel sound, especially at a high pitch level. Some can sing with relative ease; others find the singing and speaking voice equally impaired.

Long regarded by many authorities as the reflection of a deep-seated emotional disturbance, spasmodic dysphonia had been resistant to almost any form of treatment until very recent years. It now appears that there is a probable neurological basis for most cases of spasmodic dysphonia, and laryngeal **dystonia** is the term often applied. Now, through medical intervention combined with voice therapy (more about this in Chapter 9), many with this disorder are able to be helped, although not cured.

Another voice problem, *ventricular dysphonia,* will be mentioned in this section because the phonation can fade in loudness enough to impair comprehension. With ventricular dysphonia, "voicing" is produced by vibration of the false or ventricular folds, which are located just above the level of the true vocal folds. The sound often seems strangled and harsh, and you may have unknowingly produced it yourself when straining and grunting on the toilet or when lifting a heavy object. The experienced speech clinician is cautious in accepting a quick diagnosis of **ventricular phonation,** however, because it can be a misdiagnosis which arises when a client's voice is badly dysphonic and, because of tense overcompression of the false folds, the faulty action of the true vocal folds beneath them simply has not been seen. In any event, ventricular dysphonia is fortunately very rarely encountered.

Voice Quality Deviations

Vocal quality or timbre varies a great deal from person to person. There are about as many characteristic voice qualities as there are faces, which is why it usually is so easy to identify a speaker by hearing the voice. It is exceptionally difficult, on the other hand, to describe voice qualities in

Spastic dysphonia. Generally synonymous with *spasmodic dysphonia,* associated with great strain and effort in producing voice; has been referred to in the past as "laryngeal stuttering."

Spasmodic dysphonia (SD). Uncontrolled spasmodic closures (adductor SD) or openings (abductor SD) of the glottis during phonation, causing voice interruption; now believed usually to reflect the presence of a focal laryngeal dystonia.

Dystonia. Abnormal muscle tonicity due to neurologic causes; may cause spasms or writhing movements.

Ventricular phonation. Voice produced by the vibration of the false vocal folds.

words. Novelists have called voices thick, thin, reedy, shrill, sweet, rich, brilliant, grating, and even metallic, but such adjectives are rarely used by speech pathologists. Yet even the terms used by professionals are imprecise. Only a few of them are descriptive enough to have gained very wide acceptance.

One of the exceptions is the voice quality termed hypernasality. The lay person would say that a speaker with such a disorder seems to be talking through his nose too much. When most of the vowels or the voiced **continuant** sounds (other than the nasal sounds, /m/, /n/, and /ŋ/) have so much nasal resonance in them that the voice is conspicuously unpleasant, most speech pathologists would agree on the diagnosis of hypernasality. No one should have to whine when he passionately says "I love you." Not all hypernasality gives the impression of whining, however. To whine, you also usually show the upward inflection patterns of complaint combined with the excessive nasality. And some of our clients, the more neurotic ones who bathe constantly in self-pity, show this combination of pitch and quality deviations. But there are others, as we have said, who do not whine, yet show too much nasality.

In certain sections of this country there are dialectal ways of speaking that show more nasality than we find generally. Providing the Hoosier who speaks this way stays on his Indiana farm, he certainly would not possess any voice disorder at all, but he would have to reduce that nasality were he to become an actor or radio announcer in some other part of our land. (Again, we find the need always to define abnormality with reference to an individual's "speech community.") Persons from certain rural parts of New England are also said to have a nasal twang that we would hate to classify as abnormal. Indeed, most of this dialectal hypernasality seems to be due to what is termed *assimilation nasality,* which refers to the nasalization of only those sounds which precede or follow the /m/, /n/, or /ŋ/. Most of us show some slight assimilation nasality in saying such words as name, man, or mangle, the vowels being mildly nasalized.

Hypernasality is a quality commonly heard, too, in the voices of children born with cleft palates or with other impairments that make it difficult to shut the nasal cavity off from the rest of the vocal tract. Some hypernasality normally may be heard for a few weeks following the surgical removal of **adenoids**; but if the nasal resonance is great and if it does not subside, the surgery may be found to have "unmasked" a previously unrecognized palatal insufficiency.

The onset of persistent hypernasality in adulthood should be investigated with great care, we must note, for it can be an early sign of neurological disease. At the same time, of course, we would not want to unduly alarm anyone.

Another voice quality disorder that is fairly easily recognized is the **harsh** or *strident* voice. People would describe it as raspingly unpleasant, as "grating upon the ear." There is tension in it, an abrupt beginning of

Continuant.
A speech sound that can be prolonged without distortion, e.g., /s/ or /f/ or /u/.

Adenoids.
Growths of lymphoid tissue on the back wall of the throat; also called pharyngeal tonsils.

Harshness.
Voice quality usually associated with excessive laryngeal tension.

phonation, an unevenness rather than smoothness, and bits of that scratchy noise called the **vocal fry.** Try speaking aloud very harshly to see how well this description fits.

A third disorder of voice quality is the *breathy* voice. Hot Breath Harriet had one and used it as a Maine guide uses a birchbark horn to bring a lovelorn moose to the gun. In our culture, for some esoteric reason, a low-pitched husky voice in a woman sounds sexy to the vulnerable male, even though it may merely be the result of asthma or a paralyzed vocal cord or a postnasal drip. It certainly can call attention to itself and impair intelligibility in a noisy environment.

These three, the hypernasal, the harsh, and the breathy voice, can be labelled with some precision. But how about the *hoarse* voice? This quality has been defined as one that combines harshness and breathiness, and therein may lie a source of some confusion. In producing harshness we introduce substantial laryngeal hypertension; in trying to make our voices breathy, we must *reduce* tension sufficiently that the vocal folds will not completely meet during the vibratory cycle. This will appear less contradictory, though, if we remember that hoarseness can encompass a wide spectrum of possible perceptual features and that it seldom occurs in the absence of some vocal fold abnormality which alters the normal vibratory pattern. The hoarse voice can be predominantly breathy with only mild harshness, or the opposite can be true, as can any combination between the two extremes. At any rate, you should know that when a person doesn't have the flu or a cold or allergy and yet has been hoarse for a month, he or she should be referred immediately to a laryngologist because growths may be forming on the vocal folds or some other unpleasant consequences may lie in wait. Even when the hoarse voice is suspected to be the result of obvious vocal abuse and strain, it is a signal that something should be done.

Finally, we have the disorder of **denasality,** another one that is difficult to describe or define. Sometimes called the adenoidal voice because it is characterized by a lack of nasality **(hyponasality),** when you hear it you want to swallow or clear your throat and are impelled to get out of range of suspected cold germs. Denasality has also been classified among the articulation disorders because the /m/, /n/, and /ŋ/ lose some of their nasality and turn into /b/, /d/, and /g/, respectively. And, of course, assimilation nasality will be absent from this voice. If you will pretend that you have a very bad cold and say this sentence, you will probably show the picture of denasality: "My mother made me come home." Chronically enlarged adenoids can be the cause of denasality (as well as the cause of habitual mouth breathing), as can any other condition (nasal **polyps,** for example) that blocks the nasal cavity from being opened posteriorly to the mouth and throat portions of the respiratory and vocal tract. Denasality virtually always has a physical cause, however temporary and fleeting it may be.

Vocal fry. Low-pitched continuous clicking sound produced by the vocal folds; also known as *glottal fry* and as *pulse register.*

Denasality. A lack of, or reduced, nasality.

Hyponasality. Lack of sufficient nasality, as in the denasal or adenoidal voice.

Polyp. Tissue mass that may form on a vocal fold following abuse of the voice.

The speech pathologist soon comes to recognize that few voice quality disorders are free from deviances in pitch or intensity and that their abnormality is increased when these other vocal features differ from the norm. For example, an excessively harsh and also excessively loud voice is more noticeable and more unpleasant than one that is not as loud. When we find a voice that is both hypernasal and too high in its pitch level, we can sometimes bring it closer to normality by lowering the pitch. In spastic dysphonia we hear harshness, aphonia, and breathiness combined. Again, we find deviant voices wherein several vocal quality deviations are apparent, as in the harsh nasal voice. In helping our students to sort out and to remember all these features of voice, we ask them to try to produce them before applying the diagnostic labels. Why don't you try, too?

Alaryngeal Speech

Alaryngeal speech is a term often used in reference to the speaker who, typically because of cancer, has undergone surgical removal of the larynx. The surgery is known as a *laryngectomy* and the laryngectomized person is sometimes referred to as a *laryngectomee*. The restoration of *speech*, not just of voice, is needed after surgery, for air now enters and leaves the lungs through a surgically created opening (tracheostoma) in the neck rather than via the mouth and nose.

The laryngectomized individual is not able even to whisper his name or to articulate speech sounds in the manner to which we all are accustomed. Clearly, speech rehabilitation can pose a substantial challenge for this client as well as for the clinician. Happily, success in the endeavor also is especially rewarding for both. In this chapter we acquaint you briefly with three main approaches to acquiring a new voice, *alaryngeal* voice, when the larynx has been totally amputated.

One form of alaryngeal voicing is known as *esophageal* voice. As its name implies, the user of esophageal voice has learned to inject a small quantity of orally captured air into the upper part of the esophagus and then to release this "air charge" in a way that creates a rapidly vibrating sound source near the juncture of the pharynx and the esophagus. When speech articulation gestures are skillfully superimposed on this voice, with practice the esophageal speaker can become quite fluent and easy to understand.

Another approach, one that often is used while the client is learning esophageal voice (and one that many laryngectomees elect to continue on a permanent basis), involves the use of an **artificial larynx.** Many such devices are marketed, the most common of which is the electrolarynx. With an **electrolarynx** the client learns to place a small electrically driven vibrating diaphragm against his neck in a manner that allows the device's sound to be carried through body tissue into the oral cavity where it can

Alaryngeal.
Without a larynx.

Artificial larynx.
Electronic or pneumatic vibrator used by a laryngectomee to produce a voice-like sound for speech.

Electrolarynx.
Battery-operated device used by laryngectomees to produce sound as a replacement for lost voice.

be "shaped" into speech. Alternatively, an oral adapter can be used to carry this sound to the mouth via a flexible tube that attaches over the vibrator. In either case, good intelligibility depends upon, among other things, skillful and precise articulation. The *pneumatic artificial larynx,* although utilized much less frequently than its electronic counterpart, produces a sound that more closely resembles the human voice. With this device the client's own lung air is exhaled from the **stoma** opening through a hand-held reed-like vibrator and thence to the mouth through a second tube. As in traditional esophageal speech, the accurate production of certain consonant sounds while using any artificial larynx usually requires considerable practice either with a speech pathologist or, in some circumstances, with another experienced laryngectomee.

There have been many attempts over the past decades to develop surgical solutions for the surgical loss of voice (even including one known, but failed, transplantation of a donor larynx). Several procedures that initially seemed to hold promise have later been abandoned, often because of associated problems in maintaining a viable airway. One procedure involving very minor surgery, however, has come to enjoy wide success and popularity. In the "t-e (tracheal-esophageal) puncture" approach, a small opening is created between the back wall of the trachea and the front wall of the esophagus at the level of the stoma, just below the junction of the pharynx and the esophagus. When a very small one-way valve *(voice prosthesis)* is inserted, the patient can direct lung air into the esophagus while yet avoiding the risk of saliva and other material entering the airway. In essence, this enables the client to produce esophageal sound without the necessity of injecting oral air for that purpose. Speech with the voice prosthesis can be exceptionally good: fluent, naturally phrased, and easily understood. Surgeon and speech pathologist teams around the world now work closely together to implement this technique for laryngectomee speech rehabilitation.

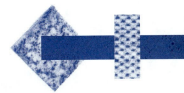

LANGUAGE DISORDERS

One of the chief fascinations about the field of speech pathology is the opportunity it presents for exploration and discovery. Humans, like the bear, must go over the mountain to see what they can see. The baby discovers her toes and babbles with delight; the child roams the fringes of his neighborhood; the adult walks gingerly on the moon. At this very moment all over the world there are people testing the boundaries of the known in astronomy, physics, chemistry, biology, and a hundred other sciences. In speech pathology, because it is a relatively new field, the unknown is very near. Every speech disorder has its puzzles, unanswered questions, and problems to be solved.

Stoma.
Opening in the neck through which the person must breathe after a laryngectomy.

Of all the disorders of communication, those of language disability most urgently need exploration. Although humans have been talking for thousands of years, language itself still holds many mysteries, and the disorders of language have many more. Language disorders are perhaps the most devastating of all communication impairments because the very substance of messages—the code or symbol system—is disturbed. All language-dependent behaviors—speech, comprehension, reading, writing, problem solving—are involved. There are two major language disorders: *aphasia* (dysphasia) and *delayed* or *deviant language development.*

Dysphasia

The term aphasia if used precisely would refer to the complete inability to comprehend or use language symbols, a condition that fortunately is rarely found, while *dysphasia* refers to a lesser degree of disability. Most working speech clinicians tend to use the terms interchangeably and so shall we. It is impossible to give you a "typical" description of an individual with aphasia because the disorder appears in many forms and levels of severity. He might show impairment in comprehending or formulating his messages or in finding ways to express them. His disability may be shown in reading, writing, or silent gesturing as well as in speaking. His speech may be so garbled as to be incomprehensible to others, or merely broken by a search for words that momentarily he cannot find. She may say "bread" when she wants to ask for "butter" or "jugga" for soup. She may nod her head affirmatively when she wants to say no. He may hold a pencil in his hand and yet not be able to copy the triangle placed before him. Dysphasia as a disorder has a thousand faces and the speech pathologist's first job is to analyze the features of the disability presented by the client. So let us here confine ourselves to brief symptomatic pictures.

One of our colleagues, a professor of biology, suffered a mild stroke and dysphasia. When he recovered, he told us what it was like during the initial stages of the disorder: "I could pick out words here and there when people talked to me, I could sense the flow of a message, but the meaning was lost. It sounded as if the nurses, my doctor, even my wife, were speaking a foreign language, or a jumble of strange sounds. It was so frustrating and caused me so much anxiety that I refused to listen when people talked to me. That's when I became very depressed and felt so isolated."

Ned Labonte, a sixty-four-year-old farmer, presented a similar albeit less severe problem in understanding spoken words. When we asked him to define the word "money" he responded: "Money, money, ah, money . . . how did you say that again?" We repeated the word. "Money, let's see, money, ah, you mean like you get 5 or 10 . . . and put it in your pocket?"

Some of our clients have told us that when trying to read, they see "a line of meaningless squiggles or scribbles" and haven't the slightest idea as to what they mean. Some of them cannot even recognize snapshots of their own faces or those of their friends.

In these examples, we see the receptive problems of aphasia, the difficulties in comprehending language symbols whether they are spoken or written. More dramatically visible is the impairment that may be shown in speech. Here is what one of our clients wrote in her autobiography after she had made a good recovery.

> When I tried to say a few things the words wouldn't come out. I got so upset! All I could say was, "Shit!" And I always detested that word. There were strange things I would say like, "I died," as if I had come back to life. As I sat at the dinner table, my family would encourage me to name foods, but I called everything "catsup" or "fish." But I thought I was talking normally.

The expressive loss often extends to writing as the same client noted in her autobiography.

> One time soon after my second operation, my sister-in-law visited me. I was trying to say something but the words would not come out, so I thought, "I know what, I will write it." So I picked up pencil and paper and expected to write, but I looked at her and said, "I can't write!" We both laughed; it wasn't funny, but we both laughed.

In treating the patient who has dysphasia, the speech pathologist ideally is just one member of a closely coordinated rehabilitation team that includes at least the physician, an occupational therapist, a physical therapist, and perhaps a psychologist or social worker. Even so, the speech-language professional often is the person who works most closely with the family of the stroke victim, helping them to understand the client's communication difficulties and ensuring that they help rather than hinder the process of rehabilitation. Perhaps no work in speech pathology is more challenging than helping the person with aphasia become able to communicate effectively again and to regain a sense of human dignity.

Language Development Problems

Problems of language development are encountered often by every worker in the field of special education as well as by the speech pathologist. A child who, for one reason or another (and there may be many reasons), does not understand what others say to him or who does not know the basic rules by which our language is structured is truly handicapped, for he cannot send or receive the messages that are essential in a society that demands constant communication. There is little doubt that language is the most important acquisition a child will ever make. Most, if not all, skills or knowledge are learned through language. Relationships with others are mediated through the exchange of messages. But language is more than a vehicle for learning and relating; it is also an instrument that shapes the way in which the user perceives and conceptualizes the world. The child with delayed or deviant language is pretty helpless in a world of words.

Especially during the past two decades, speech pathologists increasingly have responded to the challenge that these youngsters present. Surveys show that over one-half of the caseload of public school speech pathologists now consists of children with language disabilities. As a matter of fact, the parent organization of speech pathologists, the American Speech and Hearing Association changed its name in 1977 to the American Speech-Language-Hearing Association. The worker in speech pathology began to be referred to as the "speech and language clinician" at that same time.

A language problem may be defined as a disturbance in, or impoverishment of, the symbol processing system—the child's supply of concepts and use of linguistic rules is either severely limited or is significantly different from the conventional usage of his peers (see **semantics**). These disorders range from a very mild disturbance to profound or almost total absence of language. Many diagnosticians find it useful to distinguish between two broad categories of language problems: *delayed* or *deviant*. Children with delayed language exhibit symbolic functioning that would be considered normal at an earlier age; their verbal skills are, in other words, underdeveloped relative to what is expected at a given chronological age. On the other hand, some children use deviant language when they invent idiosyncratic (their own unique) rules for processing information.

Delayed Language Development. Although the child with delayed language development usually shows many articulation errors (sometimes to the point of unintelligibility), his major difficulties often lie in vocabulary deficits that restrict his speech output, in grammatical deficits that prevent him from expressing himself according to the hidden rules of communication (appropriate plurals, tense, subject-predicate, etc.), or in his inability to handle transformations, such as being able to know the difference between a statement and a question or to be able to express himself in both ways.

Anyone who wants to help a child with such a language disability must not only determine that his language competence and performance are inferior to other children of his chronological, mental, or physical age levels; he must also analyze the child's specific difficulties in encoding and decoding.

For illustrative purposes, we include a brief portion of a speech and language clinician's presentation of her diagnostic findings on a language-delayed child at a staffing conference.

Semantics.
Meaning; the relationship of symbols to objects and events.

Carol Dilworth is a five-year, one-month-old language-delayed child discovered by our preschool screening program. At that time we administered several screening tests, took a language sample, and conducted an extensive parent interview. The screening test results are as follows: (1) Gross and fine *motor skills* are delayed; Carol completed items up to the three-year-old level. (2) *Personal and social skills* are also performed at the three-year-old level. (3) With regard to *language skills,* the child is performing at a level one year behind her chronological age on all recognition and auditory comprehension items; verbal expressive skills are more severely delayed—Carol successfully completed task items up to but not beyond the normative level for twenty-four-month-old children. (4) An assessment of her syntax shows that she is still using simple two-word utterances ("Carol play?" "Want Mommy.") characteristic of children between the ages of eighteen to thirty months.

The *language sample* was taken in the Dilworth home. We showed the child twenty-five items (pictures, objects) and asked her to tell us about them. Carol's mean (average) length of response was 1.8; typically, she responded with two-word utterances. Once again, this level of language usage is appropriate for children about two years of age. A youngster of five should have a mean length of response of about 5.7 words per stimulus item.

The *parent interview* revealed a general slowness in Carol's development. For example, she sat up at eleven months, walked at nineteen months, and was toilet trained at three years, six months. Mrs. Dilworth noted very little babbling or vocal play when Carol was an infant. Reportedly, the child did not use her first word meaningfully until almost two years old.

Deviant Language.   Children with deviant language not only do not show the linguistic patterns generally found in normally developing younger children, they also use atypical or eccentric forms instead of simplifying the symbolic code. They tend to have a limited repertoire of utterances and may even have difficulty repeating simple messages after the diagnostician. They devise a strange language of their own. Let us listen in on a parent interview with the mother of identical twin boys who show signs of deviant language. A college graduate in anthropology, Mrs. Mannion kept careful records on the development of her six-year-old sons:

Clinician:	You said that Otis and Lotis had a bizarre form of communication. Could you describe what you mean?
Mrs. Mannion:	Well, almost right from the start, they seemed to be tuned into each other, perhaps through some type of nonverbal clues. Even now they can finish each other's sentences—one will start to say something and the other will complete the message.
Clinician:	Did they have special words they shared?
Mrs. Mannion:	Yes, they had several words—they called it "werry talk." When I tried to learn the meanings of their words, they

would just laugh and look at each other like conspirators. Let's see, they called the fireplace "rapabeef," shoe was "di" at first, and then they named their feet "moppy" and "pedo." My husband and I found that we were using some of the children's words: One time I gave someone directions by telling him to go downtown and turn "pedo"!

Clinician: Did they have any other unusual language forms?

Mrs. Mannion: Yes, Otis and Lotis made up their own rules for singular and plural nouns. For example, I remember that they used "clo" as singular for "clothes." And, by the way, they still do not use the word "why"—they say "what-cause" instead.

We do not have the space here to include a complete inventory of the twins' speech, but the sample we provided does illustrate atypical or deviant language development. In addition to the novel use of plurals and *wh* words and the contrived vocabulary, the children also showed unusual syntax and articulation. They had created their own special language.

These, then, are the disorders of communication with which the speech pathologist must cope. If at the moment you feel a bit overwhelmed by their number and variety, be reassured. We shall discuss them one at a time in later chapters. Our purpose here is merely to acquaint you with the scope of speech pathology.

Before ending this presentation of the classification of speech disorders, let us offer one warning: We must avoid the tendency to slip into "label language." Remember, a communication disorder does not transform a person to a state of being less than human; we treat children and adults, not lispers, cleft palates, and spastic dysphonics. The proper focus of speech pathology is the whole person.

STUDY QUESTIONS

1. What three questions must be answered in order to determine whether a person's speech is impaired?
2. Into what four major classifications do we categorize speech communication disorders?
3. What types of problems might we expect to find in the speech of a child who has been severely hearing impaired since birth?
4. How would you begin to describe the basic features of stuttering to someone who never has heard or seen stuttering? And what would you point out as major differences between stuttering and cluttering?

5. What advice or suggestions would you give to the mother and father who are concerned that their three-year-old child "may be beginning to stutter"?

6. Why may voice problems be more difficult to categorize as disorders than are other types of speech problems?

7. In the speech of a person with a voice disorder we may expect to hear deviations from "normalcy" in one or more of what three basic vocal features?

8. What is meant by "esophageal voice," and for what reason may an individual need to use this form of phonation?

9. What typically causes dysphasia in the adult, and why is it important that the speech pathologist not work with dysphasic clients in isolation from other members of a rehabilitation team?

10. What difference(s) might help you to distinguish *delayed* from *deviant* language development in children?

REFERENCES

Iglesias, A., and Anderson, N. (1993). Dialectal variations. In J. Bernthal and N. Bankson. *Articulation and phonological disorders,* 3d ed. Englewood Cliffs, NJ: Prentice Hall.

SUPPLEMENTARY READINGS

Battle, D. (1993). *Communication disorders in multicultural populations.* Stoneham, MA: Butterworth-Heinemann.

Malstrom, P., and Silva, M. (1986). "Twin talk: Manifestations of twin status in the speech of toddlers." *Journal of Child Language,* 13: 293–304.

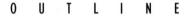
Emotional Aspects of Communication Disorders

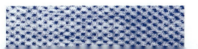

In the previous chapter we have focused on the outward symptoms of various speech disorders, but it is important to remember that each of the people who possesses them is a unique individual with a past history that may be laden with hurt. Brief examples of such emotional factors were seen in some of the clients mentioned in Chapter 1, where it was evident that current emotional reactions also can be a significant part of the problem. And the person who does not hear normally, as we will see again in Chapter 13, may be burdened as much by social and emotional consequences as by the loss of hearing. Nor is it just the individual alone who may be affected. Impaired communication, whether in a child or an adult, can impact significantly on the emotions of family members and of the family constellation itself. Our primary emphasis for now, however, will be on speech and the speaker.

To ignore the individual's history, feelings, and attitudes and merely to treat the outward behaviors is folly. If we are to hope that the behavioral changes we may help our clients achieve will persist, we must know their needs and feelings. Often we find that our clients have incorporated their abnormalities of communication into their self-concepts, and, unless we help them make essential changes in the way they perceive themselves, all of our efforts may be in vain. This is not to say that the speech pathologist or audiologist must assume the role of the professional psychotherapist. When a client's emotional problems are severe we, of course, make the necessary referrals.[1] Nevertheless, those who seek to serve persons with communicative disorders need to have some background in counseling, and they need to understand the emotional aspect of impaired communication.

It is hard for normal speakers to comprehend how difficult it is to live in a culture such as ours without possessing the ability to speak in an acceptable fashion. Perhaps a glimpse into the inner world of R.K. may help us begin to understand.

> When I really take a look at things I have done—and still do—because I stutter, it makes me want to vomit with revulsion. Stuttering has dominated my whole life. Using the telephone, especially to call girls, was a nightmare. Since I could talk fine when all alone, I once made a tape recording with which I planned to call a particular young lady. I used all the appropriate social gesture language and tried to time the pauses for her responses. It backfired: her father answered the phone! I don't go in certain restaurants, like fast-food places, because of the time pressure; I write a note with my name and phone number when I take clothes to the cleaners; and in full-service gas stations, I still sing, "Fill it up to the brim" when the attendant comes to the car window. I even picked a shy, introverted woman for a wife so I wouldn't be dragged off to parties where I might have to talk. Which reminds me, I had so much trouble talking during the wedding rehearsal, the minister suggested that I just "think" the vows during the actual ceremony. When Cindy and I have an argument, I tell her that I wasn't really thinking about "I will" when

we were married. Being a stutterer is not really funny, though. I often feel like I have a large scarlet letter "S" on my forehead.

This may seem exaggerated and distorted. Unfortunately, it is not. We have heard literally thousands of similar tales in one form or another. These people have been hurt deeply and repeatedly because they did not and could not conform to the speech standards of our society. The tragedy lies in the fact that they *could not*. They were not responsible for their defective speech, but those who hurt them acted as though they were, as though they had a choice. This assumption is the core of the problem not only of the person with impaired speech or hearing but also of the poor, the person with mental illness, the person who has **epilepsy,** those who have learning disabilities, and most of the other kinds of deviancy.

Once, on Fiji in the the South Pacific, we found a whole family of stutterers. As our guide and translator phrased it, "Mama kaka; papa kaka; and kaka, kaka, kaka, kaka." All six persons in that family showed marked repetitions and prolongations in their speech, but they were happy people, not at all troubled by their stuttering. It was just the way they talked. No hurry, no frustrations, no stigma, indeed very little awareness. We could not help but contrast their attitudes and the simplicity of their stuttering with those that would have been shown by a similar family in our own land, where the pace of living is so much faster, where defective communication is rejected, where stutterers get penalized all their lives. To possess a marked speech disorder in our society is almost as handicapping as to be a physical cripple in a nomadic tribe that exists by hunting. Western society does not suffer the speech-handicapped gladly, and the persons with whom we work come to us with a special kind of human misery.

COMPONENTS OF THE EMOTIONAL FRACTION

The pollution of human misery comes from many wells, but its composition is the same: **PFAGH.** This strange word is an acronym, a coined assemblage of letters, each of which represents another word. The *P* represents penalty; the *F* frustration; the *A* anxiety, the *G* guilt, and the *H* hostility (Figure 5-1). We invent this word to help you realize and remember the major components of the emotional fraction of a communication disorder.

Impaired speech is no asset to anyone. It invites penalty from any society that prizes the ability to communicate effectively. Speech is the membership card that signifies that its owner belongs to the human race. Those who do not possess normal speech are penalized and

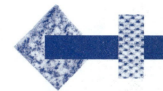

Epilepsy.
A neurological disease characterized by convulsions and seizures.

PFAGH.
An acronym representing penalty, frustrations, anxiety, guilt, and hostility.

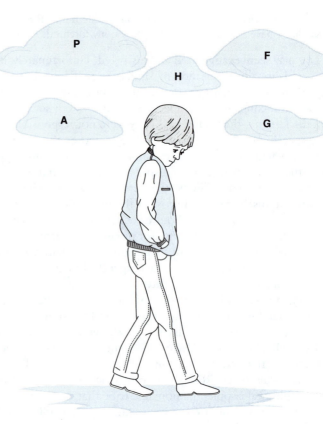

FIGURE 5-1   PFAGH:
The emotional fraction
of a communication handicap

rejected. Even the struggling speaker himself often feels this rejection is justified.

Moreover, the inability to communicate, to get the rewards our society offers to those who can do so effectively, results in great frustration. To be unable to say the word when he desires to do so, as in the case of the stutterer; to say "think" when he means "sink," as in lisping; not to be able to produce a voice at all, as in the laryngectomee; to try to say something meaningful only to find that gibberish emerges, as in the aphasic—all these are profoundly frustrating. So, too, is it frustrating to mishear spoken directions, or to be unable to hear whispered words of endearment, or to answer a teacher's question only to discover from reactions of classmates that a quite different question apparently had been asked. Anxiety, guilt, and hostility are the natural reactions to penalty and frustration. You, too, have known these three miseries transiently when you have been punished or met frustrations, but many individuals with communication disabilities spend their lives immersed in these emotions.

Penalties

Let us look at some illustrative penalties culled from the autobiographies of clients with whom we have worked.

> I hate to stutter in restaurants because the waitress ignores me and then talks to my companions. I feel like a nonperson. And when they do talk to me, they speak too loudly, slowly, and in a patronizing manner; and they never, ever look at me.

> In junior high school I got a lot of teasing about the scar on my lip and the way I talked through my nose. Once someone put a set of glasses and a big nose like persons wear on Halloween on my desk and all the kids laughed when I came into class. Even the teacher was grinning behind her workbook.

> It was quite a shock when I came to college from the small hometown where everyone knew me. My articulation is so garbled that I have to show people my name tag when I introduce myself. The worst part is the stares I get in stores. Speech is so public, so self-revealing, and I'm sure people think I'm either drunk or retarded.

> A hearing loss really isolates you, even from your own loved ones. They try not to show it, but they get so annoyed when I ask them to repeat. That's why I stay at home a lot.

These are but a few of the many penalties and rejections that any individual with an unpleasant difference is likely to experience. Imitative behavior, curiosity, nicknaming, humorous response, embarrassed withdrawal, brutal attack, impatience, quick rejection or exclusion, overprotection, pity, misinterpretation, and condescension are some of the other common penalties.

The amount and kind of penalty inflicted depend on four factors: (1) the vividness or peculiarity of the difference; (2) the person's own attitude toward the difference; (3) the sensitivities, maladjustments, or preconceived attitudes of the people who penalize; and (4) the presence of other personality assets.

First, in general, the more frequent or bizarre a speech peculiarity, the more frequently and sternly it is penalized. Thus a child with only one sound substitution or one that occurs only intermittently will be penalized less than one with almost unintelligible speech, and mild stuttering will be penalized less than severe. Second, the speaker's own attitude often determines what the attitude of the auditor will be. If he considers it a shameful abnormality, his listeners can hardly be expected to contradict him. Empathic response is a powerful agent in the creation of attitudes. Third, the worst penalties will come from those individuals who are sensitive about some difference of their own. Since some of them have parents or siblings with similar speech differences, they are often penalized very early in life by those persons.

You ask why I slap Jerry every time he stutters? I do it for his own good. If my mother had slapped me every time I did it I could have broken myself of this habit. It's horrible going through life stuttering every time you open you mouth, and my boy isn't going to have to do it.

Moreover, many individuals have such preconceived notions or attitudes concerning the causes or the unpleasantness of speech handicaps that they react in a more or less stereotyped fashion to such differences, no matter how well adjusted the speaker himself may be. Finally, as we have pointed out, the speaker may possess other abilities or personal assets that so overshadow her speech difference that she is penalized very little.

Even though some children with a speech disorder are fortunate enough to be brought up in a family and an environment where they meet little punishment for their difference, eventually they will meet the rejection that society reserves for the person who has an unacceptable difference. Indeed, some of these protected children are more vulnerable than those whose lives have been full of penalty.

A second-grade boy had been receiving speech therapy for over a year and had made excellent progress in mastering many of the defective sounds. In the third grade he met a teacher who was old and uncontrolled, who had had to return to teaching after her husband had died, and who hated the whole business. She used the boy as a scapegoat for her own frustrations. Under the guise of helping him, she ridiculed his errors and held him up to scorn before his fellows. Shortly after the fall term began, this boy's speech began to get worse, and within a few months it had lapsed to its former unintelligible jargon.

Oddly enough, penalties also can be felt—and may have devastating effects—because of *improvement*. This can occur especially if the clinician has not prepared a client for the possibility of adverse reactions. It is one of the reasons we often advise the person with a resolving voice problem to "try out the new voice" first with strangers, later with acquaintances and family.

Charles, age 15, had come to us only three weeks ago, referred by a school clinician because his persistent falsetto voice was not yielding to therapy. In the new and unfamiliar setting of our clinic, however, he had quickly learned to use his natural (and pleasantly low-pitched baritone) modal register voice at will. In spite of his delight with this newfound confirmation of his masculinity, Charles was encouraged to wait and not to use the new voice until we had done more to stabilize it in therapy. He did not come to therapy in the fourth week, nor did we hear from him or his family. When he failed to show up the following week, we telephoned the school clinician to inquire about him. As it happened, she had just talked with Charles. Fighting to hold back tears, and in his high-pitched falsetto, he told her of having used his new voice to surprise his family at the dinner table a week earlier. He noticed a smile on his mother's face, and he was not unpleased that his younger sister seemed shocked. He was not at all prepared for his father's reaction: "What makes you think you're a man?" It was only after several counseling sessions with his parents that Charles was allowed to return to therapy, and even then it was a long time before he was able to risk using his new voice, even with us.

Fortunately, experiences of the type Charles had are not terribly common, and we were able to counter it successfully. Unfortunately, Ted's experience may be more common and less easily remedied.

We had been working for three years with Ted, an eight-year-old youngster. His cleft palate had been repaired surgically; but it remained a bit difficult to close off the rear opening to the nasal passages with speed. He had improved greatly, however, and only a few bits of nasal snorting or excessive nasality remained when he talked carefully. Then one day his associates on the playground, led by the inevitable bully, began to call him "Nosey-Nosey." Within one week his speech disintegrated into a honking, unintelligible jargon, and he refused to come to the clinic for any more therapy.

Covert Penalties.   Not all the penalties bestowed upon the person who talks differently are so obvious. Perhaps the worst ones are those that are hidden, the **covert** kind. One of our clients who stuttered wrote this:

When I stutter at home the silence is deafening. No matter how much I struggle, no one acknowledges that I am having trouble talking. My mother freezes like an arctic hare and my father hides behind the *Wall Street Journal*. I feel like a family pariah. My problem is unmentionable, unspeakable. The emperor has no stuttering problem. Maybe I should walk around ringing a bell and chanting "Unclean, unclean!"

Most of the more obvious penalties are felt by children. After a speech-handicapped person becomes an adult, few people mock him, laugh at him, or show disgust. Instead, he now finds that they shun him. Their distant politeness may hurt worse than the epithets he knew when he was young. One of our cases, a girl with a paralyzed tongue and very slurred speech who was desperately in need of work so she could eat and have a place to sleep, contacted forty-nine different prospective employers before she found one who would give her a chance to exist. "Not one of them ever said anything about my speech," she told us. "Some were extra kind, some were impatient, some were rude, but all of them had some other reason besides my speech for saying no. I could tell right away by seeing how they changed the moment I began to talk. Like I was unclean or something."

Why do such things happen? Why do we punish the person who is different? Why must he punish himself? Surely Americans are some of the kindest people who have ever lived on this earth. We show our concern for the unfortunate every day. No nation has ever known so many agencies, campaigns, foundations, and private charities. One drive for funds

Covert.
Hidden; inner feelings, thoughts, reactions.

follows another. Muscular Dystrophy, the Red Cross, the United Fund, the Heart Association, Seeing Eye dogs, the coin bottle in the drugstore, the pleading on radio and television. Surely all of these activities seem to show that we help rather than punish our handicapped, but perhaps we find it easier to give our money than ourselves.

Cultural anthropologists have regarded this altruism with more than academic interest. They point out that our culture is one that features the setting up of a constant series of material goals and possessions that are highly advertised. Prestige and status seem often to be based upon winning these possessions and positions in a highly competitive struggle. We fight for security and approval, but in the process we trample underfoot the security of others. Some psychologists have felt that our need to help the handicapped is a product of the guilt feelings we possess from this trampling. Others attribute our concern for the underprivileged to fear lest someday we too will be the losers in the battle for life. They claim that we tend to say to ourselves, "There, but for the grace of God, go I," when we meet someone who has failed to find a place for himself in the world for reasons beyond his control. These organized charities do much good, but they cannot fulfill the needs of the handicapped for personal caring. Perhaps legislation such as the Americans with Disabilities Act will help in some ways.

Aggressive or Protest Behavior as a Reaction to Penalty.   Penalty and rejection may lead individuals to react aggressively by attack, protest, or some form of rebellion. They may employ the mechanism of projection and blame parents, teachers, or playmates. They may display toward the weaknesses of others in the group the same intolerant attitude manifested toward their own. In this way they not only temporarily minimize the importance of their own handicap, but also enjoy the revenge of recognizing weaknesses in others. They may attempt to shift the blame for rejection. "They didn't keep me out because I stutter—they just didn't think I had as nice clothes as the rest of them wore." In this way they will exaggerate the unfairness of the group evaluation and ignore the actual cause. Another attack reaction may be to refuse to cooperate with the group in any way, belittle its importance openly, and refuse to consider it in their scheme of existence. Finally, they may react by direct outward attack. A child, or an adult with an easily provoked temper, may indulge in actual physical conflict with members of the nonaccepting group.

> Kevin's speech was marred by several articulation errors that made him sound considerably younger than his nine years. But his left hook was worthy of a prizefighter twice his age. No one teased Kevin about his speech disorder, not even older children in the elementary school. If anyone did refer to his speech, he flew into a towering rage that ended only when the offender was bloody and bowed. The youngster refused to read aloud or recite in class. When an unknowing substitute teacher insisted

he answer a question one day, Kevin broke seven windows in the school that evening. When he was selected to go to speech therapy, he cursed the other children in his group, tore up the clinical materials, and sat sullenly in a chair. Instead of responding directly to his obvious anger, the clinician separated Kevin from the group and, without making any demands for him to talk, enlisted his assistance in assembling a large model of a sailing ship. Gradually, and it took several months, she was able to gain his confidence and eventually Kevin could tolerate direct speech therapy for his several articulation errors.

A rejected individual may spread pointed criticism of the group in a resentful manner. In any of these methods, the object of the rejection does not retreat from reality—he reacts antagonistically and attacks those who made his reality unpleasant. The more the person attacks the group, the more it penalizes him. Often such reactions interfere with treatment, for many of these persons resent any proffered aid. They attack the speech pathologist and sabotage his assignments. The inevitable result of these attack reactions is to push them even farther from normal speech and adequate adjustment.

Frustration

Frustration is always experienced when human potential is blocked from fulfillment. It is the ache of the giant in chains. All lives are filled with frustrations. We cannot live together without inhibiting some of our impulses and desires. Circumstances always place barriers in the paths we desire to take. But for some persons, the cup of frustration is filled to the brim and more is added every day. Frustration breeds anger and aggression, and these corrupt everything they touch. Those who cannot talk normally are constantly thwarted. Consider, then how a person must feel if unable to talk intelligibly. Others have difficulty in understanding the messages of the stutterer, the jargon-talking child, or the person who has lost his voice due to cancer. Others listen, but they do not, they cannot, understand. The aphasic tries to ask for a cigarette and says, "Come me a bummadee. A bummadee! A bummadee!" This is frustration.

Communication is the lifeblood of a society. When it cannot flow, the pressure builds up explosively. The worst of all legal punishments short of death is solitary confinement where no one can talk to the prisoner, nor can the prisoner talk to anyone else. There are such prisoners walking about among us, sentenced by their speech and hearing disorders to lives of deprivation and frustration.

One young client diagnosed his own problem for us. His speech was full of irregular and forced repetitions. He hesitated. He seldom was able to utter even a short sentence without having wide gaps in it. One day, after he had just beaten up our plastic-clown punching bag he confided in us. "Y-y-y-you know . . . y-y-you know whuh-whuh-what's wrrrrrong with me? I-I-I-I-I'm the llllllittlest . . . child." He was. He was the runt of the litter, the weakest, smallest, most unattractive of the eight children in that family. The others were an aggressive bunch, yelling, fighting, arguing, talking. His mouth never had an ear to hear it. When his sentences were finished, it was some brother's or sister's mouth that finished them. He was constantly interrupted or ignored. He had learned a broken English, a hesitant speech.

The good things of life must be asked for, must be earned by the mouth as well as the hands. The fun of companionship, the satisfaction of earning a good living, the winning of a mate, the pride of self-respect and appreciation, these things come hard to the person who cannot talk. Often she must settle for less than her potential might provide, were it not for her tangled tongue. Speech is the "Open Sesame," the magical power. When it is distorted, there is small magic in it—and much frustration.

We need safety valves for emotion. When we can express the angry evils within us, they subside; when we can verbalize our grief, it decreases. A fear coded into words and shared by a companion seems less distressing. A guilt confessed brings absolution. But what of those who find speaking hard, who find it difficult even to ask for bread? This wonderful function of speech is denied them. The evil acids cannot be emptied; they remain within, eating their container. For many of us it comes hard to verbalize our unpleasant emotions, even though we know that in their expression we find relief. How much more frustrating it must be for those who feel that they have only the choice of being still—or being abnormal.

Perhaps most frustrating of all is the inability to use speech as the expression of self. One of the hardest words for the average stutterer to say is his own name. Most of us talk about ourselves most of the time. We talk so people will notice us, so we can feel important. This **egocentric** speech is highly important in the development of the personality. Until the child begins to use it, he has little concept of selfhood, according to Piaget, the famous French psychologist. If you will listen to the people about you or to yourself, you will discover how large a portion of your talking consists of this cock-a-doodle-dooing. When we speak this way we reassure ourselves that all is well, that we are not alone, that we exist and belong. The person with a severe speech defect finds no such reassurance when he speaks. He exposes himself as little as he can. In this self-denial, too, lies much frustration.

Egocentric. Self-centered; pertaining to the self and its display.

For years, almost a decade now, I took a backseat because of my hearing loss. Conversation with more than two persons was impossible; I felt like such a fool when I missed the point of a story or laughed at the wrong time. Listening is so hard when you only get fragments. The whole business of talking with people took too much time and energy. Eventually, I just gave up and didn't even go to church.

One very severe frustration is the deprivation from social interaction which persons with speech disorders experience. It is not hard to understand why this occurs. Speech is the vital prerequisite for human interaction. It is the bond that unites us. When it is impaired, that bonding is disrupted. Long ago the senior author spent a week in a school for the deaf where all the students used sign language and did very little lipreading. He felt isolated, rejected, excluded from the miniature society; and it was with relief that he re-entered a speaking world. Those who cannot talk feel much the same way. They are rejected from membership. They find it hard to belong. The worse they talk the more isolated they become. Here again we find in speech pathology a miniature model of a basic evil that pollutes humanity, the same rejecting exclusion that plagues the physically disabled, the poor, the elderly, and minority groups.

Anxiety

It should not be difficult to understand why people who meet rejection, pity, or mockery would experience anxiety. When one is punished for a certain behavior, and the behavior occurs again, fear and anxiety raise their ugly heads. If penalty is the parent of fear, then we might speak of anxiety as the grandchild of penalty, for the two are not synonymous. The stutterer may fear the classmate who bedevils him, or he may fear to answer the telephone since fear is the expectation of approaching evils that are known and defined. But anxiety is the dread of the unknown, of defeats and helplessness to come. In its milder form, we speak of "worrying." There is a vague nagging anticipation that something dangerous is approaching. To observe a person in an acute anxiety attack is profoundly disturbing. Often she can find no reason for her anxiety, but it is there just the same. At times it fades, only to have its red flare return when least expected. Few of us can hope to escape it completely in our lifetimes, but there are those for whom anxiety is a way of life. It is not good to see a little child bearing such a burden.

One of the evil features of anxiety is that it is contagious. When parents begin to worry about a child's speech, the child is almost bound to reflect and share their feelings. "Will he ever be able to go to school, to learn to read, to earn a living, to get married? Who will hurt him? Will he ever learn to talk like others?" Such thoughts may never leave the parents' lips, but somehow they are transmitted to the child, perhaps by tiny gestures or facial expressions or even the holding of the breath. Once the seeds of anxiety are planted, they sprout and grow with incredible speed.

Another of the evils of anxiety is that it usually is destructive. It does not aid learning or speech therapy. It distracts; it negates. It undermines the self-esteem. The person seeks to contain it, to explain it. Sometimes she invents a symptom or magnifies one already there. When speech becomes contaminated with anxiety, the way of the speech pathologist is hard. One of the first things a student must learn is to create a permissive atmosphere in which speaking is not painful, over which no threat hangs darkly. The speech therapy room must be a welcoming, pleasant place. All of us need a harbor once in a while; *these* children need a haven often, one where for once they can feel free from penalty and frustration, where impaired speech is viewed as a problem instead of a curse. In the presence of an accepting, understanding clinician, they can touch the untouchable, speak the unspeakable. There they can learn. Anxiety does not help in learning or relearning.

Reactions to Anxiety.   Anxiety is invisible, but it has many faces. By this we mean that it shows itself in different ways.

> Edward had undergone many operations for his cleft palate, but the scars on his face and the speech that came from his mouth bore testimony of his difference. Throughout his elementary and secondary school years, he had appeared a carefree, laughing, mischievous child. He was the happy clown, and by his behavior, he had managed to gain much acceptance. When other people laughed at him, he laughed with them. His grades were poor, although he was bright. Then suddenly, in the final semester of his senior year in high school, he underwent a marked personality change. He laughed no longer; he became apathetic, quiet, and morose. Formerly very much the extrovert, he now withdrew from contacts with others. He daydreamed. He walked alone. Our intensive study of this boy revealed that he had always lived with anxiety, that his cheerful behavior was adaptive but spurious. Underneath he had always ached. The compensatory pose had brought him rewards, but it had not allayed the anxiety. When faced with the necessity for leaving school and earning a living, the anxiety flared up too strongly to be hidden, and the change of personality took place. Not until we were able to provide some hope through the fitting of a **prosthesis** (a false palate) and some information about the possibility of plastic surgery, did the anxiety decrease sufficiently to enable us to improve his speech.

One of the common methods used to ease anxiety is the search for other pleasures. By gratifying other urges we seem to be able temporarily to diminish anxiety's nagging. Some of the people with whom we have worked are compulsive eaters of sweets; they grow fat and gross. And then they worry about their weight. Others relieve their anxiety by sexual indulgences. There are others who find a precarious and temporary peace by regressing to infantile modes of behavior, trying to return to the period of their lives when they did not need to worry about speaking. We also find a few sufferers who attach themselves to a stronger person like leeches, hoping for the security of dependency. Yes, they are many ways of reducing anxiety; but unless the spring from which it flows is stopped, it always returns. That is why people with communication impairments need speech pathologists and audiologists.

Prosthesis.
An appliance used to compensate for a missing or paralyzed structure.

When the anxiety clusters about speaking, one way of reducing it is to stop talking. Some persons with speech disorders merely become taciturn; some lose their voices; other contract what is called **voluntary mutism** and do not make an attempt to communicate except through gestures. We knew a night watchman once who claimed that he averaged only two or three spoken sentences every twenty-four hours. "It's easier on me than stuttering."

There is also a curious mechanism called *displacement,* which most of us use occasionally to reduce our anxiety. We start worrying about something else besides the real problem that is causing us such distress. The shift of focus seems to bring some relief, much as a hot-water bottle on the cheek can ease a toothache. The scream of a little child in the night may reflect such a displacement, but perhaps a better example can be found in Andy.

> Andy stuttered very severely when he came to us at the age of seven. He blinked his eyes, jerked and screwed up his mouth, and sometimes cried with frustration when he was unable to begin a sentence. At times he spoke very well. But what struck us most about Andy was his furrowed brow. Whether he stuttered or not, he seemed to be constantly worried. His face always had an anxious expression. Finally we were able to get him to tell us what he was worrying about. Surprisingly, it was not about his stuttering or his parents' very evident concern about his speech. Andy said he was worrying about the moon hitting the sun. He said that if this happened, everything would blow up. He said that on those nights when there wasn't any moon, and both sun and moon were under there someplace, that they might crash together. Andy said he could never sleep on those nights. His mother and father had told him this couldn't happen, but Andy said they had lied about Santa Claus, and how did they know, anyway, that it wouldn't happen? It took a lot of play therapy, speech therapy, and parent counseling before Andy was able to surrender his solar phobia and express his real anxiety, which concerned his speech.

But there are some fortunate persons with speech disorders who are lucky in their associates and ability to resist stress, who seem to manage to get along with a minimum of anxiety. They may find themselves loved and accepted. They may possess philosophies or compensating assets that make the speech problem minor in importance.

To illustrate our point, we quote now from the laboriously written diary of an adult aphasic. (We have omitted the many errors.)

> I remember the feeling of being a "mummy" when I could barely speak. In spite of all the troubles of the past, I am happy that I'm capable of doing so many things now. I'm learning more every day and continually strive to improve my reading and writing. Above all, my numbers are coming back to me. A person has to be happy in their heart and soul. To relax and forget the past. There is always tomorrow. We get

Voluntary mutism.
Refusal to speak.

Displacement.
The transfer of emotion from an original source to another stimulus.

too impatient. To me, that is the secret of it all. I can live gracefully as an aphasic. Lately, I have been busy and I have accomplished many things.

Right now I am happy and content. It has been five years since my stroke and in the last three weeks, I feel it has been worth it. I shall be a more graceful, middle-aged woman from now on.

So let us state our caution again. If there is excessive anxiety, recognize its face where you find it, no matter how it is disguised; but do not invent or imagine its presence if it is not there!

We wish to conclude this section with a caution. Let us remember that some people with impaired speech have no more anxiety than those who speak normally. All of us have some anxiety and probably need some. A bit of anxiety in the pot of life is like a bit of salt in a stew. It makes it tastier. But too much salt and too much anxiety ruin both. We have had to describe the anxiety fraction of a speech handicap so that you will not add to it, perhaps so that you may relieve it. Those of us who come in contact with children or adults with disabilities may unwittingly make their burdens heavier if we do not understand.

Guilt

Like anxiety, guilt also contributes a part of the invisible handicap that often accompanies abnormal speech. We have long been taught that the guilty are those who are punished. Intellectually we can understand that the converse of this proposition need not be true, that those who are punished are not always those who are guilty. But let affliction beset us, and we find ourselves in the ashes with Job of the Old Testament. "What have I done to deserve this evil?" We have known many persons deeply troubled by speech disorders and other ills, and most of them have asked this ancient question. Parents have asked it; little children have searched their souls for an answer. Here's an excerpt from an autobiography.

Even when I was a little girl I remember being ashamed of my speech. And every time I opened my mouth, I shamed my mother. I can't tell you how awful I felt. If I talked, I did wrong. It was that simple. I kept thinking I must be awful bad to have to talk like that. I remember praying to God and asking him to forgive me for whatever it was I must have done. I remember trying hard to remember what it was and not being able to find it.

It seems to be the fashion now to blame parents for many of the troubles of their offspring, for juvenile delinquency, for emotional conflicts, for speech difficulties. We can blame the school if Johnny cannot read, but few parents of a child who comes to school with unintelligible speech have escaped the blame of their neighbors. The father of a child with a cleft palate often feels an urge to accuse the mother, and the mother the father, for something that is the fault of neither. When guilt enters a house, a home is in danger. Children who grow up in such an atmosphere of open or hidden recrimination are prone to blame themselves. Thus the emotional fraction of a speech disorder may grow.

Reactions to Guilt Feelings.   Guilt is another evil that eats its container. In its milder forms of regret or embarrassment, most people can handle it with various degrees of discomfort. However, when shame and guilt are strong, they can become almost unbearable. The person may react with behavior that produces more penalty or more guilt. We have seen children deliberately soil themselves, throw temper tantrums, break things, steal things, even set fires so that they could get the punishment they felt their guilt deserved. After the punishment comes a little peace!

Sometimes people punish themselves. We have seen people who stutter use their stuttering to hurt themselves, using it in much the same way as the flagellants of the Middle Ages flogged and tortured their bodies for their sins. We have known children with repaired cleft lips and palates who could not bear to watch themselves in a mirror even to observe the action of the tongue or soft palate. We have heard children cry and strike themselves when they heard their speech played back from a tape recorder. We must always be alert to this need for punishment lest they place the whip in our hands.

Here is what one adult with cerebral palsy painfully typed for us.

> Sometimes when I lie in bed pretty relaxed I almost feel normal. In the quiet and the darkness I don't even feel myself twitching. I pretend I'm just like everybody else. But then in the morning I have to get up and face the monster in the mirror when I shave. I see what other people see, and I'm ashamed. I see the grey hairs on my mother's head and know I put them there. I eat but I know it isn't bread I can earn. Oh there are times when I get interested in something and forget what I am, but not when I talk. When I talk to someone, he doesn't have a face. He has a mirror for a face, and I see the monster again.

We who must help these people must also expect at times to find apathy and depression as reactions to the feelings of guilt. It is possible to ease the distress of guilt a little by becoming numb, by giving up, by refusing to try. Again, we may find individuals who escape some of their guilt by denying the reality of their crooked mouths or tangled tongues. They resist our efforts to help them because they refuse to accept the *fact* of abnormal speech. Somehow they feel that the moment they admit the existence of abnormality they become responsible. And with responsibility comes the guilt they cannot bear. So they resist our efforts to help them. Finally, we meet persons who absolve themselves from guilt by projection, by blaming others for their affliction, by converting their guilt into hostility or anxiety. But this brings us to the next section.

Hostility

Both penalty and frustration generate anger and aggression. We who are hurt, hate. We who are frustrated, rage. Here is an example to help you understand.

> One of our former clients, a university professor, had always been a quiet, self-effacing man. Interviews revealed that no one, not even members of his family, ever heard him swear or raise his voice in anger until he suffered a massive stroke. He awoke in the hospital to find himself incontinent, aphasic, dysarthric, and paralyzed on his right side. Since he found it so difficult to chew and swallow, chopped and strained foods were prescribed. He endured all the indignities that had befallen him with stoic detachment until a nurse's aide brought his lunch tray containing three containers of baby food with the labels still on the small jars. The mild-mannered professor threw the tray at the aide and soundly cursed his wife and the patient in the adjoining bed.

Reactions to Hostility.   Hostility, like anxiety and guilt, ranges along a continuum all the way from momentary irritation through anger to intense hatred. A few of our clients have had such a huge reservoir of anger that they mistrust the motives of anyone who tries to befriend them. A young man with Gilles de la Tourette syndrome, a neuropsychiatric disorder involving involuntary movements and explosive, often obscene speech, described his distorted relationship with young women this way.

> This mixture of conflicting emotions became even stronger when I began dating. I wanted to go out with girls, to socialize, and to conduct a normal relationship. On the other hand, whenever a girl did accept a date with me, especially more than once, I invariably began wondering what was wrong with her—why would she want to go out with me?

Resentment, or remembered anger, is perhaps the worst form of hostility. As long as we are resentful of another person for some past hurt, ironically our lives are in part controlled by that person.

Some individuals with severe speech problems show little hostility; yet we have known some with mild and minor disorders to show much. One may have much anxiety or guilt but little hostility; another may reveal quite an opposite state of affairs. Some people just seem to roll with the punches and the frustrations and manage to get along with a minimum of emotional response. But often hostility and aggression are found, and so we must understand them. The experienced clinician knows that she may become the target for pent-up emotions and she does not react personally to a client's expressions of anger and resentment.

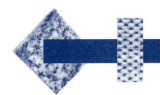

ROLE OF THE SPEECH-LANGUAGE PATHOLOGIST

Fortunately, most of the emotional conflicts shown by persons with impaired speech are not deep-seated problems such as those treated by psychiatrists, psychologists or psychiatric social workers. They are not phobias, obsessions, or compulsions. They are not neuroses or psychoses. Instead, they are related directly to the speech disorder and the ways in which others and the person himself have reacted to it. When the person gains acceptable speech most of the negative emotions disappear, though their scars may remain.

This is not to say that the speech clinician can ignore the hidden emotional handicap of the person who comes to her. Indeed, she must become highly aware of the client's history of penalty, frustration, anxiety, guilt, and hostility because any of them untreated may interfere with successful speech therapy.

The major task of the clinician in dealing with these emotional problems is to provide understanding and an opportunity for the client to ventilate feelings, feelings rarely confided to anyone. Once shared, they seem to lose their force. Let us describe some of the ways that this is accomplished.

Evoking the Expression of a Negative Emotion

It has long been known that anxiety, guilt, and hostility, when repressed or blocked from expression, tend to maintain themselves or even to increase in intensity. They thereby create other problems and certainly interfere with therapy. The healing that comes from the confession of guilt, the relief achieved by verbalizing fear or anger is well known. However, when the speech clinician is confronted by a hostile, fearful client or one who feels great embarrassment or shame, the verbal expression of these feelings is often constrained by the speech disorder itself. How can the stroke patient with aphasia verbalize his emotions when he has no language? How can a laryngectomized person ventilate her feelings when she has no voice? When speech is labored as in stuttering, or unintelligible as in delayed speech development or severe misarticulations, the ventilation of unpleasant emotions presents some real difficulties.

Establishing a Therapeutic Relationship

It is very important when working with a person disturbed by his speech that we immediately seek to create an atmosphere of safety. We reveal ourselves as nonthreatening, warm, and caring. We also show that we are competent. There are many ways of doing this, of course. Often in the first session we do much of the talking, outlining what we hope to accomplish and describing some of the procedures we may undertake. We demonstrate that we know how the client may feel about his disorder and accept these feelings. We express our faith that with our help the person can learn how to speak more normally. Often, too, in this first session we may begin our joint exploration and study of his speech disorder, stressing the fact that therapy is a joint effort. Here is a report of part of such an introductory session.

> When Joe had become relaxed after my explanation of the course of therapy, I told him that I needed to know just what happened when he stuttered. I needed to know where he was tensing his speech muscles, how he was breathing, and so on. To do so I needed to learn to stutter in the same way that he did and that he'd have to teach me. I told him I wasn't mocking him, but just trying to know what happened. Then I said, "I know that most stutterers have trouble saying their names so I hope you'll stutter when you say yours so I can have a good sample." Well, he stuttered on it and I made an attempt to imitate it. "No," I said, "I didn't get that quite right. You skew your lips to the right and I didn't. Would you mind saying it again?" It took several attempts before I was satisfied and Joe's stuttering on each was less severe. Indeed, on the final trial he didn't stutter at all. I thanked him and said I'd have to do some hard thinking about how I could best help him and that was all we did that day. I could tell, however, that he was amazed that I was willing to put his stuttering in my own mouth and could do so without having it upset me in the least.

Modeling

In the above illustration we find not only that the clinician is verbalizing the emotions of her client but also showing him that she can stutter without becoming too emotional. Modeling might be used in treating snake phobias in a similar way. The therapist plays with a live snake and seems to have no fear at all. Observing this, the client loses a bit of his fear. Speech pathologists must learn to imitate speech disorders if they use this approach.

Desensitization

Persons with communicative disabilities who have been rejected or penalized because of them often develop strong fears of speaking in certain situations. To help reduce those fears, clinicians often use the same techniques that physicians employ to desensitize their allergy patients to the pathogens that produce the allergic reactions. They inject minor doses first that do not cause the reaction, then progressively greater doses, thus building up the patient's tolerance. In speech therapy there are occasions where we create progressive hierarchies of speaking situations, and after getting the client to maintain a state of relaxation in each one, we have him attempt the next most difficult task. For example, with the client who panics at the thought of making a telephone call we may set up the following hierarchy: (1) Pick up the telephone and hold it to your ear; (2) Dial a number, then hang up immediately; (3) Dial another number and wait for the person to answer before hanging up; (4) Dial another number and say a few words, but hang up before the listener responds, and so on. At each step on the hierarchy, however, the client must be able to remain calm and relaxed.

Reducing the Penalties and Rejections

The speech pathologist is often called upon to consult with the families, associates, and teachers of a speech-impaired child to remove some of the stress caused by misunderstanding or teasing. Many parents who need basic information on how to react to such a child's speech difficulties will willingly cooperate when they know what to do and what not to do. The mockery on the playground often ceases when the ringleader is brought in, the problem explained, and when he is given the role of protector. Teachers can be taught how to handle the child's speaking opportunities in the classroom so that she will not react with anxiety, shame or anger.

Most important of all is the relief that comes from having hope that the person can, with the clinician's help, overcome his speech problem. In the therapy room he finds a safe place and a person he can trust, someone who not only knows how to help him, but someone who cares.

Play Therapy

Even normal-speaking children find it hard to put their unpleasant feelings into words, and therapists have found that play often provides a useful way of providing release. Brought into a playroom with various materials such as toys, clay, crayons, and other materials the child will often reveal the feelings that disturb her. She may curl up under a table and suck on a baby bottle to relieve her anxiety. She may smear not only paper but herself with finger paint, often in the area of the mouth when she feels her speech is shameful. She may smash her toys angrily. Sometimes the clinician will verbalize feelings for her; at other times he may merely let the child act out frustrations or other emotions. Always the clinician is accepting and permissive. "Let the bad stuff come out," he seems to say. By so doing, he helps the child understand stressful feelings and, most importantly, know that someone else can share them without being upset. This report may illustrate our point.

> Peter is only in the fourth grade but has been a holy terror always. His school file is full of accounts of asocial and destructive behavior, fighting, truancy, and even attacks on some of his teachers. He has no friends

among his classmates because they fear him. There is an unconfirmed report of parental abuse. His speech problem consists of many inconsistent articulation errors at times so severe that he becomes unintelligible, though most of the time I can understand what he says, which isn't much. Though our first session went fairly well, subsequent ones did not. He hated me, often refused to cooperate, and generally showed his hostility to my attempts to befriend him. Soon it became obvious that we were getting nowhere. Finally I felt that somehow I must find a way to relieve that hostility, so I began every session with activities that would allow him to vent his rage. I had him make clay figures and smash them with a mallet; I drew pictures that he could scribble over. I gave him my photo and let him cut it into little pieces with some scissors. I contrived many such activities and the first part of each therapy hour was spent doing them as I tried to verbalize his feelings. Only then did we begin to work on his speech. As a reward for each achievement I let him bang a gong as hard as he could. The result was almost unbelievable. Peter lost his hostility and became friendly and most importantly, began to speak much better. I'm no psychologist but I know that he needed that opportunity to express his anger without getting punished. Anyway it worked, I think he likes me and trusts me now.

Adult Therapy

With adults whose speech is intelligible enough we generally use client-centered, nondirective procedures to reflect our understanding of what the person is saying as he tells us of his past history or hurt and frustration. Often this is preceded by getting a written autobiography with special emphasis on experiences where attempts to communicate have been painful.

But again we often find individuals who find talking so difficult or unpleasant that the free expression of feelings is almost impossible. When this occurs the speech pathologist has to do the talking for the client. This skill is not easily learned and demands much sensitivity on the part of the clinician. You may be interested in a strategy used many years ago by the senior author to sharpen his own sensitivity.

At first I sought to gain as much information as possible about my clients, using autobiographical material and such, but that proved to be only minimally helpful. I still wasn't able to walk in their moccasins, to understand their innermost thoughts and feelings. And so I began to train myself in **empathy.**

Initially I sought to increase my alertness to my client's body language by closely observing his postures and facial expressions and by scrutinizing his movements. That helped—but not enough. Only by covertly assuming and duplicating his body language did I discover what he was feeling. Day after day, yes, year after year, I practiced reading the body language of others, not just with my eyes but with my whole body. I

Empathy.
The conscious or unconscious imitation or identification of one person with the behavior or feelings of another.

tilted my head as they did; I adjusted my eyebrows and eye openings. I assumed their facial expressions, their smiles and how they held their mouths. I made my own body match their arm and leg movements, their gestures, even how they crossed their legs. I even tried to breathe as they did though often that was difficult. Above all, I tried to duplicate any areas of tenseness wherever they occurred.

I learned how to echo and shadow my client's speech, though of course I did it silently. By echoing, I simply waited until the client paused, then said to myself what he had uttered trying not only using the same words but the same pacing and intonation. The latter proved to be very revealing about how my client was feeling. After some practice I could do this almost automatically. Often I found I could silently finish his unfinished sentences for him and knew when he was lying or telling the truth.

If this self-training seems unduly laborious, I should say that I did it intermittently, in little bits and snatches, never continuously. It demands an alertness that cannot be sustained very long. Often at first I found my silent mimicry was inexact, that my hidden postures, movements and speaking were not true to my model. With further practice, however, they always came closer and closer, and soon I knew I was on target. One always realizes when he is truly in tune. I have found this training in reading the body language of others not only useful in therapy but also in general living. Through these hard won skills I have found my life greatly enriched. They have enabled me to become one with others, to live not only my own life but theirs, too.

Most speech pathologists do not subject themselves to such a program, but all become highly aware of those features of body language that signify acceptance or rejection. They need this information throughout therapy as they verbalize their client's feelings. Sometimes these clues are merely the vertical head nods, the yeas and nays, but often they are more subtle, such as holding the breath or closing the lips tightly for *no,* and the widening of the eyes for *yes.* All clients have their own ways of showing agreement or negation. Some clinicians become very skillful, and their clients often feel amazed at their understanding. One way or another, the clinician does manage to help the person he is trying to help ventilate his anxieties, shame, or anger.

Most of this "psychotherapy" is informal and takes place during the speech therapy itself. When frustration or resistance occurs, the clinician verbalizes the client's feelings and encourages the client to do the same. When a task arouses anxiety, the clinician shows that she understands.

I think you're about ready to tackle telephoning for the first time. You've always avoided doing that in the past and you're afraid the listener may hang up when you stutter or perhaps laugh when you stutter. Still feeling you just aren't up to it? OK, let me do the phoning and I'll stutter severely. Listen in on the other phone and let's see what happens.

We could provide many other examples of the way speech clinicians cope with the emotional conflicts associated with their client's communicative difficulties. They just cannot ignore these problems; they interfere too much with successful treatment. Take just the common problem of trying to motivate a child to confront the fact that he has a hoarse voice, or cannot make the correct *r* sound in his name "Robert," or makes strange faces when he stutters. Such confrontations can be very unpleasant and the client may refuse to cooperate. He just can't bear to touch the untouchable, the thing he feels is shameful, or the behavior he fears. Of course he will seem unmotivated and uncooperative.

We close now with excerpts from an eloquently but anonymously written commentary that arrived in the senior author's mailbox one day without any explanation, though we believe it was written by one of our more insightful students. If it has been printed elsewhere (other than in our departmental journal), we're sorry, but we still think it's worth reading. And it provides food for thought which is particularly appropriate as we end this discussion of the emotional aspects of communication disorders.

> Don't be fooled by me. Don't be fooled by the face I wear. For I wear a thousand masks, masks that I'm afraid to take off, and none of them is me. Don't be fooled, please don't be fooled! I give the impression that I'm secure, that all is sunny and unruffled with me, within as well as without, that confidence is my name and coolness my game; that the water's calm and I'm in command, and that I need no one. But don't believe me. Please.

> My surface may seem smooth, but my surface is my mask. Beneath lies no complacence. Beneath dwells the real me in confusion, fear, and aloneness. But I hide this, I don't want anybody to know it. I panic at the thought of my weakness and my fear of being exposed. That's why I create a mask to hide behind, to help shield me from the glance that knows. But such a glance is precisely my salvation. My only salvation. And I know it. That is, if it's followed by acceptance, if it's followed by love. It's the only thing that will assure me of what I can't assure myself, that I am worth something.

> But I don't tell you this. I don't dare. I'm afraid your glance will not be followed by acceptance. I'm afraid that deep down I'm nothing, and that you will see this and reject me. And so begins the parade of masks. I tell you everything that is really nothing and nothing of what's everything; so when I'm going through my routine, do not be fooled by what I'm saying. Please listen carefully and try to hear what I'm *not* saying, what I'd like to be able to say, but what I can't say.

> I dislike hiding. I'd really like to be genuine and spontaneous, and me, but you've got to help me. You've got to hold out your hand, even when that's the last thing I seem to want. Each time you're kind and gentle and encouraging, each time you try to understand because you really care, my heart begins to grow wings.

You can help me to break down the wall behind which I tremble, to remove my masks. Please do not pass me by. It will not be easy, I know, for a long conviction of worthlessness builds strong walls. I fight against the very thing I cry out for. But I am told that love is stronger than walls, and in this lies my hope.

Who am I, you may wonder. I am someone you know very well. For I am every person you meet.

Our concern, first and foremost, always must be with the *person* who has the communication disorder. Truly, speech pathologists and audiologists are more than mere trainers of tongues and dispensers of hearing aids.

STUDY QUESTIONS

1. What do the authors mean by "premature referral" of a client for psychotherapy, and why do they proceed cautiously in making such referrals?
2. For what does the acronym *PFAGH* stand?
3. The amount and type of penalty associated with a communication disorder tend to vary as a function of what four factors?
4. What are some of the types of behaviors that may reflect a client's reaction to penalty?
5. Why might frustration be a common feeling among persons who have communication disorders? Why might this feeling be shared by members of their families?
6. How does anxiety differ from fear? Which is the more debilitating and persistent emotion, and why?
7. For what reasons may the clinician find himself the object of hostile reactions from a client? In that circumstance, how should the clinician react?
8. Why must the clinician be sensitive to the possible needs of a client to express repressed emotions?
9. Give an example, other than the one in this chapter, of how you might go about desensitizing a client to a feared situation.
10. What types of nonverbal behavior can help us to understand the feelings that a client may be experiencing?

ENDNOTES

[1]We make such referrals with caution and sensitivity, and always with careful preparation. Sometimes even a person who already recognizes the need for seri-

ous psychological help may be unable as yet to acknowledge that need. Perhaps coming to our clinic is a first step in the appropriate direction for such individuals, however, and a step they are able to take because they may perceive speech therapy as less threatening than psychotherapy. In such cases, premature referral can dissuade the client from continuing to seek *any* help, including our own.

SUPPLEMENTARY READINGS

Andrews, J., and Andrews, M. (1990). *Family based treatment in communicative disorders: A systemic approach.* Sandwich, IL: Janelle Publications.

Benjamin, A. (1981). *The helping interview,* 3d ed. Boston: Houghton Mifflin Co.

Emerick, L. (1988). Counseling adults who stutter: A cognitive approach. *Seminars in Speech and Language,* 9, 257–267.

Hejna, R. (1960). *Speech disorders and nondirective therapy.* New York: Ronald Press.

Luterman, D. (1984). *Counseling the communicatively disordered and their families,* 2d ed. Austin, TX: Pro-ed.

Rogers, C. (1961). *On becoming a person.* Boston: Houghton Mifflin Co.

Schum, R. (1986). *Counseling in speech and hearing practice.* Rockville, MD: National Student Speech-Language-Hearing Association.

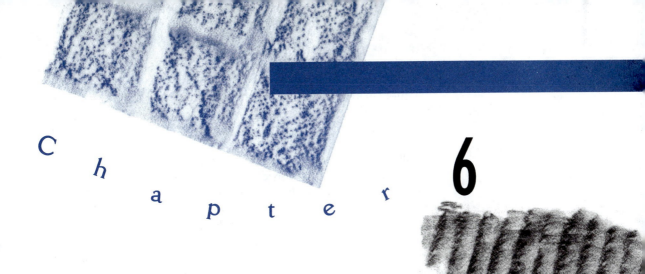

C h a p t e r **6**

Developmental
Language
Disorders

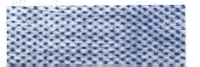

Unfortunately, not all children progress easily in acquiring speech and language skills. It is estimated that two to three percent of preschoolers and about one percent of school-age youngsters have language disorders (National Institute of Neurological Disorders and Stroke, 1988). Indeed, the bulk of the caseloads of school speech pathologists are children who have not mastered various aspects of our language. Similarly, many professionals who practice in hospitals or community clinics deal daily with clients who have language problems, often of organic origins.

Why have these children failed to learn words and sounds and the rules for combining them? What are the causes of these language disabilities? It seems wiser to speak of deterrents rather than causes. Language disability is not a disease but a failure to learn, and there can be many reasons why certain children have trouble learning the hidden rules that govern our language. In some cases the origin of a specific language impairment remains forever unknown, but we do know some of the deterrents: mental retardation, hearing loss, brain injury, impaired motor coordination, severe emotional problems, illness during the early years, and the lack of a caring, nurturing parent to serve as a model (experience deprivation). These are not causes in the medical sense, but they create obstacles that some children find difficult to surmount.

Children with language disabilities come with a wide range of differences. Some, as in profound mental retardation, appear to have learned none of the rules of our language, and their vocalizations have little meaningfulness. The profoundly deaf, however, may have substantial language skills, but they are expressed through sign language or the written word. There are nonverbal children who possess language but who do not use it in speaking. The variety seems endless. But the great majority of children with language impairments just show delay in language development. For one reason or another they are a year or more behind those who develop normally. Some seem stuck in the babbling or jargon stages; some have learned to speak in single words or noun and word phrases but seem unable to progress further. Still others show marked delay in acquiring the phonology, the sounds of our language, and cannot be understood.

And there are some children who show not merely delayed speech and language but also deviant forms. They seem to have invented not only their own words for things and actions but also their own ways of combining them. They have invented a language of their own, and if the parents learn their language, they will never learn ours. However, as Curtiss, Katz, and Tallal (1992) have shown in their longitudinal study, most language-impaired children show delay rather than deviance.

Before proceeding, we must note, as we did in Chapter 4 (and as we will mention elsewhere, especially in Chapter 7), that a *difference* is not necessarily a *disorder*. As the "minority" proportions of our country's population change, it is increasingly important that the professional practitioner be sensitive to linguistic and cultural variabilities. We will be seeing increasing numbers of children in whose homes English is not spoken, not spoken much, or in which some dialect other than Standard American English is used preponderantly. In some instances, they and their families also may have attitudes or beliefs—about testing, for example, or about disorders of any type, or about interpersonal communication—that are different from those prevailing in the clinician's own culture. And, needless to say, the English proficiency of these children may differ (or may appear to differ) noticeably from that of other children at comparable developmental stages.

To paraphrase Wiener (1986): In deciding whether a child's limited proficiency is a difference, a delay, or a deviance, we must determine whether it is due to exposure and experience or due to a basic problem that affects both the child's native and nonnative languages. The clinician's decision obviously is an important one with far-reaching implications.

> Considering that an underlying language disorder impedes academic performance for children in the short term and their future employment potential in the long term, . . . language assessment . . . is recognized as an essential step toward improving school achievement in English, social emotional development and access to equal employment opportunities. (Wiener, 1986, p. 41)

The presence of a difference does not rule out the possibility that a disorder also may exist, of course, so clinicians will need to become familiar with linguistic rules and developmental features associated with the languages and dialects that are found in their geographic regions. Nor may they ignore divergent cultural values with impunity. You will find these matters discussed by Battle (1993) and Nelson (1993) and in the additional references to which they will lead you.

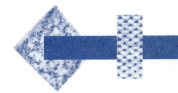

NONVERBAL CHILDREN

Although they may be delayed in speaking, most language-disabled children do acquire some verbal facility. A few, however, fail to talk at all and the impact is enormous. They are lost souls, in the world but not of it.

> Burke's parents brought him to the speech clinic because, at age three and a half, he still had not said his first word. His total communicative repertoire consisted of an expressive grunt (the vowel /ʌ/) and simple gestures. He frequently led his parents by the hand and pointed to items of food or toys that he wanted. But mostly he was silent and *very* active.
>
> We were not sure how much Burke understood language since he did not seem to attend long enough to discern our instructions. He was in constant motion from the moment he entered the room. Despite his obvi-

ously poor motor coordination and a peculiar shuffling gait (he seemed to sway from side to side when fleetingly standing still), Burke dismantled our office. He removed every book from a shelf, opened one, grunted in seeming dissatisfaction, and tossed it aside. When the child burrowed into the bottom drawer of a metal file cabinet leaving a shower of manila folders in his wake, his mother finally restrained him on her lap.

"I'm tired to the bone," she told us. "This little whirling dervish gets up early each morning and roams the house until late at night. He pokes and prods into everything. He seems driven, almost like he was searching for . . . something. Worst of all, I can't talk to him and he can't tell me what's bothering him or what he wants. Sometimes when the tension builds up, he explodes in a tantrum."

Blake describes two seven-year-old boys, Jim and Ted, neither of whom had usable speech. We will use them here to show the marked variability in these problems of delayed language. Ted had been diagnosed as having been brain damaged; Jim had congenital heart disease. They differed markedly in personality, Ted being extremely hyperactive and aggressive, while Jim was shy and well controlled.

At the beginning of therapy they both seemed to comprehend some spoken language fairly well, as demonstrated by the ability to follow simple instructions, understand simple gestures, and play with and relate to objects and by their response to other informal tests. Neither had adequate voicing in his attempted vocalizations. Ted's vocal quality was hoarse and extremely breathy, whereas Jim's vocalization attempts were whispered. Neither child was classified as verbal. Ted's main attempt at vocalization at the beginning of therapy was a rhythmical oronasal production of "k-k-k, k-k-k, k-k-k." He did attempt an approximation of *mama,* which was vocalized as [a-a], with no attempt at labial (lip) closure or valving at the lips for the [m]. The word *daddy* was also approximated as [æ-i]. The words *yes* and *no* were vocalized as [hʌ] with the appropriate head gesture for each. This was the observable extent of Ted's intelligible vocabulary.

Jim's mother described him as a child who seemed to understand what was said to him but who made very little or no attempt to verbalize on his own. His only intelligible vocabulary approximation was observed (and confirmed by his mother) to be a whispered production of "mama." (Blake, 1969, p. 364)

These two boys might appear to the casual observer as being hopelessly lost. We know that once the most favorable age of readiness for the acquisition of language has been passed—it is usually felt to be during the second to fifth years—the prognosis is poor. Nevertheless, Blake's experience and that of many of us who have worked intensively with these children may provide hope. Here is what he reports.

Both Ted and Jim have developed functional speech far beyond the expectations of their parents and the clinician. Their vocabularies are continuing to grow, and they use sentences with as many as seven or eight words now. They use functional speech in appropriate context and show promise of developing more complex speech and language skills. After one year of therapy, which has included two 30-minute sessions of language stimulation per week, Ted and Jim speak in sentences with an average length of four words. (pp. 368–369)

Not all of these children are so restricted in their verbal utterance. Some of them vocalize almost constantly, but they speak a gibberish that no one can understand. It resembles the jargon that many young normal children use. The utterances are full of inflections and are accompanied by gestures so that one almost believes that they are truly trying to communicate, but we have analyzed many of their vocalizations and have been unable to find any consistency that might indicate a self-language.

Some of these children for various reasons may never learn to speak. Nevertheless, some of them can be taught enough language to enable them to communicate through the use of a communication board, signing, or the written word.

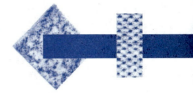

CHILDREN WITH DELAYED OR DEVIANT LANGUAGE

Much more frequently found are children who do have some useful language and can communicate to some extent, but where it is clear that marked emotional problems or linguistic deficits are present. All these youngsters exhibit some delay or disturbances in grammar, in using words conceptually, and in using language appropriately for social interaction. There are some other features which, while common among our language-disabled clients, are not universal. These include a late onset of speech, disturbance in the comprehension of speech, and a restricted MLU (mean length of utterance). Finally, we often see a constellation of behavioral abnormalities, such as a short attention span, distractability, **perseveration,** and lack of self-monitoring.

But now let us present some clinical examples of children with delayed and deviant language. Wood describes a **hyperactive** and possibly schizophrenic boy named Paul with various difficulties.

> Paul had developed speech, but failed to communicate ideas through speech. He usually talked at inappropriate times and on inappropriate subjects. He might begin with a specific idea, which he apparently wished to discuss, but his speech would wander away from the subject and he would include things which had occurred in the past, or objects which he had seen in his surroundings, or people's names which he seemed to remember suddenly. His conversation sounded something like this: "I saw a dog—ah—the chalk mama put to the desk—ah—on the

Perseveration.
The automatic and often involuntary continuation of behavior.

Hyperactivity.
Excessive and often random movements as often shown by a brain-injured child.

picture pinned there—have you seen the car? My name is Paul. I am eight years old. Goodbye." (Wood, 1964, p. 109)

This speech indicates some comprehension of the rules of the language, yet in the sentence "the chalk mama put *to* the desk," we note just one small indication of deficit. In the following description, we find the telegrammic speech of early language development. Many of the function words are absent. The British girl who spoke this passage was eight years old. Hers was a disorder of language, not of speech.

> I went to Reading, See, see bus. Long time. Went swimming. Mummy. Me. And the black man by. Mummy job. Down a stream. Quiet. Married. Long way. Very long way. Church. When I went there, fell I did. And I went soon, soon. Know her, she bride. Went to Reading, bus. Went to seaside. Not. Only next. Next. See the bridge. Way to holidays. (Renfrew, 1959, p. 35)

Many children with delayed language are not so impaired, but the flavor of the telegram with its omitted words is always present. The syntax is limited. Some of these children have not mastered the use of question words, the appropriate pronouns, plurals, or the use of verb tense. Others can use noun or verb phrases, but fail to combine them into subject-predicate sentences as in this sample of the speech of a five-year-old boy.

> Me Go. [Pause.] Outdoor. Mama in car now. Firsty [thirsty]. Dink Tommy cup. No dink now. Go Mama now. Tommy bed. [Was he trying to tell us he was tired?] Car. Car now. Dink mama car now. [He wanted to go home.]

Jennifer, a girl the same age as Tommy, spoke much better, but she too showed language difficulties. She was telling us what she was doing with our playhouse.

> Here the kitchen and stove is there and Jenny cook stove eggs for breakfast. Um and Jenny go sleep here by bed. See! Oooh, bathtub. Soap no um in in a bathtub? [Questioning inflection.] You get soap for wash feet? Me like bathtub. Spash [splash] on water all over.

The examples we have given, of course, are those of children whose language ability is very poor.

Finally, let us present a group of school children who are not as profoundly handicapped yet still have language problems.

> Five-year-old Gary with normal hearing caught the teacher's attention, and pointing to his mouth said, "Another one coming in back a tooth." Teacher looked in his mouth expecting to find a missing tooth. Instead, a six-year molar was just appearing through the gum.

> John, age four, with hearing impairment, put his ideas in improper sequence when asked what he did after school. His answer, "Buy toys and go store."

Matthew, age five, with hearing impairment, was asked to tell what he remembered of the Thanksgiving party. His reply, "Teacher sit in the chair watching the children. The children all eating dinner. The children sitting down in the chair. Some of the children didn't ate all their supper. And the children went to get a drink of water in the cup and they was all quiet. And they came back in the room. Then they ate, and then they went back home. That sure is a long story."

A group of six-year-old children without hearing impairment were drinking their milk. John finished, looked up, and noticed Kerry had also finished. Instead of saying "We tied," John commented: "Me him beat together." (Bangs, 1968, p. 13)

Children Who Have Had Language but Lost It

You will also encounter some children with language disabilities who have suffered brain injuries due to trauma or illness, and others with a history of acquired rather than **congenital** deafness or severe hearing loss.[1] Some of these have retained only the rudiments of their former language; others demonstrate their problem only in the use of occasional odd locutions. The range of language impairment in these clients is very great and, in most instances, depends upon the level of language development achieved by the child before the interruption. Although it is difficult to present any representative or typical case examples, we include a brief résumé shared by a colleague in special education. Despite her heart-rending grief and feeling of total helplessness, Maggie Watson followed the course of her daughter's decline with professional objectivity.

> When Cindi was two years and eight months old, I began to notice subtle changes in her behavior. She had talked early, used complex sentences at two and a half, had good motor control, and was an alert and very bright child. Then, I noted the signs that concerned me: apathy, a slight muscular weakness in her lower limbs, frequent complaints that she was tired. Our family doctor examined Cindi, found nothing wrong, but prescribed a vitamin supplement for her. Three months later, I knew something was wrong, very wrong with her: She dragged her feet in the later afternoon and evening; complained that she had difficulty seeing; did not want to play "mother" to her nine-month-old sister, Amy; and her speech was slurred. We took Cindi to a famous Midwestern medical clinic where, after exhaustive testing, they diagnosed Schilder's disease, a rare, apparently hereditary demyelinating disorder. The disease strikes young children and is progressive. The physicians offered little hope except temporary remissions. In less than six months after the onset of the disease, Cindi was virtually blind, incontinent, and reduced to one-word, holophrasic speech. A year later, our daughter died—blind, paralyzed, helpless, speechless. During the last few months she was in a vegetative coma. Three days after Cindi's funeral, I saw the same early symptoms of Schilder's disease in Amy.

Congenital.
Present at time of birth.

This second case illustration is a bit more representative of the type of child we see in therapy.

> Nine-year-old Tom fell from a tractor and fractured the left side of his skull. One month after the accident, the youngster could only say three words, "mother," "water," and "Puuko" (the name of his cat). His memory span was severely limited, and he found it difficult to comprehend even simple messages. When he could not speak or understand, he cried, cursed, and withdrew. Gradually, after several months of intensive therapy, Tom's vocabulary increased, he spoke in short, but well-formed sentences, and his comprehension was nearly normal. Even now, one year after the accident, he still omits articles and prepositions, confuses certain prefix and suffix rules, and has considerable difficulty with word retrieval. Tom is able to read only very simple material, and his writing is nonfunctional at this point; this is particularly frustrating to the child because he had been an avid reader and had excelled at all forms of language arts in school.

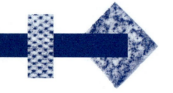

DETERRENTS TO LANGUAGE ACQUISITION

While it is clearly evident that failure to master our language is often found in the seriously mentally retarded, the congenitally deaf, the brain injured, or in some children with severe emotional problems, we cannot be sure that these conditions *cause* the language problem. Rather it would seem wiser to view the relationship as deterrent or obstacle-creating. Severe hearing loss makes communication difficult rather than enjoyable, and it prevents a child from perceiving the models he needs to do the learning he must do. Mental retardation makes it hard for a child to recognize or recall meanings and relationships, and both, of course, are vital to language learning. The emotionally disturbed child may reject the models or the interactions involved; the brain-damaged child may find it hard to concentrate his attention on language stimuli or to see their patterning.

Any one of these children, because of the way he was labeled or treated, may simply have learned not to learn. Tragically, all of them have been deprived in some way from having the crucial experiences for acquiring language which most children get over and over again. Whatever may be the conditions that have deterred or prevented language learning, the job of the clinician is to help the child master the language code, both in comprehension and in output.

Nevertheless, to commence helping a child overcome a language disability, a speech clinician tries, in concert with the parents, the audiologist, the special education teacher, the physician, the psychologist, and other treatment team members where possible, to determine why the youngster is not using words appropriately.[2] When we identify the obstacles, or combination of obstacles, it provides a broad direction to the therapy—a child who is deaf needs a form of treatment different from that for one who is autistic or mentally retarded. In some instances, this careful search for deterrents to language acquisition assists in eliminating or minimizing agents that are still operating, such as environmental deprivation.

Mental Retardation

Learning to talk is a complicated business. It is not easy to achieve the proper blend of message content, form, and appropriate social use. Since mentally retarded children find it difficult to learn even simple skills, we should not be surprised to find them slow to develop language. Indeed, mental retardation is the most prevalent problem associated with disordered language development. The acquisition of language, as we stressed in a prior chapter, depends upon cognitive antecedents—the capacity to see relationships and solve problems, in general, the ability to operate conceptually.

Retarded children are arrested or delayed in their development, and the consequences are pervasive. They are slow in all areas—motor skills, social behavior, self-care, language—in all forms of intellectual and adaptive behavior. In fact, a key identifying feature of mental retardation is an *even slowness* in all phases of development. We have seen some cases, however, particularly children suffering infection or injury during early childhood, who retained small islands of normal or near normal functioning.

A number of factors—infection, trauma, metabolic disorders, genetic abnormalities—can cause mental retardation. The cause may occur prenatally, at the time of birth, or at some point in an infant's early development. In some instances, for example, in Down's syndrome, a chromosome defect (Trisomy 21), a distinct physical symptom pattern accompanies the intellectual deficit.

There is a wide range in the extent of retardation, from mild or borderline deficiency to profound impairment. All aspects of language—phonology, grammar, semantics, and pragmatics—are affected, and the degree of involvement is related to the severity of the retardation. To illustrate the range of language impairment in mental retardation, we present brief clinical portraits of four clients.

> *Borderline or mild mental retardation* (I.Q. 75 to 90). Debbie Harkinen is fourteen years old. Her I.Q. is 82. She is currently in a special education program and is working on academic material at about the sixth-grade level. She is described as a "slow learner" by her teacher and parents. Debbie's vocabulary and sentence structure seem adequate, but she has difficulty using language meaningfully to understand and express abstract ideas. The sentence types she uses are very redundant and limited in variety. Additionally, she uses a number of general words—"one," "some," "thing," "this," "that"—in the place of specific ones. Debbie

takes longer to catch on to humor and does not comprehend expressions with double meanings or plays on words. She substitutes /d/ for /θ/ and distorts the /s/ and /z/ phonemes.

Educable mental retardation (I.Q. 50 to 75). Tim Kunze is eight years old and has an I.Q. of 60. He is a Down's syndrome child. Onset of speech was very late (twenty-six months). At the present time, Tim is learning grammatical inflections (possession, past tense) and vocabulary. The length, complexity, and structural variety of his sentences are limited; syntactically, he is operating at the four-year-old level. He often shows difficulty with subject/verb agreement. Phonologically, the child omits or substitutes plosives for most fricatives; the /r/ and /l/ sounds are distorted. He is judged to be about 60 percent intelligible. Tim's voice is low pitched and very husky, which makes him difficult to understand even when his articulation is accurate. He is very affectionate and has made an excellent social adjustment educationally.

Trainable mental retardation (I.Q. 20 to 50). Eleven-year-old Romain Dunchan is in a special education program for the trainable retarded. He is being taught self-care skills (food, safety, cleanliness) designed to make him semi-independent. His intellectual functioning (I.Q. 38) shows an even performance across all psychometric tasks. Romain has limited but functional use of language; he can comprehend and express messages that relate to his basic needs. His syntax is very limited; he omits articles and uses simple noun phrase expressions. His vocabulary is restricted to concrete items. Additionally, the child is echoic and exhibits some surface language; that is, uses words as labels, not as concepts; he utters a few words and short phrases that he has been taught in a mechanical, rote fashion. By and large, Romain does not mediate experience via language. He seems to *think* in gestures and postural symbols rather than in words; he appears to code his perceptions in a "body English" rather than in language.

Custodial or profound mental retardation (I.Q. below 20). Psychologists found it impossible to measure Max Nielsen's intelligence, but it is their clinical judgment that he is severely retarded. He was a victim of congenital syphilis. For the last nineteen of his thirty-three years, he has been a resident of a regional hospital for the profoundly mentally retarded. Max has no functional oral language. Oral expressions are limited to cries, groans, and a few barely intelligible obscenities taught to him as a "joke" by male attendants. Max responds to signals that relate to his food and bathroom needs, although he is still incontinent. He is incapable of self-care.

Hearing Impairment

Most children who have hearing problems are not totally deaf. They have various degrees and kinds of hearing loss, topics addressed more fully in Chapter 13.

If a child cannot hear the words and sentences of his parents or play-mates, or hears them distortedly or faintly, he will find great difficulty in learning the language skills necessary for speech. Children who are born totally deaf never speak entirely normally, no matter how conducive the environment or how skillful their teachers. They can be taught language through signing and many learn to read and write well, mastering their morphology, syntax and semantics, but have real trouble producing the sounds they have never heard.

By hearing loss we mean that some usable hearing still exists. The person can hear certain sounds at a certain loudness level. He may hear some of what you say. He may be able to hear sounds that are low in pitch yet fail to hear the high-frequency sounds.

There are two major kinds of hearing losses: **conductive** and sen-sorineural. By the first, the *conductive*, we mean that the loss is caused by some defect in the outer or middle ear. There may be wax in the ear canal; there may be fixation of one of the tiny bone transmitters in the middle ear behind the eardrum. There are many possible reasons for conductive loss, but the important thing to remember is that the lower- and middle-frequency tones are usually heard as being more muffled or fainter than they should be. Children with conductive loss usually learn to speak, though some problems may occur. They may show articulation errors of substitution and omission. More seriously for a child's academic future, even temporary episodes of conductive hearing loss may produce secondary effects—reduction in language skills, auditory perceptual problems—that persist after the middle-ear pathology is medically corrected (Kavanagh, 1986).

The other type of hearing loss is *sensorineural*. It may be due to an injured or malfunctioning cochlea in the inner ear, or to a damaged nerve, or to injury to the brain itself. Of the two types of hearing loss, this is usually the more serious for speech learning or maintenance, because it introduces distortion as well as muffling of sound. Most children with sensorineural loss have a harder time hearing the high-pitched sounds than they do those lower in pitch. Sounds such as $/s/$, $/\theta/$, $/f/$, $/t\int/$, and $/t/$ are some of the high-frequency sounds. If you could not hear the announcer on the television because you had such a loss, turning up the volume wouldn't help you much because the low sounds would seem to be blasted out so much louder proportionally. The tiny high-pitched overtones would still be lost. A person with a high-frequency loss can never hear normal speech as it really is.

But even more important is the difficulty that children with auditory disorders experience in figuring out the structure of language itself. The child with normal hearing is provided with a wealth of speech samples from which she can find the combination rules that are acceptable; the deaf child is impoverished. However, even when taught very carefully in a

Conductive hearing loss.
Hearing impairment due to middle (or outer) ear problem; cochlea and auditory nerves are not involved.

highly favorable environment, the profoundly deaf child seldom seems able to overcome completely the handicap of sensory deprivation.

The human hearing mechanism is uniquely designed and finely tuned to facilitate the acquisition of language. We learn to talk because we have the capacity to hear—and listen to the right things. When a child's hearing is impaired, the extent of her language disability will depend upon how severe the sensory loss, when the loss occurred, how early it was detected, and at what point treatment was started. Early detection is of critical importance. We include now some guidelines for identifying deviation from normal development of auditory perception. Keep in mind that development is gradual and receptive skills emerge over a period of time rather than at a specific age level.

Age	Hearing and Understanding
0–3 months	Responds to sounds by ceasing activity ■ most responsive to speech ■ low-frequency sounds inhibit distress, increase motor activity ■ high-frequency sounds increase distress, inhibit motor activity
4–7 months	Responds to noise and voice by turning head to locate source Distinguishes between friendly and angry talk Listens to own voice
9–12 months	Vocalizes in response to adult speech Responds to name "Listens" to people speaking Responds to simple commands: "Want more milk?" "Give it [an object] to me"; "No-no!" (sometimes)
18 months	Comprehends up to 50 words Enjoys nursery rhymes, songs Points to pictures when named Recognizes names of family members, pets, objects Points to body parts (2–4) when named
2 years	Listens to stories read and wants them repeated over and over Comprehends up to 1,000 words; figures out meaning by how words are used in sentence Follows two-step directions Distinguishes one from many Comprehends prepositions "in" and "under"
2½–3 years	Listens to longer, more complex stories Identifies action ("running," "swinging") in pictures Comprehends 2,000–3,000 words

- understands some opposites ("go-stop," "give-take," "push-pull")
- understands past and future

4 years   Follows three-step directions with objects, pictures

Has number concepts to 3, 4

Identifies several colors

Understands most of what is said to him or her

Deprived of the auditory experience of their own speech attempts and those of others, many children who do not hear often lose heart and make little effort to communicate except on the most primitive levels. Why try to talk when other people do not seem to understand? Why try to understand when others present only the picture of silent, moving lips? Confused and frustrated, they often retreat into a restricted, isolated, as well as silent world. Finally, because these children have been severely limited in language growth and have had to rely primarily upon visual and tactual concepts, they tend to have great difficulty with abstractions. Their concepts tend to deal with the concrete. They have trouble with most relationships that cannot be seen or felt, and language involves many of these.

We would like to stress the fact, however, that the deaf and severely hard of hearing (unlike the mentally retarded) *do* have the same basic symbolic resources as the child who can hear. They are capable of learning language—not necessarily speech—if proper stimulation can be channeled into their system through an alternate route (see, for example, Chomsky, 1986). We must help the individual to *compensate* for the sensory deprivation. Let us be more specific: *We* believe that it is absolutely essential to establish an early visual language system for the deaf child, not only to enhance cognitive growth, but more basically as a way in which to communicate with persons in her environment.

Contrary to what advocates of oral methods for the deaf predict, there is no evidence that signing interferes with speech development. Quite the opposite. Nonoral or augmentative language systems actually *increase* a child's efforts to use speech.

Brain Injury

Growing up often involves running a gauntlet of hazards that can produce brain injuries that make the learning of language very difficult. Even just being born is such a hazard, for there are children who suffer that damage while entering our world. All speech clinicians encounter children with cerebral palsy and other motor disorders that interfere with speech acquisition because of the intricate coordination required by normal speech. They have the disorders of articulation called *dysarthria* and *apraxia;* we shall discuss them in a later chapter because they are not in themselves language disorders.

But there are children with **closed head injuries** stemming either from birth trauma or from automobiles or other accidents who show the characteristic features of *aphasia*, a disorder in which not only speech but also reading and writing and other skills such as handling mathematical symbols are affected. These children find difficulty

> in formulating their thoughts in words, in expressing them verbally, or in comprehending what others are saying. It's hard for them to send messages or, less frequently, to receive them. Formulating, expressing, comprehending, these are the functions that trouble the person who is aphasic. Some aphasic children have more difficulty with visual symbols; others, more trouble with symbols involving sounds. Some who cannot read (alexia) can write or copy the symbols they see on the printed page. Others can read but cannot write (**agraphia**). There are many varied disabilities lumped under the name of aphasia, but we hope that we have made our point—that aphasia refers to the difficulty in using symbols meaningfully; it is a disorder due to brain damage.

There is no doubt that aphasia can occur in children who have had speech and then lost it as a result of brain injury.

> Walter had been speaking very well, indeed much better than most children his age, when the automobile accident occurred on his fifth birthday. Thrown from the wrecked car, his head had struck a concrete abutment, and he was unconscious for over a week. When he was able to leave the hospital, he was almost mute, although occasionally a snatch of jargon would pass his lips. He had difficulty recognizing his parents and sister, but a gleam of recognition came when the family dog nuzzled him once they were home. His first word was "Tiber," which he used for the dog's name (which was Tiger). Even his gestures were confused at first. He shook his head sideways for "Yes" and vertically for "No." He had forgotten how to cut with the scissors or to hold a crayon. Emotionally, he now appeared very unstable. He cried a lot and had uncontrollable outbursts of temper. It was difficult for him to follow directions or to remember. Occasionally he would come out with swear words his parents had never heard him speak. Gradually the speech returned, aided by our patient tutoring and the parent counseling that was so necessary. At the present time, four years later, he is speaking very well but has a marked reading, writing, and spelling disability.

Closed head injury.
Traumatic brain injury.

Agraphia.
Difficulty in writing due to brain damage.

There exists some argument among certain speech pathologists concerning the concept of congenital or developmental aphasia. These terms refer to disabilities in the *learning* of symbols or language as contrasted to the *loss* of ability previously learned, which is what we find in true aphasia. Our own position, based upon our clinical experience, is that such congenital or developmental aphasias do exist. These aphasic children present different problems from those whose delay in speech is due to mental retardation or hearing loss, although they may not become apparent until after some speaking has been learned.

The Minimally Brain-Damaged Child?

There are some children who have no history of cerebral injury or any discernible neurologic signs that indicate brain pathology and yet who show many of the same behaviors and difficulties in acquiring language that the aphasic children demonstrate. No truly satisfactory term for them has yet been accepted, but generally, they are classified as "brain-injured," "perceptually handicapped," "minimally brain-damaged" children. Sometimes their problem is labeled "attention deficit disorder"; in older children "**dyslexia**" may be an expression of similar difficulties. The diagnosis is based upon an analysis of the child's behavior rather than upon any of the methods used by **neurologists** to reveal true lesions. These children do not seem to have hearing losses; they are not mentally retarded; they do not resemble the emotionally disturbed. Their labeling and their diagnosis is therefore based upon inference and presumption; but these children exist and present real problems to parents and teachers.

This is the general picture they present.

1. They clearly have an inadequate ability to regulate or control themselves, as shown by hyperactivity, great distractability, perseveration, violent shifts in emotionality, incoordination, and impulsivity.
2. They show an inadequacy in being able to integrate sensory information as demonstrated by perceptual difficulties involving awareness, discrimination, figure-ground relationships, sequencing, retention and recall, and many other similar deficits. They also show difficulties in forming concepts, in categorizing and classifying, in handling abstractions.
3. They have disturbed self-concepts and disturbances in laterality and in self-identification. They have small tolerance for frustration, little sense of past or future. They are often controlling, negativistic, and very hard to live with, for they do not perceive the needs of others. They do not relate well.

Not all these children fail to acquire language, but it should be obvious from their characteristics that they may do so with difficulty; and some continue to show marked disability later on when faced with the other language skills of reading and writing. There are also some whose lack of self-control, inability to integrate, or inadequate sense of self are just too overwhelming to enable them to learn the language system. Perhaps the many frustrations experienced by an intelligent brain-damaged child who tries to live meaningfully in a world full of words often make him seem hyperactive and excessively irritable. In working with these children, you often have to do speech therapy on the wing. They are on the move con-

Dyslexia.
Reading disability.

Neurologist.
Physician who specializes in diagnosis and treatment of disorders of the nervous system.

stantly. It's hard for them to sit still, to concentrate, to be patient. Their frustration tolerance may be abnormally low, but we suspect it is only that they are overloaded with frustration. Occasionally they may go berserk, and show what in the adult aphasic is termed the "catastrophic response." One such boy, who had been working quietly, suddenly began to scream, ran around wildly, tearing his clothes, and shuddering. It was not a seizure. We held him firmly but soothingly for a while until he calmed; then he went back to his work. If these children find it harder to inhibit emotional displays than the normal child, we must understand and help.

Can they be taught to talk? Or read, or write, or understand speech? We feel that the answer is yes, although we have had enough failures with some children to say the word hesitantly. It's so hard to get through to a child who cannot talk, who sometimes cannot understand. Perhaps the best way of putting it is to say that many of these children can be taught if given the proper help at the proper time. And, of course, not all such children are identically or equally impaired.

> When Charlie Eastman was in school more than thirty years ago, none of his teachers recognized his academic difficulties as a learning disability. They blamed him for his failures. Charlie was lazy, they concluded; he could learn to read better if only he would apply himself more diligently. In point of fact, the boy had tried, but in spite of his best efforts, the letters on a page remained a mysterious jumble. By the time he was in the fourth grade, Charlie was three years behind his peers. Each year thereafter he fell further and further behind his peers. Junior high was a nightmare for him. Viewing his grossly deficient reading skills as willful resistance to school discipline, the teachers imposed the worst possible penalty: endless drills in reading. Pep talks, admonitions, and finally threats followed until finally he withdrew into a sullen rage and chronic truancy. On his sixteenth birthday, Charlie quit school, and even now as an adult he remains bitter and resentful about teachers and education.

Fortunately, educators today are much more sophisticated about identifying children who cannot learn by conventional classroom instruction. We have come a long way in preventing the loss of human potential of school-aged children who have difficulty learning (often termed specific learning disabilities).

A learning disability is characterized by *core elements*—which form the nucleus of the problem—and a variety of *associated features*. The core elements include (1) disturbances in basic psychological processes, such as perception, attending, sorting and sequencing, and memory, and (2) deficits in language-dependent behaviors, listening, mathematical calculation, and, in particular, reading and writing. A child with a learning disability may show one or several of the following associated features: impulsivity and hyperactivity, negativism, emotional liability, mixed dominance, difficulty with spatial and time relationships, and poor motor control and coordination.

In general, treatment efforts focus on the basic psychological processes involved in understanding and using language—attending, memory, sequencing, and so forth. The best programs we have seen concentrate on making the child aware of his thought processes; they show him how to plan, solve problems, and evaluate his performance using all sense modalities. They also take into account the changing types and forms in which the child's difficulty may find expression as the child grows. So they provide for careful follow-up and monitoring. Even when the child may seem to have "caught up" with her peers at a given age level, she later may be confronted with new and different demands with which she is unprepared to cope (Damico, 1988).

Working in the area of language-learning disorders is very demanding, although it also can be very rewarding. But to work effectively with these youngsters requires a breadth and depth of knowledge and experience unlikely to be possessed by any single clinician or teacher. Therefore, a team approach is most important. Ongoing collaborative consultation among professionals from diverse disciplines (see Nelson, 1993), as well as family support, are essential ingredients if the child is to realize optimal benefit.

Emotional Problems

All of us have difficulty putting our deepest emotions into words, and perhaps only the poet manages to do so. Some unfortunate children experience almost constant storms of emotion, and it is easy to understand why they would have trouble learning to talk. When we speak we enter into a relationship with our listener; if most of our unpleasant emotions center in that listener, we find it hard to talk to him. Emotionally disturbed children cannot find the words to express the surges of unpleasantness that flood their beings. Perhaps their private world of protective fantasy has few words in it. When there are no words for communicating the incommunicable and when one fears or hates his listeners, why try to speak the unspeakable?

The range of problems encountered in this category is wide. In it we find children who are psychotic or autistic at one extreme, and children who are emotionally immature or negative at the other. They do not learn to talk because, perhaps, they fear the communicative relationships that speaking demands or because their flood of inner emotional static prevents them from hearing the models they need. Some of these children live in a world of their own. Others find their *lack* of speech a powerful tool for controlling others. There are children who find the awaiting world of adult life too unpleasant a prospect after they hear their parents screaming at each other, and so they prefer to remain infants all their days. What better way than to refuse to talk? Why should a child wish to put something into his mouth if it is unpleasant or painful? Why should a child speak if speaking puts him in contact with someone he fears or hates? Speaking is revealing; there are children who cannot bear the exposure.

Childhood Schizophrenia.   The child with this type of mental illness may show normal language development until the ages of two or three and probably does not belong in the category of delayed language. In fact, of all the etiological categories described to this point, the emotionally disturbed are most likely to exhibit *deviant* language. However, they are truly delayed in using the language competence they may have achieved to communicate and relate to others. Josh Greenfeld, novelist and playwright, provides a very graphic description of the changes that took place in his own son.

> At the age of four Noah is neither toilet-trained nor does he feed himself. He seldom speaks expressively, rarely employs his less-than-a-dozen-word vocabulary. His attention span in a new toy is a matter of split seconds, television engages him for an odd moment occasionally, he is never interested in other children for very long. His main activities are lint-catching, thread-pulling, blanket-sucking, inexplicable crying, eye-squinting, wall-hugging, circle-walking, bed-bouncing, jumping, rocking, door closing, and incoherent babbling addressed to his finger-flexing right hand. But two years ago Noah spoke well over 150 words, sang verses of his favorite songs, identified the objects and animals in his picture books, was all but toilet-trained, and practically ate by himself. (Greenfeld, 1972, p. 4)

When overheard, the verbalizations of the psychotic child are bizarre. Here is one sample.

> Big train ... under bed [screams] ... I eat um up ... and go toidy [toilet] ... hurt hurt ... [screams] ... choo-choo-choo-choo ... was dirty ... I big house ... green house and red and black and blue and ... Mama, you go bed now.

All of this speech was uttered while playing with a truck on the floor; the child's voice was flat and expressionless. These children live in a private world, one often full of terrors and hallucinations perhaps, but yet better than the intolerable world of reality.

Some of them show very little verbal output. They are so mute that they often are thought to be deaf. Their refusal to speak is compulsive rather than voluntary. In the histories of some of our cases of delayed speech, we find that at one time they had begun to talk not only in single words but also in sentences. Then something happened, a shock, an accident, a frightening experience, a separation from the mother, a stay at the hospital—and the child stopped talking.

Autism.   The schizophrenic child often talks more to himself than to other people, but he will communicate with them at times, though his speech often reflects his obsessions. The autistic child—a very strange child—resists verbal interaction with others. If you saw the movie *Rainman* you've seen an excellent portrayal of the adult version of this disorder. He won't answer questions and he rarely asks one. If he does reply to a demand it is a perfunctory reply, often an exact but monotonous repetition of what was said to him, and often it appears three or four minutes afterward. Although, according to Rimland (1964), whose work is a classic on the subject, about half of all autistic children are mutes and remain so all their lives, we personally have been able to evoke considerable speech from some of them. It is strange speech, full of exotic words at times, or unusual metaphors, sometimes interspersed with odd snatches of singing. But what strikes the observer especially is that the speech sounds dead, lifeless. There is no emotion or inflection in it. Here is a picture of one who spoke very little until treated.

> Kipper's parents' complaints were that "he can't pay attention," has "no speech," shows "inconsistent hearing" and "other unusual behavior." In particular, his unusual behavior consisted of periods of "finger flicking" (strumming the index or small fingers of his left hand with the index finger or four fingers of his right hand), and periods of sitting very still and "staring off at something."
>
> He was essentially unresponsive and inactive during our initial evaluation. He sat where placed without moving. He showed no response to his name. When eye contact could be achieved, his face remained expressionless ("masklike"), giving the impression of a "blank stare." He was heard to utter only a few random sounds. When tickled he made only a slight flinching movement. As far as could be determined, he showed no response to auditory stimuli or social reinforcers. (Schell, Stark, and Giddon, 1968, p. 43)

The cause of early infantile **autism** is unknown. Most contemporary authorities now doubt, however, that it arises solely from atypical parent-child bonding. Does an autistic child have a defective nervous system that renders him incapable of processing and organizing reality (Schopler and Mesibov, 1987)? Does he have a chromosome abnormality (Sigman, 1985) or a biochemical imbalance (Launay et al., 1987)? Does he play the repetitive, self-stimulating games to impose some order on his experience? Is he bizarre because he lives in a peculiar topsy-turvy world (Bourgondien, Mesibov, and Dawson, 1987)?

The autistic child is sometimes very intelligent. It almost seems as though he is too hypersensitive to be able to bear the barrage of stimulation in which our children must live. Alexander Pope once wrote of the sensitive soul who "dies of a rose in aromatic pain." Austistic children are threatened by too much noise (and even a little noise is too much), too much color, too much movement, too many people—and sometimes even one parent is too much. They build walls around themselves, barriers to stimulation. Some of

Autism.
Disorder resulting in a detachment from environmental surroundings; almost complete withdrawal from social interaction.

them do not seem to hear because they refuse to listen. Some of them sing the same little nameless tune over and over again to mask out the sounds and speech that can overwhelm them. Certain autistic youngsters concentrate on puzzles or mathematic manipulations to keep the world's fingers out of their lives. They may rock back and forth interminably to keep everything the same. Some of them do not talk at all or talk to themselves in a strange tongue. Other autistic children will talk a little, and even answer questions, but always in a detached and perfunctory fashion with a minimum of meaning and little feeling. They are strange children, not of this world. We have worked successfully with a few of them and have failed with more than a few. They require time and devotion that few of us can afford (Wetherby and Prutting, 1984; Paul and Cohen, 1985).

Since autistic children who acquire language skills have a more favorable prognosis of recovery, early intervention is of critical importance (Gillberg and Steffenberg, 1987; Prizant and Wetherby, 1988). Treatment programs that focus on mastery of prelanguage skills—eye contact, nonverbal imitation, memory span (Bloch, Gersten, and Kornblum, 1980)—seem to enjoy greater success than programs instating rote speech by behavior modification (Lovass, 1977). Some clinicians report better responses from these children with pragmatic or naturalistic treatment regimens. Only time and further investigation will tell, but some workers advocate the use of manual signs, symbol boards, and other augmentative devices to facilitate communication with the autistic (see Mirenda and Schuler, 1988).

Negativism.   Our culture demands much of its young. At the very time that the child is learning to talk, a hundred other demands are put upon him. He must learn how to eat at the table, how to control his bowels, how to be quiet, how to pick up his toys, how to behave himself. And this is the age at which we find out that we are *selves*, not objects, and that we are important in our own right. This is the "bull-headed" obstinate age, when the child learns how to say that favorite word to his parents: "No!" There are children who fiercely resist the constant pressure to conform, who fight a gallant but losing battle against incredible odds. And there are a few children who actually win, by discovering the one way they can refuse and get away with it. They refuse to talk.

You can't *make* a child talk. The tenacity with which some children resist their parents' efforts to eliminate thumb-sucking is minor compared with that shown by some children who triumph by not speaking. It's a tough problem to handle, once it seems to be focused on speech alone. First, we must convince the parents and associates of the child to stop making the usual demands that he say this and say that, and inhibit their complaining expressions of anxiety. We must remove the rewards brought by negativism. Here is one brief account of a child who had but one word in his vocabulary.

The teacher said to the child in a rather peremptory tone, "Johnny, you go this very minute and get yourself an ice cream cone!" The child answered "No" and the teacher asked another child, who accepted and returned to eat the ice cream under Johnny's regretful nose. Such a program soon brought a discriminatory answer to requests and commands, and when reward for positive response was added, together with humorous attitudes toward the negativism, the child's whole attitude changed, and his speech soon became normal.

We sometimes find a tendency to familial shyness and reservation when taking case histories on children who are mute outside the home. Some lived in socially isolated conditions. More than half the children exhibiting voluntary mutism we have seen in a school setting had severe articulation defects; they kept quiet to avoid teasing.

Many of these children profit from a change in environment—placement in a nursery school—where they can learn from other children that speaking can be more pleasant than refusing to speak. By puberty almost all cases of voluntary mutism, even children not seen for therapy, begin to communicate normally.

If we are to summarize these observations about the role of emotional disorders in the delay of language and speech, we would say first of all that most unpleasant emotionality involves human relationships. Communication also involves these relationships, and it therefore is dependent upon them. If the very young child is immersed in negative emotion, he will have little inclination to learn language. If he is older when reality becomes unbearable to him, he will not use language enough to realize its fullest potentials.

EXPERIENCE DEPRIVATION

Some children are born into homes where conditions are unfavorable to speech development. There are silent homes where the parents rarely talk to each other. There are homes so confused with the noise and distraction of other children, or so preoccupied with other matters, that the harried parents have no time to create the relationship out of which speech comes.

> Timothy, aged four and a half, was brought to us by the social worker who had discovered him in the course of her other duties. "Tim has very little speech and language and his mother is concerned about what will happen when he soon will have to enter school. He seems bright enough, has normal hearing, seems to understand what others say to him, but he says only a few words or phrases. Usually a silent child, he talks a lot to the farm chickens, goats, and pigs, or so his mother says. He's an only child and has no contact with other children. I can arrange to bring him and his mother if you could give us an appointment."

One of our graduate students was assigned to play with Tim and to get as many samples of his speech as possible while we interviewed the mother. Another student observed and recorded the interview.

Timothy's mother gave us this information. He had been ill most of his first two years and had done very little babbling or vocal play. When later his first two words appeared, they were "tikka" for chicken, and "mih" for milk. There were some others that she'd forgotten. He now could name many objects and activities when pressed to do so, and he had said a few simple sentences such as "Pail fell down" and "Go potty now" but often she could not understand what he tried to say. She had tried to get him to repeat after her, but he refused to try again. He did seem to understand most of what she said to him and could follow simple directions. That was about all she could tell us about Tim's speech except that she kept insisting, "He's not dumb. He's smart enough but he just can't talk." She was very worried about what might happen when he had to go to school.

She also provided some other significant information. Her husband was a farmer making a poor living by growing sod for garden centers and doing odd jobs in town during the winter. They managed to survive on produce from a big garden, eggs, goat milk, and a pig or two that they butchered every fall. The nearest neighbors were about a quarter of a mile away and Tim had no playmates. Because she often had to help her husband, and with all her other chores, she really had little time for Tim. She felt guilty about it. It would be impossible to bring Tim to the clinic for therapy. She wept a little, helplessly.

What to do? We gave her information and suggestions but it was obvious that they would be insufficient. Another lost child?

The student who had been with Tim reported that he had been cooperative and she gave us the language samples she had elicited. There were thirty-one comprehensible words, mainly names of objects or activities, several noun phrases and verb phrases and a few telegrammic sentences such as "Me hay give goat." He did seem to comprehend most of what she said to him.

As the three of us later discussed our findings, the graduate student who had observed the interview volunteered to go out to the sod farm three afternoons a week as part of her practicum experience. She would keep a daily account of each session and bring him to the clinic once every other week.

And that is what the student did. Space limitations here do not permit more than a brief summary of the therapy. She began by joining Tim when he showed her around the farm and by joining him as he talked to the chickens. He loved the attention. For the first time he had a listener and an adult playmate who did interesting things. Soon his speech output began to increase dramatically and by the end of the second month Tim was speaking in sentences of increasing complexity. By the end of the semester Tim had acquired enough mastery of his language skills to permit him to attend a preschool in town after she and the social worker had found a volunteer to provide the transportation.

Sick children are slow to talk, and there are sick homes too. Some children hear little but angry speech. Often we have seen speech decay and disappear when a child was shuffled from one foster home to another or when a youngster has been separated from his parents by a long hospitalization. When two languages are spoken in a home, one by the children and the other by the parents, some children get too confused to talk.

If a child is to talk, there must be some identification with the care giver. Models are very important.

We knew one little girl whose mother was a drunkard with whom no child could identify as she staggered around the house, dirty, cursing, and in half collapse. We have worked with children too hungry, too weak, or too tired to talk and had to take care of these basic needs before they had a chance to learn. The county sheriff once brought us three almost-wild children from a hut in a swamp only a few miles from Kalamazoo. The father was retarded and a junk scavenger who fed them when he could. The mother had abandoned them. The tale is too incredible to put in a textbook, but these three nonspeaking children in the observation room were animal children. Yes, there are environmental conditions that deter speech development.[3]

ASSESSING THE CHILD'S LANGUAGE

Since this is an introductory text, we shall not discuss assessment or diagnosis in any detail. Extensive reviews of evaluation principles and procedures can be found in many publications, including Lund and Duchan (1993), Nelson (1993), Peterson and Marquardt (1994), Shipley and McAfee (1992), and Wallach and Butler (1984, 1994).

Clearly, the diagnostic mission will vary depending upon how much language the child has: Is she nonverbal, at the single-word level, at the multiword level, or does she manifest disordered syntax? Generally, however, we seek information in at least four domains: (1) a thorough case history, including a parent interview; (2) informal observations and samples of the child's language; (3) an inventory of the child's receptive and expressive language by means of formal tests; and (4) an evaluation of the role of various deterrents to language acquisition.

The Case History

As a general rule, the younger the child and the more severe the language problem, the greater the importance of the parent interview. The clinician seeks the parents' help—as the best informed source—in determining who the child is and what is his problem. Typically, the following topics are explored:

■ The mother's pregnancy and the child's birth and neonatal history
■ History and composition of the family
■ The child's medical history
■ The child's developmental history, including motor, self-care, and communicative skills
■ How the child uses receptive and expressive language at home
■ How the family has attempted to help the child develop speech

The clinician will also scrutinize medical and school achievement records for relevant information.

The Language Sample

One of the first things we try to do is to collect a sample of the child's utterances *representative* of his problem. Although there is no universally accepted procedure for eliciting speech from a child, we prefer an unstructured play situation (see Figure 6-1) using appropriate toys or pictures (Fujiki and Brinton, 1987). In some instances, we may observe the child's speech behavior while she is interacting with her parents or sibling. The goal is to obtain *typical* behavior from the child.[4]

If the child is mute and completely nonverbal, the clinician tries to learn his gesture language, if any, or to scrutinize his vocalizations for any intonations that might indicate meaning. The clinician hunts for any evidence of comprehension of the speech of others. If the child has only a few words, she tries to ascertain whether they are true one-word declarative, imperative, or interrogative sentences or merely stereotyped meaningless parroting of adult utterances and used only for display. The clinician also tries to judge how sophisticated the child is in terms of communicative function: Does he understand listener perspective and the rules of discourse? If the child has progressed further and is combining words into real phrases and sentences, the clinician records and categorizes these to determine what the child has mastered and what he has not. Then she assembles the latter findings into a sequential **hierarchy** of targets for her training.

Testing

Hierarchy.
A series of items graded according to difficulty.

The clinician also has a wide array of tests that can be used to assess both expressive and receptive language in a child who has sufficient language for analysis. Some instruments are designed as screening tests and allow for rapid comparison of the client's performance with established norms. Clinicians also may administer more comprehensive "diagnostic" tests to

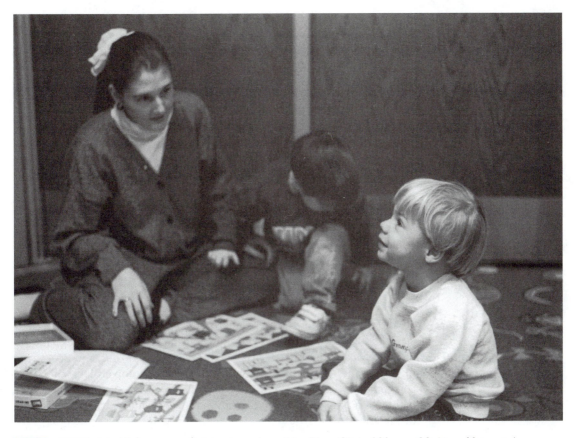

FIGURE 6-1   A language clinician in action *(Van Riper Clinic, Western Michigan University)*

assess both receptive and expressive language, and various tests have been devised to assess children's understanding and application of specific linguistic rules (e.g., rules of morphology or of syntax) and knowledge of semantics. Numerous formal tests of language are commercially available, but relatively few of them have been well standardized. In even fewer cases has test reliability or validity been sufficiently demonstrated; and, of course, language tests often tend to be culturally biased. In brief, test results must be interpreted with caution and sensitivity, and *interpretations must be based upon a complete and precise understanding of basic principles of measurement.*

A growing number of clinicians advocate the use of nonstandardized approaches—as a supplement or an alternative to tests—for assessing language-disabled children.

Most standardized tests are *norm-referenced,* which means that they compare an individual's behavior to that of others of the same age, sex, socioeconomic level, etc. *Criterion-referenced* tests, on the other hand, delineate the contents of an individual's performance; they reveal the particular developmental stage at which the child is functioning and provide more relevant guidance for therapy planning.

A child may not give his best performance, it further is reasoned, when he is frightened or unsure of the strange clinic environment, testing tasks, and examiner. Testing can be an artificial, contrived, unnatural situation for evaluating how a youngster *really* communicates. Although it may be more time consuming to obtain a spontaneous speech sample (in a child's home or classroom, for example, rather than in a clinic setting), it gives us a richer, more descriptive, and hence more accurate picture of his language performance. Nevertheless, formal testing has its place when correctly used, and readers who wish more information about particular tests will find the references cited at the beginning of this section to be useful sources.

Evaluation

In addition to history taking, language sampling, and testing, the clinicians will try to determine such contributing deterrents to language acquisition as hearing loss, deficits in reception, organizing, and processing of information, inadequate cognitive skills, and impairment of motor coordination. To illustrate the type of information assembled when evaluating a language-disabled child, we now present brief segments of a diagnostic report:

Background Information: Hannah (age 4.1) is the youngest of three children. She was born prematurely and is described as delayed in all aspects of development by her parents. Her first word was uttered at twenty-two months. At the present time the child has a very limited vocabulary (less than fifty words); her verbal output is limited to one-word utterances and gestures.

Language Comprehension: Attention span is erratic and very brief. The child performed six of ten tasks requiring her to listen to and follow simple directions.

Semantics: Mean length of utterance (for twenty-five items) was 1.1. Hannah is using a few simple action-agent and agent-object sentences. On a measure of receptive vocabulary, she achieved a mental age score of 3.2, which places her at the ninth percentile.

Syntax: The child scored at the tenth percentile on a measure of syntax comprehension.

Associated Functions: Hannah has normal hearing acuity. Administration of a screening test of gross and fine motor skills showed that the child is capable of accomplishing tasks up to but not exceeding the three-year-old level. A scale that assesses basic conceptual skills (numbers, spatial, etc.) was administered and showed that Hannah is one year behind her chronological age in fundamental conceptual development.

This very cursory review is far from comprehensive, but it indicates the complexity of the factors that may play a part in language disability. Nevertheless, once the clinician has achieved a preliminary understanding of the presented problem, she begins language therapy.

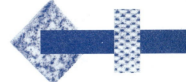

LANGUAGE THERAPY[5]

We are not sure that language can be *taught*—at least in the same sense as the mathematical tables, organic chemistry, or social studies—but we are convinced that a child can *learn* it. The clinician serves as the guide and facilitator in this learning. Based upon her knowledge of the form and content of language, she attempts to provide experiences that are relevant to the child's needs. Then, she helps the youngster narrate the experiences in such a way that he can discover the underlying rules for generating accurate messages. It is demanding work, even with children having only a mild disorder. You can imagine the greater challenge presented by children with greater language disabilities. Unfortunately, there are many of them who may be placed in your professional hands, and so you'd better know what to do and how to begin.

The Sequencing of Language Training

Most clinicians make some attempt to follow what they believe to be the normal course of language development in their language training even though the research on this topic leaves much to be desired. First, they seek to elicit vocalization as a response to stimulation if this is not shown by the child. Then they try to get him to acquire a few sentencelike words. These should be chosen with some care so that they can be easily combined with other words to make noun and verb phrases, can be used with intonations and gestures, may be truly useful in the child's communication, and finally, are not too difficult to say. Once the child has acquired these "sentence words," the clinician stimulates him with simple noun phrases and word phrases and tries to get the child to say them in meaningful context.

Next the language clinician tries to get him to expand these and other sentencelike single words into noun phrases and verb phrases with their modifiers. Following this, the clinician helps the child to generate simple sentences of various types by combining the noun and verb phrases to reflect the subject-predicate or designative or actor-action relationships.

Once these simple sentences have been acquired, the clinician seeks to have the child combine, expand, or modify these sentences through the use of conjunctions, prepositional or adverbial words, and phrases. She then might work on the transformations and the changes in word order that express questions, negatives, and commands. Or she might instead set up as the training targets those constructions that reflect pluralization, amount, time, place, verb tense, and so on until most of the complex structures of adult speech have been mastered. In the later stages of training the appropriate priorities are difficult to determine, and most clinicians "teach to the deficits," selecting as their targets those grammatical structures that seem most needed or are most easily taught.

The Linguistic Approach: Discovering Hidden Rules of Language

Speech-language pathologists whose basic orientation is linguistic view their essential role as being that of a provider of simplified language models so that the child may discover the basic patterns and rules that seem to have escaped him. These workers insist that the goal is not to have the child, through imitation, simply repeat the clinician's modeling of phrases and sentences of increasing complexity. Instead, they desire that he discover how words and phrases can and must be joined together to express meanings.

Modeling

If you were to overhear a speech pathologist of this persuasion talking to a severely language-deviant child as she played with dolls or doll furniture, you might hear her using only noun phrases in her commentary (if this is the structure she wanted the child to discover): "Dollie . . . big dollie . . . more dollie"; "Mama dollie . . . baby dollie" . . . or, many weeks later on, using simple subject-predicate models such as "Dollie jump" . . . "Dollie sleep" . . . or, in later sessions, using such transformations as the negative "Dollie no eat" . . . or the interrogative "Where Dollie?" . . . "Where bed?" . . . or even exploring the possessive, "Where Dollie's bed?" What this clinician is using here is not the itsy-cooing kind of baby talk with which some silly persons bedevil their babies or their poodles, but a carefully programmed kind of simplified language stimulation so formulated that the child has a very favorable opportunity to discover how words can be joined together to code or decode meanings. By using these models at the very instant that the child is perceiving or experiencing what is being referred to (about that dollie), the child learns how to comprehend language structure and how to use it. Moreover, the clinician often finds that, once he has been exposed to the models sufficiently, the child spontaneously begins to use the simplified models without being asked to imitate them, and to use them in generating untaught phrases or sentences of his own.

Expansions.   When the child shows (by the new phrases or sentences he formulates by himself) that he has mastered the target constructions, the clinician moves onward to more complex ones, usually those characteristic of the next step in normal language development. Thus, if the child has moved from the one-word sentence stage to the mastery of noun phrases and verb phrases including modifiers, she may next elect to stimulate him with commentary on what he is doing, perceiving, or feeling at the moment with new target sentences. Or she may use what are called *expansions,* echoing his utterances but providing a model of a more highly developed construction. Thus if the child says, "Timmy go in doggy house" the clinician might say "Timmy go in doggy's house," if there were two houses, one for dolls and one for dogs (and if Timmy is at the stage for acquiring the rules governing possessives). In these "expansions" the clinician repeats what the child has said, but in a changed form, the change reflecting a more advanced construction (Schwartz et al., 1985).

Extensions.   This term refers to the procedure whereby the clinician or parent responds to an utterance of a child, not merely by expanding it into a more mature construction by filling in the words he has omitted or misused, but by adding other phrases or sentences that make his meaning clearer. For example, if the child says, "Johnny bye-bye," the expansions might be "Johnny go bye-bye" or "Johnny wants to go bye-bye." But if instead the clinician or parent says, "Johnny wants to go bye-bye in the car. Johnny likes to ride in the car," he or she is using extensions, providing not just revisions of his simple utterance but models of how his meaning might be even better expressed.

Correction.   Probably the most frequently used technique for helping a child learn the rules of the language is simple correction. All parents use it—and often abuse it. It can certainly be overdone. We have known children to stop talking altogether after being corrected too much, especially when the correction model is accompanied by parental irritation. "Oh, stop talking like a baby. Don't say, Timmy see one, two, three car! People don't talk that way. They say, Timmy sees three cars. That's how they say it. Now say it right!" And then, if the boy says, "Timmy see three car," the parent might say, "No! Three cars. CARSZZ! Lord, won't you ever be able to talk right?" Sometimes it's hard to be a little child trying to learn his language.

The Modeling of Self-Correction.   A much better way is to have the clinician or parent provide models of self-correction. For example, suppose that the child needs to discover how past tenses are coded in our language. When describing what happened when the toy dog drank some play milk before hiding under the dollhouse bed and the boy had said, "doggy drink milk and hide bed" the clinician might say, "The dog drink the milk . . . No, I mean, the dog drinked his milk and hide under bed."

She is not too worried about the improper use of the *-ed* ending here for the past tense of the verb. He can learn "drank" later. And she will feel good when he says "goed" for "went" so long as he is saying "banged" or "showed" or "tickled" to demonstrate that he is beginning to catch on to the way in which some verbs must be changed to indicate the past tense. The important thing is that he has seen that big people can correct themselves too, that there is a right way and a wrong way to say what he means.

If an older child is having trouble with prepositional phrases and never seems, for instance, to use the words "over" or "under," the clinician and child may do a lot of crawling over and under the tables in the therapy room or putting things under or over others as she verbalizes the shared experiences, expanding on his inadequate utterances such as "Go table" by saying "Go *under* table," or perhaps using his inadequate phrases or sentences before correcting them; "Put dollie chair, no, no, I mean 'put the dollie *under* the chair.' " Or the clinician may even ask him to say it correctly, "Timmy, say: 'put dollie *under* the chair.' " Again, if the child's pronouns are all askew, we show him the differences between the correct and incorrect usages by making his error first and then correcting it. Thus the clinician might say, "Me go outdoors now . . . No, *I* go outdoors now" before indeed doing so. You might possibly feel that the clinician should never use models that are linguistically defective even though they are simplified. Should the clinician ever speak "childrenese"? The answer seems to be yes, since research shows clearly that simplified models as compared with standard ones are more effective in language training.

With an older child, we may work more directly, confronting him with his mistakes and providing the standard model as soon as the error occurs. We play "Catch me!" games in which we deliberately make the mistakes, and they are his usual mistakes, which he is to identify in order to get rewards. By "catching" these mistakes and having to show why they were mistakes and what the correct forms would be, most of these children learn the rules of the language very swiftly. They need help and they need careful teaching, but it is surprising how quickly they get the insights they need once the language task is simplified. Also, it has seemed to us that often the child appears to have already acquired the necessary linguistic competence but has not been able to convert it into performance until we provide this focused sort of language stimulation.

> We were helping a four-year-old child who, among other problems, had shown great difficulty in getting his past tenses straightened out. After some prompting and error recognition activities, which he enjoyed hugely, we were trying to get him to discriminate between "growed" and "grew." Suddenly, he grinned at us and said, "I growed-grew, knowed-knew that all the time. I knew it but now I got it." Unfortunately, the English language has many traps for the unwary, and we had to

straighten out some tangles when he overgeneralized and told us how he "shew" his mother how well he could ride his tricycle. In Chaucer's time, he would have been correct.

Some speech pathologists who use the generative grammar approach that we have been describing tend to downplay imitation, drill, or requesting the child to repeat sentences spoken by the clinician. They don't want a simple parroting of their stimulus phrases or sentences. They want the child to be able to generate phrases and sentences of his own, which are coded appropriately, and used meaningfully. Often an observer might hear very little speech being produced by a child during a therapy session, the clinician concentrating rather upon understanding and comprehension. For example, the clinician might be commanding, "Put car *in* bed," showing the child what he should do, or telling him instead to "Put car *under* bed," or finding picture cards that show not only "the toy car in a bed," but also a "bed in a car" to test his comprehension. Concepts are provided before they are coded.

Having the Parents Help.

A child who is severely deficient in language will require much help at home as well as in the therapy room, and so the parents and even the siblings must be brought into the program. We have found it wise to let the parents observe our sessions for a period of time before asking them to join us in helping the child acquire language. And we rarely try to acquaint them with linguistic theory. Instead, we ask them to stop asking the child questions and to stop drilling him or trying to get him to repeat the inappropriate things they usually demand that he imitate. We train them to use what we call "self-talk" and **parallel talk,** for these are techniques that they readily understand and will use.

Nelson (1993) describes how she used a language-delayed boy's sisters.

> In our university clinic, this is what we did with a child, Stephen, who at the age of three was nonspeaking and showed many symptoms of autism. We knew that Stephen's sisters played "house" with him at home, so we brought them in to play house in a play kitchen in the language preschool area at the university clinic. As they made pretend cupcakes and played dolls, we encouraged Stephen's sisters to include him in their play. We also taped some of Stephen's favorite songs and taught the sisters the accompanying motions so they could repeat them with him at home. When the activity was conducted in the clinic, Stephen watched his sisters closely, imitating their actions, and interacting with them.

Self-talk.

By **self-talk** we mean that the parents should talk aloud to themselves so the child can overhear them verbalizing very simply what they are seeing, hearing, doing, or feeling. Here are some samples of a mother's self-talk.

Parallel talk.
A technique in which the therapist provides a running commentary on what the client is doing, perceiving, or probably feeling.

Self-talk.
An audible commentary by a person describing actions, perceptions, or feelings.

Where cup? Oh, I see cup. Cup on table. Here cup . . . . Milk in cup . . . .
Mummy drink milk . . . . Johnny want cup? . . . . OK . . . . Johnny
drink . . . . Milk all gone . . . . Give Mummy cup . . . . Mummy wash
cup . . . . Here water . . . . Here soap . . . . Give cup bath . . . . All
clean . . . . Where towel? Here towel . . . . Wipe, wipe . . . . Give, Johnny
cup . . . . Put on table . . . . Johnny good boy.

This child was only making a few vowels, grunts, and gestures at the
time but he was alert and interested. Note the mother's simple speech,
within reach of the child's ability. Note the commentary accompanying
what she did or saw. Note the recall and prediction. Here there is no demand for display speech. Here is self-talk used as verbalized thinking. It
wasn't long before the boy was talking to himself, too. Mothers and clinicians must learn to talk this way for the time being, to build the bridge
between where the child is and where he should be in language usage. He
cannot jump the chasm. As he begins to talk, they can gradually increase
the complexity of their models. We have to begin where the child is. We
must join him before we can lead him.

A surprising bit of behavior comes when we get to the early sentence
stage. If we occasionally fumble a bit, leave a self-talk sentence hanging
uncompleted in midair, omit a key word, the child will often say it for us.
When this occurs it is unwise to make much of an issue of the achievement. Just feel good and use the technique more often. If we put words
in his ears he will find them in his mouth.

Parallel Talking.   If the clinician will demonstrate, a parent can also learn
to use what is called parallel talking. This technique does not require the
child to say anything, thus freeing him from the usual bombardment of
parental commands to "Say this" and "Say that." And it relieves some of
the parent's anxiety.

In parallel talking, the parent verbalizes not his own thoughts but
those of the child. He tells the child what he is doing, what he is feeling.
If he appears to be predicting that Jack will jump out of his box, he might
say, "Jack pop out, pretty soon." If he is about to turn off the light, he
says, "Light go away now." When the child tumbles from the chair, he
says, "Johnny fall down. Ow, ow. Hurt foot. Ow!" Emotions can be expressed in self-talk and parallel talk too.

This parallel talking is fascinating stuff. Ideally, we should say the necessary word or phrase or sentence at the very instant that the child should
be needing it. Practically, we seldom get the timing so precise. It is a skill
that develops with use. We have known parents to become wonderfully
adept after a little practice. It requires careful study of the child and a lot
of guessing, imagination, and the ability to identify with the youngster.
Every speech clinician should learn the art, for it is very useful in treating
the adult aphasic as well as the child who cannot talk. Training in empathy is vitally important in speech pathology.

We have spoken earlier of the importance of speech as a magical tool for controlling others. Nowhere do we see this so clearly as in delayed speech. As soon as we possibly can, we teach this function. We have used puppets, dolls, even ourselves as our victims. We command these beings. We tell them to fall down, to cry, to clap hands, and they must obey! The child watches us and sees the power of speech. Soon he is commanding too. Our knees still creak from a session with a little boy who insisted that we get "Unduh taybo!" thirty-seven times by actual count. This spontaneously achieved command had been preceded by much self-talk on our part, commanding first a puppet and then ourselves to follow orders.

We also use self-talk to set models for egocentric speech, for the expression of the self. Yesterday, with the same little boy, we crouched on the floor and said, "I'm little . . . . I baby . . . . " Then we got up on all fours, and said, "I kitty . . . meow!" Then we stood up and said proudly, "I big man . . . big as a house." The boy liked the display and gestured that he wanted us to do it again. We looked puzzled, paused a bit, then said, "More! . . . You want more?" He grunted. So we did it again and again, and soon he was imitating first our postures and our animal noises, and finally a little of our speech. He climbed aboard the table, stuck out his chest and arms and crowed, "Man . . . bih MAN!" This was the beginning of speech as the display of the self.

We teach speech as communication a little later. Often it begins to come in by itself, once speech as thought and speech as social control are activated. Usually, we combine it with command at first. "Mummy blow bubble . . . . Big bubble . . . Oh, oh . . . No more bubble . . . . All gone . . . . Go ask sister for soap. . . . Sssssssssoap . . . . " If he's interested enough he might just possibly do it.

Direct Language Teaching

Not all language clinicians are content merely to stimulate the child with simple models of the constructions he needs and to wait until he discovers and begins to use them. Feeling that his chances of discovering them are better when they appear in his own speech productions rather than in the expansions or models that they present, they train the child deliberately to imitate their utterances. Thus, if the child is having difficulty in using the perpendicular pronoun "I" in contrast to the word "me" in discovering the variant forms of the subject versus object relationship, they would try to get the child (repeating after the clinician) to say such sentences as "I hit dollie" as he does so; or to say "Dollie hit me," in unison when this is acted out. Also, many clinicians, as we have said before, resort to direct correction. When the child says, "Me go car" they respond by saying "*I* go car" and then insist that the child repeat what they have said. This procedure probably reflects the kind of parent-child interaction that has failed in the past to help him discover the difference between the two pronouns, but when the clinician repeatedly focuses on the problem and reinforces the correct one, it often does facilitate the discovery that must be achieved.

The Operant Conditioning Approach: Behavior Modification Procedures.
You should know that there are other speech pathologists who feel that the best way of helping a child to acquire language is through operant conditioning, and several studies have been reported in the literature wherein autistic or mentally retarded children have made considerable gains in language through careful programming and reinforcement. These workers believe that language is learned, not discovered, and that when a child has failed to master the proper linguistic codings for his thoughts, he can be taught (conditioned) to do so.

Suspecting that most of you have a basic knowledge of operant conditioning, we only describe it briefly. The basic principle of operant conditioning is that most behaviors, including language behaviors, are affected by their consequences. Some consequences increase the probability that the behavior will reoccur in the future and are therefore termed *reinforcing;* others, called *punishers,* decrease that probability.

The operant language clinician's task, then, is to define the behaviors he wants the child to emit more frequently, to carefully devise a serial program of successive objectives, and to provide and apply contingently the reinforcements according to an appropriate schedule. The criteria of successful achievement at each step of the program must be met before the child goes to the next successive step. If the child cannot meet the criterion for a given step, the program is revised, or the reinforcements are increased, or help in the form of "prompts" is given until success is obtained. Sometimes, because the desired response is too complex or does not exist (even intermittently) in the child's repertoire, a program of successive approximations called *shaping* is used. In this shaping, the clinician at first reinforces a response that may have very little similarity to what must be learned. But as it occurs again and again, however, some variability is usually shown and when it appears the clinician contingently reinforces only those behaviors that increasingly resemble the target behavior.

Conditioning the Nonverbal Child.
If the child has no verbal language at all, the operant clinician devises programs to establish imitative behaviors. For example, **contingent reinforcement** may be used when a child first looks at the clinician whenever the clinician makes a sound. When this behavior is being consistently shown (perhaps 80 percent of the time), the reinforcement is faded out for simply looking but it is given again when the child looks and also opens his mouth as the clinician makes a sound. If this is unsuccessful, the clinician may insert an additional

Contingent reinforcement. Following as a consequence of some preceding behavior.

smaller step of reinforcing the child when he imitates her head shaking or hand clapping. If she accomplishes this, the clinician may return to reinforcing the imitative mouth opening or even use the prompt of opening the child's mouth with her hands as a response to her stimulation. Usually, the child will emit some sounds in the course of the interaction, and through reinforcement, the rate of this imitative sound production can be greatly increased.

Then the clinician may move on to establishing the imitation of a few target words (names of objects or pictures or activities). In order to prevent mere parroting at this step, the clinician may insert a substep into the program wherein the child must imitate the clinician's pointing to the object or picture as it is being named by both. Then the clinician would probably point to the picture but provide the name herself only occasionally (thus fading out her prompting), and usually the child will finally be able without help to point and name often enough to get the reinforcement.

The Cognitive Approach

Although the linguistic discovery and direct teaching approaches are probably those used most frequently at the present time, the cognitive method of language therapy seems to be gaining favor. Its basic tenet is that the use of language is based upon thinking and that the focus of therapy should not be on verbal output but, rather, on the underlying concepts that must be coded in language. In other words, language emerges from general intellectual growth and is, all throughout its development, dependent upon this nonlinguistic base. Clinicians of this persuasion insist that thought and comprehension are basic, and they stress acquisition of the meanings that underlie the grammatical structures the child must discover. Treatment sessions are designed to assist a child in exploring how to use various semantic functions, such as *possession, location, recurrence, negation,* and others.

Other cognitive workers concentrate on concept formation and development following the outlines laid down by Piaget and Vigotsky. They use puzzles, conservation tasks (showing how the same quantity of water or clay may take disparate forms), symbolic play, and ways-means activities. The Montessori schools, which feature graded activities involving perception as well as initiative and coordination, have been very successful in teaching language to some intellectually deprived children or those whose home environments have deterred more normal development.

Another example of the cognitive approach is found in the tutorial system of training preschool children in abstract thinking. Rather than working on developing language structures in these socially disadvantaged children, the clinicians train them in selective attention, categories, imagery of future events, inner verbalization, cause and effect relationships, and many other such processes (Thompson and Hixon, 1984).

The Pragmatic Approach

A current trend in language therapy involves structuring sessions so that they focus on communication in the social sharing of information. The *intent* of the speaker and the interpersonal *functions* that oral communication fulfill for him are the salient considerations in planning a treatment program. Advocates of the pragmatic approach try to devise activities in which a child must use real, not contrived, language. They maintain that the therapy session should be a natural version of, and a model for, real-life communicative situations.[6]

Perhaps the popularity of pragmatics is a backlash to behavior modification programs that pervaded the literature for years. How communicative are requests to "Say this . . . ," "Repeat after me," or "What's this object?" Clearly, all these tactics violate the naturalness and sincerity of the verbal interaction. They are demands, not communicative overtures. Furthermore, they tend to disrupt rather than facilitate a child's opportunity to discern the underlying rules of language. Reinforcement is irrelevant if the child is participating in a genuine exchange of messages; in fact, external rewards actually may decrease motivation and undermine internal or self-controls.

Pragmatic clinicians select classes of behavior—expressing intentions, initiating and maintaining a conversation, gaining awareness of listener perspective, and appreciating the situational context—as targets for treatment.

> Lori, age three, possessed only a limited repertoire of strategies for requesting information. She cried, whined, or poked others to get their attention. The clinician set up a series of play activities using the child's own toys so that Lori had to ask for an item in order to complete the task. Puppets were used to model the appropriate verbal behavior at the outset.

Every effort is made to employ language and situations that will be useful in a child's life. Clinicians who favor the pragmatic approach point out that people talk differently in different situations and that the constraints of the context are important in shaping speech behavior. They recognize several features as essential for a treatment session:

- Creating an interpersonal context *(process-orientation)*
- Following the child's lead in terms of interests and language *(child-directed)*
- Working in the child's own environment *(naturalistic)*

■ Using functional reinforcement *(intrinsic reinforcement),* rewards that flow from the child's own feeling of successful communication.

We have only scratched the surface of a vast new body of information about pragmatics. But we are cautiously optimistic that this approach will prove to be pivotal in the treatment of child language disorders because it integrates and synthesizes all the features of language (form, content, and function) into a meaningful context.

Which Approach Is Best?

Language therapy is still in its infancy. There are many problems still to be resolved, and so this question cannot be answered at the present time. Perhaps an eclectic combination is best. The grammatical stimulation-discovery, cognitive-semantic, and pragmatic approaches have been shown to help some children acquire some language ability. Behavior modification is very useful for teaching a child to attend to the clinician and for reducing certain negative or off-task behaviors. We find it particularly effective as a means of instating simple routine behaviors in very young children. While operant conditioning can be used to induce a child to vocalize, even to utter words and simple sentences, it tends to produce reactive, contrived speech, not true language.

Most of the language clinicians we know use all these approaches; they are very eclectic in their work (Figure 6-2). Any teacher of language-impaired children needs to know the rationale and application of not just one but all possible methods of treatment. The child's needs and difficulties and capacities—not fragmented views of language, clinician bias, or administrative regulations—must determine how he is to be helped (Damico, 1988).

Unfortunately, there is still only limited evidence regarding the effectiveness of any therapy currently being used. The pragmatic approach has an intuitive appeal because it focuses on the client's life circumstances and this in turn seems to enhance the transfer or generalization of acquired skills. Finally, early identification and intervention are critical, since age is the strongest predictor of improvement in children with language disorders: the younger the child, the better prospects for improvement (see Sparks et al., 1990).

Children with language disabilities will have a rough time of it in school and out. Their parents may be ashamed of them and they can come to feel that way about themselves also. Not only speaking, but reading and writing skills, will be affected. If many people think they are mentally retarded (even if they aren't), they eventually come to believe those others and respond accordingly. These children need understanding and expert help. We hope that you will see that they get it.

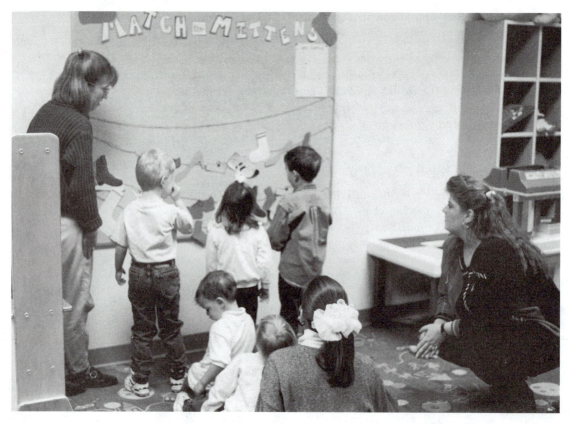

FIGURE 6-2   Youngsters with language disorders in group therapy session *(Van Riper Clinic, Western Michigan University)*

STUDY QUESTIONS

1. How widespread are language disorders among children?
2. Why do the authors prefer the term *deterrent* to the term *cause,* and what are the major known deterrents to normal language development?
3. What is meant by "telegrammic" speech?
4. Explain in your own words why it is important that we not confuse the terms "difference," "delay," and "deviance" in describing children's language.
5. What types of observations may lead us to suspect that a child's language difficulties are due to mental retardation?
6. Of the two basic kinds of hearing loss, which is the more likely to be a serious deterrent to language development?

7. How would you advise the parents of a deaf child who ask if their child should be allowed to learn signing?
8. What characteristics are we likely to observe in a child who has a learning disability?
9. What would be your response if asked to describe the behavioral features that are particularly likely to be found in autism?
10. Why do speech-language clinicians not rely entirely upon norm-referenced standardized tests to assess children's language development?

ENDNOTES

[1]It has been estimated that about two children in every 1,000 suffer head trauma each year and that the annual incidence of stroke in children may be almost three in 100,000 (National Institute on Deafness and Other Communication Disorders, 1991). And about one in 1,000 children develops a sensorineural hearing loss severe enough to interfere with language acquisition (National Advisory Neurological and Communicative Disorders and Stroke Council, 1989).

[2]Early identification of potential language-disabled children is of critical importance. Infants with low birth weight, respiratory or feeding problems, and other high risk factors should be monitored closely. See Sparks et al. (1990) for a discussion of infants at risk for communication disorders.

[3]For a complete account of these three nonverbal "near-wild children" see Van Riper (1979).

[4]We realize that "typical" behavior may not easily be elicited or accurately recognized. It may vary from one context to another, and it may be wise to do sampling in a variety of situations. And if the child is reasonably verbal, the analysis of samples can be laborious. Hopefully, however, we will continue to see advances in computer-assisted language analysis programs such as those of Miller and Chapman (1985) and Shriberg (1986).

[5]In earlier days, some of our colleagues feared that the use of medically derived terms such as "therapy" and "diagnosis" would imply subservience to physicians. Accordingly, such terms acquired a mild taboo and terms such as "intervention," "remediation," and "assessment" gained favor. In this book we sometimes use the older terms because we feel that the independence of speech-language pathology has become pretty well established. Besides, remediation implies remedies as in medicine. Intervention sounds like interfering rather than helping (and assessments are flavored with tax increases). Selah!

[6]The advocates of pragmatics owe a large debt to the conversational method devised by Backus and Beasley (1951) nearly half a century ago!

REFERENCES

Backus, O., and Beasley, J. (1951). *Speech therapy with children*. Boston: Houghton Mifflin.

Bangs, T. (1968). *Language and learning disorders of the pre-academic child*. Englewood Cliffs, NJ: Prentice Hall.

Battle, D. (1993). *Communication disorders in multicultural populations.* Stoneham, MA: Butterworth-Heinemann.

Blake, J. N. (1969). A therapeutic construct for two seven-year-old nonverbal boys. *Journal of Speech and Hearing Disorders, 34,* 362–369.

Block, J., Gersten, E., and Kornblum, S. (1980). Evaluation of a language program for young autistic children. *Journal of Speech and Hearing Disorders, 45,* 76–89.

Bourgondien, M., Mesibov, G., and Dawson, G. (1987). Pervasive developmental disorders: Autism. In M. Wolraich (ed.). *The practical assessment and management of children with disorders of development and learning.* Chicago: Year Book Medical Publishers.

Chomsky, C. (1986). Analytic study of the Tadoma Method: Language abilities of three deaf-blind subjects. *Journal of Speech and Hearing Research, 29,* 332–347.

Curtiss, S., Katz, W., and Tallal, P. (1992). Delay versus deviance in the language acquisition of language impaired children. *Journal of Speech and Hearing Research, 35,* 373–383.

Damico, J. (1988). The lack of efficacy in language therapy: A case study. *Language, Speech, and Hearing Services in Schools, 19,* 51–66.

Fujiki, M., and Brinton, B. (1987). Elicited imitation revisited: A comparison with spontaneous language production. *Language, Speech, and Hearing Services in Schools, 18,* 301–311.

Gillberg, C., and Steffenburg, C. (1987). Outcome and prognostic factors in infantile autism and similar conditions: A population-based study of 46 cases followed through puberty. *Journal of Autism and Developmental Disorders, 17,* 273–287.

Greenfeld, J. (1972). *A child called Noah.* New York: Holt, Rinehart and Winston.

Kavanagh, J. (1986). *Otitis media and child development.* Parkton, MD: York Press.

Koegel, R., O'Dell, M., and Koegel, L. (1987). A natural language teaching paradigm for nonverbal autistic children. *Journal of Autism and Developmental Disorders, 17,* 187–200.

Launay, J. et al. (1987). Catecholamines metabolism in infantile autism: A controlled study of 22 autisitc children. *Journal of Autism and Developmental Disorders, 17,* 333–347.

Lovass, O. (1977). *The autistic child: Language development through behavior modification.* New York: Irvington.

Lund, N., and Duchan, J. (1993). *Assessing children's language in naturalistic contexts* (3rd ed.). Englewood Cliffs, NJ: Prentice Hall.

Miller, J., and Chapman, R. (1985). *SALT: Systematic Analysis of Language Transcripts—Users manual.* Madison, WI: University of Wisconsin, Language Analysis Laboratory, Waisman Center.

Mirenda, P., and Schuler, A. (1988). Augmenting communication for persons with autism: Issues and strategies. *Topics in Language Disorders, 9*(1), 24–43.

National Advisory Neurological and Communicative Disorders and Stroke Council. (1989). *Decade of the brain: Answers through scientific research* (NIH Publication No. 88–2957). Bethesda, MD: National Institutes of Health.

National Institute of Neurological Disorders and Stroke. (1988). *Developmental speech and language disorders: Hope through research* (NIH Publications Pamphlet No. 88–2757). Bethesda, MD: National Institutes of Health.

National Institute on Deafness and Other Communication Disorders. (1991). *National strategic research plan for balance and the vestibular system and language and language impairments* (NIH Publication No. 91–3217). Bethesda, MD: National Institutes of Health.

Nelson, N. (1993). *Childhood language disorders in context, infancy through adolescence.* New York: Merrill.

Paul, R., and Cohen, D. (1985). Comprehension of indirect requests in adults with autistic disorders and mental retardation. *Journal of Speech and Hearing Research, 28,* 475–479.

Peterson, H., and Marquardt, T. (1994). *Appraisal and diagnosis of speech and language disorders.* Englewood Cliffs, NJ: Prentice Hall.

Prizant, B., and Wetherby, A. (1988). Providing services to children with autism (ages 0 to 2 years) and their families. *Topics in Language Disorders, 9*(1), 1–23.

Renfrew, C. (1959). Speech problems of backward children. *Speech Pathology and Therapy, 2,* 35.

Rimland, B. (1964). *Infantile autism.* Englewood Cliffs, NJ: Prentice Hall.

Schell, R., Stark, J., and Giddon, J. (1968). Development of language behavior in an autistic child. *Journal of Speech and Hearing Disorders,* 33, 42–47.

Schopler, E., and Mesibov, G. (eds.). (1987). *Neurobiological issues in autism.* New York: Plenum Press.

Schwartz, R. (1985). Facilitating word combination in language-impaired children through discourse structure. *Journal of Speech and Hearing Disorders,* 50, 31–39.

Shipley, K., and McAfee, J. (1992). *Assessment in speech-language pathology: A resource manual.* San Diego, CA: Singular Publishing Group.

Shriberg, L. (1986). *PEPPER: Programs to Examine Phonetic and Phonologic Evaluation Records.* Madison, WI: Software Development and Distribution Center, University of Wisconsin.

Sigman, M. (ed.). (1985). *Children with emotional disorders and developmental disabilities.* Orlando, FL: Grune and Stratton.

Sparks, S., Clark, M., Erickson, R., and Oas, D. (1990). *Infants at risk for communication disorders: The professional's role with the newborn.* Tucson, AZ: Communication Skill Builders.

Thompson, R., and Hixon, P. (1984). Teaching parents to encourage independent problem solving in preschool-age children. *Language, Speech and Hearing Services in Schools,* 15, 175–181.

Van Riper, C. (1979). *A career in speech pathology.* Englewood Cliffs, NJ: Prentice Hall.

Wallach, G., and Butler, K. (eds.). (1984). *Language learning disabilities in school-age children.* Baltimore, MD: Williams and Wilkins.

Wallach, G., and Butler, K. (eds.). (1994). *Language learning disabilities in school-age children: Some principles and applications.* New York: Merrill.

Wetherby, A., and Prutting, C. (1984). Profiles of communicative and cognitive-social activities in autistic children. *Journal of Speech and Hearing Research,* 27, 364–377.

Wiener, F. (1986). The non-native speaker: Testing and therapy. In F. Bess, B. Smith Clark, and H. Mitchell (eds.). *Concerns for minority groups in communication disorders: ASHA Reports 16.* Rockville, MD: American Speech-Language-Hearing Association.

Wood, N. (1964). *Delayed speech and language development.* Englewood Cliffs, NJ: Prentice Hall.

SUPPLEMENTARY READINGS

Adler, S., and King, D. (eds.). (1994). *Oral communication problems in children and adolescents.* Boston: Allyn and Bacon.

Cole, L. (1989). E pluribus pluribus: Multicultural imperatives for the 1990s and beyond. *Asha,* 31, 65–70.

Duchan, J., and Weitzner-Lin, B. (1987). Nurturant-naturalistic intervention for language-impaired children. *Asha,* 29, 45–49.

Gullo, D., and Gullo, J. (1987). An ecological language intervention approach with mentally retarded adolescents. *Language, Speech, and Hearing Services in Schools,* 18, 301–311.

Prutting, C., and Kirchner, D. (1987). A clinical appraisal of the pragmatic aspects of language. *Journal of Speech and Hearing Disorders,* 52, 105–119.

Romski, M., Joyner, S., and Sevcik, R. (1987). Vocal communications of a developmentally delayed child: A diary analysis. *Language, Speech, and Hearing Services in Schools,* 18, 112–130.

Warren, S., and Rogers-Warren, A. (eds.). (1985). *Teaching functional language.* Baltimore, MD: University Park Press.

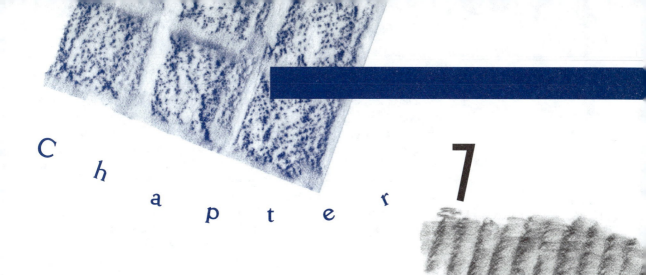

Articulation and Phonological Disorders

Deviant speech sound production is the most common type of communication disorder found among school-age children. In school settings, then, where a majority of speech-language pathologists are employed, a relatively large portion of the clinician's caseload may consist of children who are having difficulty with speech sounds. For one reason or another, these youngsters have failed to learn how to produce certain phonemes, especially motorically complicated sounds such as /s/, /l/ and /r/.

Some have other error sounds, too, of course, and a child's failure to produce a phoneme in the expected manner does not necessarily reflect the presence of a motor coordination difficulty. Nor does it necessarily reflect any detectable anatomic, motor, or sensory limitation affecting the production of a specific speech sound.

A child trying to master the phonology of her language may find that certain distinctive features of some sounds are difficult to perceive or to produce. As a result, she does the best she can, by omitting or simplifying or substituting sounds that she hears or makes more easily. Such strategies are called *phonological processes*. There are many such processes, but the most common are *fronting, stopping, deleting, voicing, gliding,* and *cluster reduction*.

We shall look more closely at phonological processes a bit later in this chapter. For now, however, we merely observe that the two terms *articulation disorder* and *phonological disorder* sometimes have been used interchangeably, even though they do not represent synonymous concepts. The distinction offered by Elbert and Gierut (1986) represents the view of many current writers.

> We can generally describe "articulation disorders" as difficulties with the motor production aspects of speech. . . . The term "phonological disorders," on the other hand, (views) speech sound . . . production and use as part of the total language system, on a par with other aspects . . . such as syntax, semantics, pragmatics, and morphology. (pp. 9–10)

In making this distinction, clinicians tend to label speech sound disorders as "phonological disorders" whenever no obvious anatomic or neurophysiologic cause is present. On the other hand, when such causes *are* evident, the problem tends to be labelled as an "articulation disorder" or, by some, as a "phonetic disorder."

The differentiation, however, may not always be as clear-cut as it first appears. For example, along with others we note that "a phonological disorder of unknown etiology may be caused by one or more subtle organic, learning or environmental factors" (Bernthal and Bankson, 1993, p. 2). Moreover, it clearly is possible for both motor (phonetic) and cognitive or linguistic (phonologic) factors to be impeding an individual's articulation skills.

In any event, why does the speech pathologist work with these children whose speech sounds are deviant? Why can't she wait, for example, and allow phonological or motor maturation to take place? The basic reason is that these errors can become so firmly embedded in the child's language that he will never become able to correct them unless he gets her help. Each time an articulation error occurs, it gains strength and indeed is rewarded by the consummation of communication. When a child asks for "tandy" and gets candy, the substitution of /t/ for /k/ will become more firmly fixed. With rare exception, we don't "outgrow" our faulty phonemes; we learn to utter the standard ones that others use. Unfortunately, parents don't know this and most of them do not even begin calling the errors to the child's attention until he is about to enter school. At most they just ask him not to say "thoup," but to "Say soup," and the child, if he does respond, answers, "But I did thay thoup."

This child's statement reflects another feature of phonemic errors. He is usually unaware that he has uttered an incorrect sound because the /θ/ has become an integral part of the morpheme /sup/. That liquid in the bowl is /θup/ to him. In addition, an individual sound hidden in a word within a fleeting sentence is hard to recognize or recall. We listen to meanings, not to phonemes. After years of use, the error sound is familiar, not strange. Proprioceptively, it feels right. Indeed, as one of our clients told us after he had learned to produce the correct /r/, "It sounds okay but it feels wrong." We must remember that articulation errors are not mispronunciations in which the person fails to use a speech sound that he can otherwise say. They are inabilities, not mistakes. One mother told us that her son, in response to her efforts to correct his distorted /r/, wailed, "But I don't know how to say it!" Therefore, our job is to teach him how to do so. Parents who simply demand that the child correct his errors will merely add to his and their own frustration. He needs the help that only a professional speech pathologist can provide, and he should get it before the error becomes habitual or he will never be able to talk normally.

To provide just one illustration of the impact felt by an adult whose only troublesome sounds were the /r/ and /ɝ/ we recount what he told us.

> From the time I first entered school I have been mocked and hurt by others. They nicknamed me "Wudolf the Wed Nosed Weindeer." They teased me so unmercifully I became afraid to recite, yes, even to talk. When I did I tried not to say words with R sounds in them. As a result I became withdrawn and was excluded from many activities. Teachers corrected me in vain. I just couldn't say those sounds right no matter how hard I tried. Even when I became an adult I felt ashamed and hated the little looks I got when others recognized my mistakes. Job interviews were disasters. I even legally changed my first name from Rudolph to William, which helped, but there are too many R words you need to say. I never even asked girls out for fear of rejection. Those damned R sounds have spoiled my life.

Before continuing our discussion of articulation and phonologic disorders, we must point out that the definition of "disorder" in this context is not always as simple as once it may have appeared to be. Among the many factors to be considered is the multicultural nature of our population.

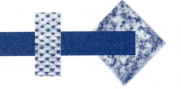

DIALECT DIFFERENCES

As we mentioned in Chapter 4, racial, ethnic-cultural, and linguistic diversities have become ever more apparent in our country in recent years. It is generally projected, moreover, that our present "minority" groups, taken together, may well become the "majority" of our population in the next few decades. Whatever their extent, shifting demographics have important implications for the helping professions, including speech-language pathology and audiology.

The impact of increasing diversity already is being felt by many clinicians, especially those working in locales where languages other than English and dialects other than Standard American English are commonly encountered. And it is our recognition of present and future population characteristics that has stimulated an increasing emphasis on cultural and linguistic variations in the course and practicum experiences of students who are preparing to become speech-language pathologists or audiologists.

In an introductory text we must limit our discussion to selected linguistic variations, and even then we can touch only briefly just on the topic of dialects. The term *dialect* typically is used in reference to the variations in a spoken language that are associated with particular geographic regions, cultures, or social classes. Probably a dozen or more variations of English are spoken by rather substantial numbers of people in the United States, including Standard American, Black, Southern, Eastern, Appalachian, Mexican Spanish, and others. And the differences among these dialects include variations of pronunciation and phonology, as well as variations in syntax, semantics, and pragmatics (Figure 7-1).

Not all members of a population speak its dialect, while others may be adept at code switching, choosing to use the dialect in some situations but not in others. Nevertheless, dialectal features are as integral a part of a population's identity as are its geography, history, and traditions.

For our purposes, the fundamental concept that must be borne in mind is simply that dialectal differences are not disorders. Nor is a dialect "defective" or "wrong" simply because it differs from the dialect that may predominate in a given region or socioeconomic context. Even so, the speech-language clinician may be called upon to assist an individual who wishes to modify his or her dialectal speaking pattern. In such instances,

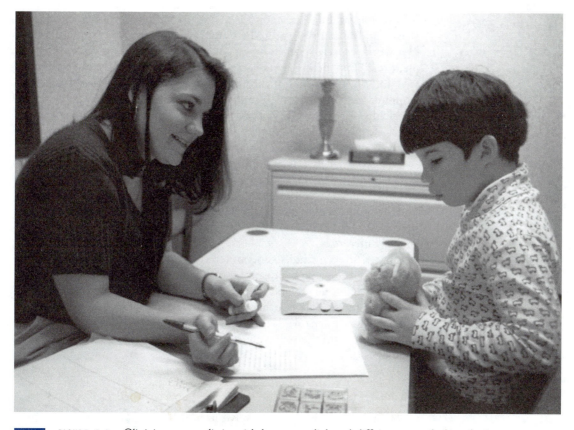

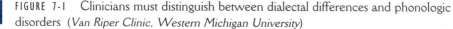

FIGURE 7-1   Clinicians must distinguish between dialectal differences and phonologic disorders (*Van Riper Clinic, Western Michigan University*)

however, as in the instance of a school system seeking to teach all children to speak Standard American English, "such instruction should not be confused with . . . rehabilitation of a communication disorder." (Taylor, 1994, p. 58)

It is equally important to remember that the presence of a dialect difference does not rule out the possibility that a disorder also may exist. Thus, to deal appropriately with individuals whose dialect varies from their own, clinicians must be sensitive to the fact that linguistic rules differ from one dialect to another. For some clinicians it can be essential even today to be familiar with specific rules that underlie the use of particular dialects. In years to come, such knowledge will be even more widely applicable.

In order to assess the phonology or articulation of children or adults whose dialect differs from their own, clinicians obviously must be able to separate phonological characteristics from speech sound errors. According to Iglesias and Anderson (1993), for example, a normal speaker of Black English can be expected to simplify a consonant cluster at the end of a word, especially when an alveolar consonant is involved (for example, "test" may be spoken as /tɛs/). Similarly, such features as the substitution of /f/ for /θ/ at the end of a word (/bæf/ for "bath") and the stopping of /ð/ at the beginning of a word (/diz/ for "these"), or the devoicing of final stops (/pɪk/ for "pig") are among the major phonological features that distinguish Black English from Standard American English (p. 149).

Moreover, it is not just phonological variations that complicate our task. Certain grammatical features also might be misinterpreted by the uninformed clinician. For example, the absence in Black English of a present tense, third person marker (as in "he play" for "he plays") might be misperceived as the omission of /z/ by a clinician who is not sensitive to dialectal differences. And, of course, Black English is just one of several variants of spoken English encountered by the practicing professional.

It is not possible to include more detailed information in this book, but we would urge interested students to review the thorough discussions of Black English and of other common dialects found in Battle (1993), Iglesias and Anderson (1993), and Proctor (1994). We close our own brief section with the following excerpt from Proctor's advice for speech-language pathologists.

> A phonological disorder is diagnosed after the SLP has accounted for presence/absence of structural and neurological problems . . . and has considered dialectal variations and/or the influence of another language. A disorder is present when the (speaker):
>
> 1. is unintelligible or displays reduced intelligibility to native speakers of the same speech community; (or)
> 2. misarticulates phonemes that are pronounced the same in (Standard American English) and the first dialect or language; (or)
> 3. produces idiosyncratic patterns that are not representative of the processes normally found in the first dialect/language, SAE, or as a function of borrowing or code switching. (1994, p. 216)

To this advice we would add only the reminder that, whatever the dialect may be, a speaker's own feelings about his or her speech pattern never are ignored by the true clinician.

TYPES AND CAUSES OF ARTICULATORY DISORDERS

There is a feeling of helplessness and inadequacy that appears when a person tries repeatedly to say sounds correctly and cannot. We vividly remember a woman who had spoken correctly all her life until being fitted with dentures that resulted in a high-pitched, shrill whistle every time she produced an /s/ sound. Each session used up a half box of our tissues as she wept her way through therapy. The dentist had done his utmost to revise the dentures to eliminate the strident lisp, but it was not until we taught her to anchor her tongue tip against her lower teeth as she made her sibilant sounds that the piercing whistle disappeared and she was unreluctant to go to the grocery store again.

Children, especially the younger ones, do not seem to be as sensitive, for our society tolerates more deviant sounds in a child than in an adult. Indeed, one of the major problems in helping children with articulatory errors, as we shall see, is that they do not recognize their mistakes. Nevertheless, there are some children who have been hurt very deeply by their jeering playmates or by parents who have "corrected" them blunderingly or cruelly and then rejected them when the inevitable failures occurred.

Disorders of articulation vary widely in severity, from speech that is almost entirely unintelligible to a tiny transitional lisp in which a *th* /θ/ sound precedes or follows the /s/ as in *sthoup* /sθup/ or *yeths* /jɛθs/. Generally, the more defective sounds that are exhibited by the client, the more severe will be the speech handicap. An articulatory error on a single sound can be quite noticeable, but when many standard sounds are defectively produced, there is also a marked decrease in intelligibility and this compounds the problem greatly.

As you will recall from Chapter 4, there are three basic ways in which speech sounds may be misarticulated: *omission* of sounds ('oup for soup), *substitution* of one standard sound for another (*th*oup for soup), and *distortion*, the substitution of a nonstandard sound for a standard one (a slushy, unvoiced /l/ for /s/). Some regard *addition* (/kəlin/ for clean) as a fourth way. The three more common types of sound errors, however, may be surface characteristics of delayed or deviant usage of underlying phonologic rules. They may reflect the incorrect way in which a child employs the various properties or features (distinctive features) that comprise speech sounds. From this point of view, individuals with articulation defects do not have "broken-down" sound production facility; on the contrary, careful phonologic analysis reveals that many do have coherent principles by which they organize speech sound production. Let us illustrate, by presenting a brief analysis of the most common of articulatory errors, the substitution.

Although on initial inspection, substitution errors may seem random, further observation usually will reveal a definite regularity. Which phoneme is substituted for another depends, in part, on how alike the sounds are—how much they *sound* alike and how much the *movements* that produce them are similar (see Figure 7-2). Rarely, for example, will the /z/ sound be substituted for the /w/; the /l/ is seldom replaced by the plosive /p/.

Articulation errors also exhibit regularity in another way: Not all phonemes are misarticulated with equal frequency. Those sounds that are

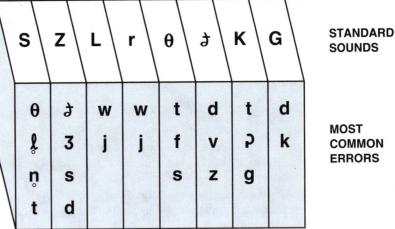

FIGURE 7-2
Common consonantal errors (most frequent substitutions)

more difficult motorically to utter, such as /s/, /θ/, /r/, and /l/, are among those most frequently in error. The sibilant sounds—/s/, /z/, /ʃ/, and /ʒ/—seem to be particularly difficult, and disorders of these phonemes are termed *lisps.* Clinicians recognize five types of lisps: (1) *frontal* or *interdental,* characterized by substitution of the /θ/ for /s/; (2) *lateral,* which features the substitution of an unvoiced, slushy /l/ for the sibilants; (3) an ***occluded lisp,*** the substitution of a /t/ sound for the /s/; (4) replacement of the /s/ with a nasal snort, a nasal lisp, and (5) a *strident, piercing whistle* in the place of the sibilant sounds.

But most workers prefer to look beneath the labels to see how an individual is using the sound system of the language. In this frame of reference, two main types of articulation disorders are recognized.

Phonetic disorders. The person cannot produce sounds acceptably because of anatomical, motor, or sensory impairments.

Phonological disorders. The person is capable of producing sounds but uses them inconsistently or not at all. Sound errors are due to incomplete learning of the rules of usage, and thus are linguistically or cognitively based.

As we have pointed out, it is sometimes difficult to differentiate phonetic from phonological disorders. Phonological or "functional" sound errors among school-aged children historically have absorbed a considerable portion of speech pathologists' professional energy. Consequently, in the next sections on cause, assessment, and treatment, we focus primarily upon these often enigmatic and difficult-to-remedy developmental disorders of articulation.

Occluded lisp.
The substitution of a /t/ or a /ts/ for the /s/, or the /d/ and /dz/ for the /z/.

Causes of Articulatory Disorders

Learning to produce phonemes correctly is just one aspect of language learning, and the causes or deterrents we have discussed in Chapter 6 are also present in disorders of articulation. It is difficult for the mentally impaired to do this learning. Hearing losses (even temporary ones) may prevent children from perceiving the models of the phonemes they need if they are to master them. Neurological damage, as in cerebral palsy, may lead to deficiencies in motor control that make the mastery of such motorically complicated phonemes as /r/, and /l/ a formidable task. Emotional problems, isolation, or the lack of a caring parent can also interfere with the necessary learning.

Structural Factors

Most of the research (Weiss, Gordon, and Lillywhite, 1997) seems to indicate that organic deviations of the tongue or other oral structures do not play an important part in the problems presented by most children with defective phonemes. Nevertheless, the speech pathologist finds some clients who seem to present an exception to this general rule. One of them was a child who had filled his mouth with lye, resulting in speech that was so slurred as to be almost unintelligible. His clinician noticed, however, that the child could elevate the middle and back of the scarred tongue to some degree. Accordingly, she formulated a therapy program in which the child was taught to speak with his teeth held together and to use the bulging middle of his tongue to produce pretty fair facsimiles of the front consonants. If you will try to talk with your teeth together and the tongue tip flat in the mouth you will see that it is possible to speak intelligibly this way if you speak very slowly and carefully, though some muffling occurs. Later therapy activities allowed the child to open his mouth more widely and took care of that problem.

In Figure 7-3 we see another child, one with a **frenum** so short that he found difficulty in learning his /l/, /r/, and /s/ sounds since he was unable to raise the tip of his tongue. This so-called "tongue-tie" is rarely found to play a part in an articulatory problem, but when it does the speech pathologist, of course, notes it on his diagnostic report and refers the client to a physician for surgery or plans a program for teaching compensatory ways of producing the sounds that are made incorrectly.

Figure 7-4 shows another person, a girl with a different organic problem, a severe **malocclusion,** who presented several error sounds, notably distortions of the /s/, /z/, /r/, and /l/, along with some unseemly facial contortions as she vainly tried to compensate for her extreme overbite. Underbite and openbite, two other common abnormal dental closures, are shown in Figure 7-5. One young adult with a severe underslung (prognathic) lower jaw made the /f/ and /v/ sounds by placing his lower in-

Frenum.
The white membrane below the tongue tip; also called frenulum.

Malocclusion.
An abnormal bite.

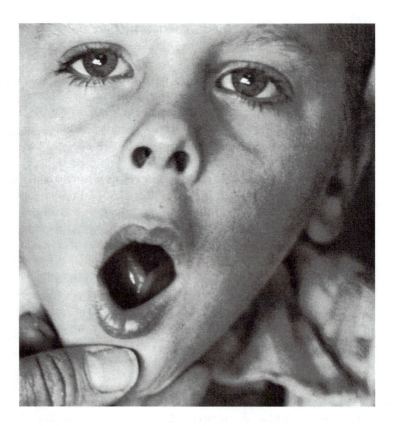

FIGURE 7-3   Tongue-tie
(ankyloglossia)

cisors on his upper lip. Try it while watching yourself in a mirror. It sounds
perfectly normal but looks grotesque. Although there is no systematic,
one-to-one relationship between malocclusions, missing or jumbled teeth,
and sound errors, clients who misarticulate—particularly lispers—seem to
have more dental abnormalities than do normal speakers.

Occasionally, speech pathologists have to work with clients who, because of cancer surgery, accident, or paralysis, have lost much of the tissue
or use of their tongues. These are often difficult clients to work with, but
we have found that they achieve good articulation when taught to compensate for their disabilities.

In addition to these abnormalities of the tongue or jaw we also have
the effects of clefts of the lip or palate. Palatal clefts in particular can result in articulation errors such as the "nasal lisp" and can also cause difficulty with other phonemes that require the momentary stoppage or
constriction of oral airflow. We will look more closely at oral clefts in a
later chapter.

Finally, although not a structural anomaly, *tongue thrusting* should be
mentioned. This type of swallowing behavior once was thought to be a

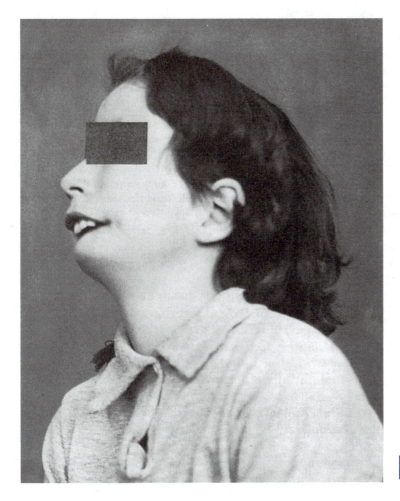

FIGURE 7-4
Distocclusion (overbite)

FIGURE 7-5   Other malocclusions:
(a) openbite, and (b) underbite or
mesiocclusion

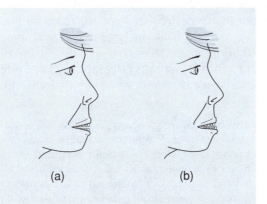

(a)   (b)

significant causal agent in the failure of many children to master their speech sounds. At the present time, however, few of our workers feel that tongue thrusting has much direct effect on speech, except perhaps when, in combination with other factors, it may contribute to sibilant difficulties in some youngsters.

Perceptual Deficiencies

As we have mentioned, many misarticulating children do not seem to recognize their errors and so they cannot correct them even when they are called to their attention. Does this mean that they have some basic deficiency in auditory perception? For example, do they have too short an auditory memory span?

To test for auditory memory span, the clinician speaks a series of digits, sounds, or nonsense syllables, then after a short period of silence asks the child to repeat what he has heard. His performance is then compared with the norms of normally speaking children. In our experience, very few of our clients have shown such deficiency and we know of no research that shows that it is an important factor.

Auditory Discrimination

Another possible perceptual deficiency that could interfere with the mastery of speech sounds involves the ability to recognize the essential differences between them. Much of the early research in auditory discrimination sought to discover whether misarticulating children possessed a general inability to distinguish between pairs of words that differ in one phoneme. "Tell me if they are the same or different: red, red; red, bed; red, led; red, red;" and so on.

The research indicates that no such general discrimination deficiency is characteristic of misarticulating clients but that they may have trouble telling the difference between their error sounds and the correct ones. Monnin says flatly "these children did not exhibit a general speech sound discrimination deficiency but showed a deficiency specific to their misarticulation" (1984, p. 6). Bernthal and Bankson agree that speech sound production errors in some children appear to be related to their faulty auditory perception of certain phonemic contrasts (1993, p. 102) and offer the following summary after thoroughly reviewing years of research in this area.

A relationship appears to exist between speech sound perception and articulation in subjects with impaired phonology although the precise nature of the relationship has not been determined. Self-monitoring of error productions would appear to be an important skill, but instruments to assess such a skill are lacking. Further data are needed to better understand the relationship between discrimination errors and articulation disorders. . . . (But) when perceptual deficiencies are present, perceptual training would seem appropriate (1993, p. 176).

How can this be? Why does the child have no general problem in phonetic discrimination but still cannot recognize his own articulatory errors even when they are brought to his attention? We feel that the answer is a simple one. The child does not recognize his errors because they have become habitual. They have become so automatic they have little stimulus value. His errors have become bound to the morphemes in which they are embedded. They are now integral parts of his words. We listen to the meanings of our utterances, not to the sounds we produce when speaking. Moreover, any phoneme lasts only a brief part of a second. For these reasons we are not surprised to learn that he has a specific, rather than a general problem in phonetic discrimination. Indeed, when we begin to help him, we will need to make that discrimination one of the first targets of therapy.

Developmental Factors

For a long time, speech clinicians suspected that functional articulation disorders might be associated with a more extensive language disability. In exploring a child's history, they sometimes found not only that he was delayed in the onset of the first words but also that he was a very quiet youngster showing little babbling or vocal play, or that his normally developing speech was suddenly interrupted by an extended plateau, or that he regressed to gesture or jargon or even became mute for a time. They observed, too, that many of the children in their caseloads were having difficulty in school with language-dependent skills—reading, spelling, and vocabulary comprehension. It was even more apparent that a common factor was involved because quite often both the articulation errors *and* other language skills improved with speech therapy.

So it came as no surprise to clinicians when research confirmed that many children with phonological disorders, especially those with multiple sound errors, did indeed have disturbances in syntax, vocabulary, and comprehension (Stoel-Gammon and Dunn, 1985). Since phonology is one facet of language, and since all the linguistic subsystems are closely interrelated, we might expect that developmental sound errors would be reflected in other aspects of language. There may be causal agents, perhaps intellectual or cognitive, that are common to all types of language disabilities, including phonological disorders.

As we have pointed out before, some sound errors, rather than stemming from inability to produce phonemes, are systematic rule-based behaviors. If there is no organic factor, then it may be rewarding to search for when and how a client's acquisition of the rules for phoneme use was disrupted. A speech clinician conducts this search by reviewing key developmental factors—a child's history, family situation, and psychosocial adjustment.

Since disorders of phonology have their origin in early childhood, we must know something of a child's past if we are to treat her intelligently. As we interview her parents, we are alert for environmental factors that could have hampered—or that still impede—a child's acquisition of speech sounds. To illustrate some of the case history data that a speech clinician assembles, we provide the following brief survey.

Parental and Family Influences

Names. The child's consonant productions might possibly be related to imitation of a parental dialect or to the learning of similar consonants belonging to another language. Family names may be a clue.

Age. When the age of the parents seems somewhat unusual in terms of the child's age, certain emotional factors may be influencing the latter's speech development. Thus, Peter, age seven, had parents aged twenty-two and twenty-four and (as we found out by following the clue) was an unwanted child, neglected, unstimulated, and untrained. His articulatory errors were easily understood against this background. Or consider Jane, who astonished her forty-nine-year-old father and forty-five-year-old mother by being born. Their excessive attention and demand for adult standards drove the child too early into a negativism that made her reject their constant corrections and persist in her errors.

Parental models. Imitation may be a causal factor in articulation, but we must be sure that the symptoms are similar. The father of a ten-year-old lateral lisper asked us to "fiksh up hish shonsh shpeech" with the same slushy sibilants shown by the child. It is often wise to explore to ascertain whether the parents had possessed a speech defect in their own childhood, since such an event would affect their attitudes toward the child's difficulty. What about the rate and complexity of the parent's speech—do they provide a model which is possible for a child to imitate? We overheard one parent, father of a kindergarten child with multiple sound errors, answer his son's inquiry (about a CB radio) with this response: "It is a polyelectronic communication device."

Home conditions. A knowledge of the home conditions, the tempo of the life lived therein, and the attitudes of family members is often vital to the understanding of the articulation problem. Conflicts between one parent and the other, or between parent and child, may create an unfavorable environment for speech learning. Speech development is not fostered by a critical, demanding environment or by one that fosters overdependence.

Development History

Physical development. When we learn that a child was delayed in sitting alone, in feeding himself, in walking, we usually probe to discover whether speech development was similarly retarded. Almost any factor that retards physical development also may retard speech. Many youngsters with sluggish tongues and palates have histories of slow physical development.

Illnesses. These have importance according to their severity and their aftereffects. Certain illnesses may so lower the child's vitality that he does not have the energy to learn the difficult skills of talking correctly. Prolonged illness may result in parental attitudes of overconcern or overprotection. The parents may anticipate the child's needs so that he learns to talk relatively late. If illness occurred during the first years of life, the child may not have had the necessary babbling practice.

Intelligence. Although mentally retarded children tend to have many articulation errors, within the range of normal mental ability there is only a limited relationship between intelligence and phonological disorders. Nevertheless, speech clinicians explore an individual case's intellectual capacity by testing and by investigating his performance in school.

Play. Children adopt the consonant errors as well as the grammatical errors of their playmates. In one instance, children from three different families in the neighborhood acquired a lisp by identification and imitation of a dominant older boy.

Emotional problems. There is no characteristic or typical personality disorder exhibited by individuals with developmental articulation problems. But we have seen individual cases whose speech sound errors stem from emotional immaturity. The list of emotional problems given in the case history can give us some indication of a child's reaction to his speech defect. The child who is always fighting, hurting pets, setting fires, or performing similar aggressive acts must be handled very differently from one who withdraws from the challenges of existence.

Patterns of Causation

It is very difficult to pin down the actual cause or causes in a specific case of articulatory disorder. Who can really know what happened long ago in a child's development that caused him to fail to learn the standard phonemes of his language? The many investigations dealing with causation have compared groups of persons with normal speech with those who exhibit misarticulation; but the cases were examined long after the errors became habituated, and all sorts of articulation problems were lumped together in the defective groups. However, the speech clinician must always investigate these causal agents in his clients because the lack of *group* differences does not always reflect the impact of certain factors in an *individual* case. For example, although children with articulation disorders generally cannot be distinguished from their normal-speaking peers in terms of tongue thrusting, we have seen a few youngsters whose sibilant distortions did seem to stem from such an abnormal swallowing pattern.

All things considered, the best advice we can offer is this: Rather than try to identify a single causal agent as the basis for a child's sound errors, look for a *pattern* of factors that have combined to disrupt the maturation of articulatory performance. An example from our clinical files illustrates this.

> Michael, age eight years, was evaluated recently and found to have multiple articulation errors. At the present time, his hearing is normal, he is doing well in school, and his home situation is unremarkable. The only suspicious finding is that the child scored on the slow end of normalcy with respect to oral motor skills. When we reviewed his history, however, it was noted that (1) Michael's father was absent from the home for almost a year when the child was three; (2) during his time his mother worked and an elderly relative, described as having "poor English," took care of him; and (3) he had a chronic middle-ear infection from the age of three until almost five. It is possible that the three factors mentioned, in combination with the slow normal oral motor function, interfered with the child's acquisition of speech sounds during the formative years between three and five.

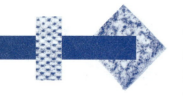

ANALYZING MISARTICULATIONS

Before any therapy begins, the client's repertoire of speech sound productions must be described in detail and then carefully studied for clues about possible causal factors and for information that can help us to design effective therapy strategies. Perhaps a first thing the experienced clinician will do, even as the relationship is being established, is to observe informally exactly that sounds are being omitted or incorrectly produced. A bystander might fail to recognize that this is going on as the clinician skillfully evokes enough speech to enable her to get a pretty good idea of the person's articulatory disability. We have been amused at the amazement expressed by student observers when at the end of such a casually conducted exploratory session, the clinician was able to identify not only all the defective sounds but many of the phonetic contexts in which the usually defective sound was uttered correctly. "How does she do it?" they ask us, and we answer by saying that as she was talking to the client her well-trained "phonetic ear" was probably scanning the client's speech against an internalized phonetic inventory of the common errors.

Nevertheless, no matter how skillful or experienced she is, the clinician administers more comprehensive and systematic tests as soon as she accepts the client for therapy (see Morrison and Schriberg, 1992). There are just too many sound combinations to assess through casual conversation alone, and a phoneme may be defective in one combination or phonetic context when it is correct in another. This is important information, since if the client is already able to produce the standard sound in some word positions or contexts, these can be used in treatment.

The Articulation Inventory

Although some speech pathologists construct their own test materials, we now possess several widely used instruments for determining proficiency in articulation. All of them employ pictures of common objects to elicit spontaneous speech. The pictures are chosen to test each of the English phonemes in the various positions within the word. In addition, most of these tests provide either sentences to be read or repeated or stories to be retold, and they include other materials that will elicit samples of connected speech.

Diagnostic articulation inventories are not really tests, but sets of pictures, words, nonsense syllables, or reading materials that can be used to elicit speech samples to be analyzed for error. Both spontaneous and imitative responses may be demanded, because if a child can match the clinician's model through imitation and thereby produce a correctly articulated sound or word that he usually misarticulates, the prognosis seems to be better than if the child does not seem to profit from such stimulation. The test items present each phoneme as it would occur in the initial (the beginning) position of words, as well as the medial and final positions. In most of these tests, there are sufficient items containing the phonemes most frequently misarticulated (the /s/, /l/, /r/, /θ/, and their blends) so that if the client happens to say a specific phoneme correctly on a given test word but makes errors when it occurs in others, this can be ascertained. It's good to know that he can say it right on the test word, but we must also make sure that his mastery of the phoneme is complete. Almost anyone could administer these articulation tests, but it takes training before one is able to identify the inconsistencies and recognize and record the kinds of errors that are produced. The real test, in a diagnostic sense, refers to the evaluation process of the listener, not to the stimulus pictures. The clinician is the diagnostic instrument.

Description of the Errors.   Following the administration of an articulation inventory, the clinician next undertakes a phonemic analysis. This procedure identifies three things: (1) the sounds that are in error, (2) the type of errors—omissions, substitutions, distortions, or possibly additions—and (3) the location of the errors—the initial, medial, or final positions. Figure 7-6 presents an articulation inventory record sheet summarizing some of the findings of an evaluation done with a nine-year-old boy.

Generally, the more defective phonemes shown by a client the more she will be handicapped, and so the speech pathologist's report of the diagnostic examination will always show how many there are and what they are. When a child has not mastered eight or nine of the phonemes of our language, the clinician knows that a lot of work is ahead. Nevertheless, she is also vitally interested in the kinds of errors that have been revealed by

Phoneme	I	M	F
k	√	√	√
g	√	√	√
l	√	√	√
d	√	√	√
t	√	√	√
j	√	√	√
f	√	√	√
v	√	√	√
s	t	θ	—
z	d	ð	ð
r	×	×	×
ʃ	s	s	s
ð	d	d	d
θ	t	t	t
ʧ	ʃ	ʃ	ʃ
ʤ	d	d	d
ɝ	×	×	×

√ = The sound was produced correctly
— = The sound was omitted
t/s = Substitutions are recorded phonetically
× = The sound was distorted

FIGURE 7-6 Articulation Inventory Record Sheet

her testing since certain types of errors are more difficult to eradicate than others. The distorted sibilants of lateral lisping, for example, are usually more difficult to correct than the substitution of a *th* /θ/ for the /s/ in a child with an interdental lisp. The same holds true for the distorted /r/ and /l/ sounds, which are usually difficult to remedy. A child who substitutes a /t/ for the /k/ should have less trouble conquering that error than one who replaces the /k/ with a little coughlike glottal fricative. It is necessary, therefore, to scrutinize and analyze the articulatory errors.

In the analysis of misarticulations the clinician first defines the *nature of the error*. Is it one of substituting another phoneme for the correct sound? For example, does the child use a /t/ for the /k/, saying /tæt/ instead of *cat*? Or does he produce a distorted /s/, saying it with the slushy, nonstrident sound of the lateral lisp? Or does he omit a sound that should be present, saying /kul/ instead of *school*? Or, perchance, does he insert a sound that should not be present, as in /bəlu/ for *blue*? Again, these are the major types of articulation errors, *substitution, distortion, omission*, and occasionally *addition*.

Consistency of the Errors

Speech sound errors are not always consistent by any means. Sometimes the client may misarticulate a sound only when it begins (releases) a syllable but not when it ends (or arrests) the syllable. One of our clients was unable to get the first /s/ right in the word *sauce* but always said the final /s/ correctly. We knew then we could use that syllable-arresting /s/ as a nucleus of therapy. When a child already makes the sound correctly in certain words, or syllables, or in certain phonetic contexts, it is much easier to help her than if she always misarticulates that sound. Interestingly, we've found error sounds being produced quite correctly in words that had been added to the child's vocabulary more recently than were the earlier-acquired and usually misarticulated words.

Phonetic Context

The speech pathologist is always alert to notice whether an error sound may be spoken correctly when preceded or followed by certain other sounds. Adjacent sounds influence each other, sometimes quite dramatically, because the posture and other features of a phoneme are adjusted in the direction of the posture and other features of the phoneme that precedes (and/or follows) it. Accordingly, a child may be able to produce /k/ more correctly in the syllable /ku/ than in /ki/, because the /u/ requires the lifting of the back part of the tongue and so does the /k/.

By discovering such nuggets of correctly produced sounds, the clinician knows that he can use them in deciding that of them he will use as first "targets" and what types of nonsense syllables or what words will be easier for his client to master.

An instrument that sometimes has been used for locating these facilitative phonetic contexts is McDonald's *Deep Test of Articulation* (1968). Two pictures are shown to the child, who is asked to name them. Then he is asked to make a "funny big word" by combining them (for example: mouse, tree, mou*setr*ee; cat, sun, ca*ts*un). The two words are to be said without pausing between them. Sixty such pairs of pictures provide enough sampling so that a favorable phonetic context often can be identified. The procedure followed in this test can be useful, even if the test itself is not employed.

Stimulability

Some children are able to correctly pronounce their error sounds when they are strongly stimulated to do so, especially when saying those sounds in isolation or in nonsense syllables. Therefore, the speech pathologist al-

Deep testing.
The exploration of an individual's ability to articulate a large number of words, all of which include one specific sound, to discover those in which that sound is spoken correctly.

ways tests to see if the child can do this. She may also find that certain nonsense syllables will elicit the correct sound when others will not primarily because the phonetic contexts are favorable. Thus one child was able to repeat the syllables, *seeta* /sitə/, *saeno* /sæno/, and *eensi* /insi/, correctly though others such as *cass* /kæs/ and *musay* /muse/, were not correctly spoken. In general, if the isolated error sound can be correctly produced, after strong stimulation, or in many nonsense syllables, the prognosis is very favorable and the client should make rapid progress.

Conditions of Communication

The clinician seeks to determine if certain conditions of the communication increase or decrease the probability of misarticulation. She examines the speed of utterance, since many children produce more errors when speaking rapidly. She investigates to see if they have fewer errors in oral reading. Does the verbalization of negative emotion show more error? Does the child show fewer misarticulations when talking to authority figures such as the teacher than he does in conversing with his playmates?

Kinetic Analysis of Errors

It may not be difficult for the clinician to recognize errors of substitution, omission, distortion, or addition; but especially when the client produces distortions, we must do more than simply record them as such. The speech pathologist makes an analysis of the articulation errors themselves, a **kinetic analysis.** It is important to know that sounds are being misuttered, but we need also to know *how* they are being produced. The label "lisp" is a *phonetic* term; the modifying adjectives "lateral," "occluded," "interdental," or "nasal" are *kinetic* terms. They describe how the error is being made.

Let us consider the distorted /s/ sounds characteristic of the lateral lisper. Acoustically, they lack the stridency of the correctly produced /s/ sound. They sound slushy yet they are not /ʃ/ sounds. Motorically, the tongue fails to make the narrow groove down which the airflow goes to the teeth. In one type of lateral lisp the groove is just too wide; in the other, the tongue tip is anchored to the alveolar ridge and the air flows around both sides of the tongue. Hissing noises are produced by either action but the hiss is not high enough in its pitch. The clinician uses diacritical marks in recording these differences. For the distorted /s/ produced by too wide a groove, she records the distortion as /ŝ/; for the one where the air flows around the side of the upraised tongue she records it as /ḻ/, the tiny circle underneath the /l/ meaning that the sound is really an unvoiced, breathy /l/ sound.

Distortions are really allophones of the standard sound, but ones that lie beyond the boundaries of that standard sound. Any sound has many

Kinetic analysis.
The analysis of error sounds in terms of their movement patterns.

variants, but as long as they remain within the boundaries of that sound, they are permissible. Lateral lisps are allophones of the /s/ but they deviate too far from the norm to be acceptable.

Other phonemes, notably the /r/ and /l/ sounds, are also distorted by some of our clients, but the basic analysis is similar. The clinician analyzes how the distorted sound is produced and records it by diacritical marks.

Each of the speech sounds can be incorrectly produced in several ways. The most frequent error of such *stop plosives* as k and g seems to be due to (1) the wrong location of the tongue contact. Other errors include (2) the wrong speed in forming the contacts, (3) the wrong structures used in contacts, (4) the wrong force or tension of the contacts, (5) too short a duration of the contacts, (6) too slow a release from contacts, (7) the wrong mode or direction of release, (8) the wrong direction of the air stream, and finally, (9) sonancy errors in which voiced and unvoiced consonants are interchanged. Examples of these errors are described below.

1. The child who says "tandy" for "candy" is using a tongue-palatal contact, but it is too far forward.
2. A breathy k sound [xki] for [ki] results when the contact is formed so slowly that fricative noises are produced prior to the air puff.
3. A glottal catch or throat click [ʔæt] for [kæt] is often found in cleft-palate cases. These people make a contact, but with the wrong structures.
4. Insufficient tension of the lips can result in the substitution of a sound similar to the Spanish *v* for the standard English *b* sound.
5. When the duration of the contact is too short, it often seems to be omitted entirely. Thus the final k in the word *sick* [sɪk] may be formed so briefly that acoustically it seems omitted [sɪ].
6. Too slow a release from the contact may give an aspirate quality to the utterance. *Kuheep the cuhandy* [kʰip ðə kʰændɪ] is an example of this.
7. The lowering of the tongue tip prior to recall of the tongue as a whole can produce such an error as *tsen* for *ten* [tsɛn] for [tɛn]. In this error the client is not inserting an *s* so much as releasing the tongue from its contact in a peculiar fashion.
8. Occasionally the direction of the airstream is reversed and the plosion occurs on inhalation. Try saying "sick" with the k sound produced during inhalation, and you will demonstrate this error.
9. The person who says "back" for "bag" illustrates a sonancy error.

Most of the errors in making the *continuant* sounds are caused by (1) use of the wrong channel for the airstream (using an unvoiced *l* for the *s*), (2) use of the wrong construction or constriction ("foop" for "soup"), (3) use of the wrong aperture, (a lateral lisp), (4) use of the wrong direction of the airstream (nasal lisp, inhaled *s*), (5) too weak an air pressure (acoustically omitted *s*), (6) the presence of nonessential movements or contacts (*t* for *s*, occluded lisp), and (7) cognate errors (*z* for *s*, or vice versa).

Most of the errors in making the *glide* sounds are produced by combining the types of errors just sketched. They may be generally classed as movement errors. They include (1) use of the wrong beginning position or contact ("yake" for "lake"); (2) use of the wrong ending position [fɪʊ] for [fɪr]; (3) use of the wrong transitional movement in terms of speed, strength, or direction [rweɪd] for [reɪd]; (4) the presence of nonessential contacts or positions [tjɛloʊ] for [jɛloʊ]; (5) **cognate** errors [wɛn] for [hwɛn].

It is helpful to analyze any given articulation error according to this scheme to understand its nature. It is not sufficient merely to start teaching the correct sound. We must also break the old habit. Many of our most difficult articulatory cases will make rapid progress as soon as they understand clearly what they are doing wrong. Insight into error is fundamental to efficient speech correction.

Patterns of Errors

Finally, the clinician looks over the inventory of misarticulated phonemes to see if she can discover patterns of usage. If she finds this pattern: s/z, f/v, k/g, and so on, it shows that all these errors are alike in one respect. The child is substituting the unvoiced sound for its voiced counterpart. This is important information because once the child learns the contrasts of voiced and unvoiced sounds, he should be able to correct not just one but all of these errors.

Similarly, the clinician may find that many of the child's errors involve the substitution of a stop plosive for a continuant sound, saying /tup/ for *soup*, /bælɛtaɪn/ for *valentine*, /tu/ for *shoe*, and /pæn/ for *fan*. His basic error may not be that he cannot produce the sounds he misarticulates but that he fails to recognize the fact that some sounds must be prolonged to be correct. He needs to learn the contrasts between stops and continuants.

These are but two of the many error patterns that may be discovered. Especially in a child who has multiple phonemic errors or is barely intelligible the speech pathologist performs what is termed a linguistic analysis.

Linguistic Analysis

Linguistic analysis shifts the focus from the child's specific error sounds ("surface errors") to a much more detailed exploration of patterns and underlying rules by which the child's phonology is organized. This exploration, which looks closely at *distinctive features* and *phonological processes*, is undertaken when there are so many error sounds that child's speech is

Cognate.
Referring to pairs of sounds that are produced motorically in much the same way, one being voiced **(sonant)** and the other unvoiced **(surd)**. Some cognates are /t/ and /d/, /s/, and /z/.

Sonant.
A voiced sound.

Surd.
Unvoiced sound such as the *s* as opposed to its cognate *z*, which is voiced or sonant.

largely unintelligible. There is little if anything to be gained by doing such detailed analyses when a child has only a few misarticulated phonemes to be corrected; but when the disorder is more severe, the results of linguistic analyses can help us to devise more efficient therapy strategies.

Here we can take only a brief look at this topic, but many writers, including Hodson and Paden (1983), Bernthal and Bankson (1993), and Lowe (1994), provide detailed discussions of linguistics-based analyses.

Distinctive Features. Speech sounds are composed of a number of properties that linguists call *features*. Here, for example, is a partial list of features that comprise the phonemes /s/ and /z/.

/S/	Features	/Z/
(−)	*nasal* (nasal resonance)	(−)
(+)	*continuant* (minimum blockage of air stream)	(+)
(+)	*strident* (friction sound)	(+)
(−)	*voice* (vocal cords function)	(+)

Note two things: (1) The features are binary, either present (+) or absent (−), and (2) the phonemes /s/ and /z/ differ by only one attribute—voicing. When particular features serve to differentiate one speech sound from another, they are said to be distinctive.

When a child shows multiple sound errors, the speech pathologist is interested in their patterning, for she knows that many of them may reflect the child's failure to discern or to produce certain of the distinctive features that characterize the phonemes he does not produce correctly. Pollack and Rees (1972, p. 453) describe the phonological analysis in terms of four questions: (1) Is a specific feature totally absent from the child's repertoire? (2) Does a feature appear in combination with one or more other features but not in combination with a different feature or set of features? (3) Are all the features present but inappropriately incorporated into the child's phonemic system depending upon positional variables within a morpheme or word? (4) Are all the features pertinent to a specific phoneme present in one phonetic context (independent of position within the morpheme or word) but absent in another?

Let us give just one example of the usefulness of this sort of analysis.

One of the children with whom we worked never uttered any of the following phonemes correctly /s/, /z/, /θ/, /ð/, /f/, and /v/. Instead, she used various stop plosives as their replacements or omitted them entirely. For the sibilants, she substituted a /t/ or /d/; for the labiodentals she used /p/ or /b/; for the affricates she substituted a /k/ or /g/. A distinctive feature that was missing in all these misarticulations was that of stridency, so instead of teaching one sound after another, we concentrated on teaching the girl to hiss and whistle and buzz, then to recognize the stridency feature in our own speech as we prolonged these sounds when we talked with her. Then we asked her to imitate us and to talk as we did in this peculiar way. As soon as she could do so with some adequacy, we then concentrated first on the /f/ and /v/ sounds and next on the /s/ and /z/ until when she spoke carefully she could speak words containing these sounds without error. Progress was very rapid thereafter and we never did have to teach her how to make the other phonemes. Once she had gotten the idea that some sounds had to have the little noises of stridency in them if they were to be spoken correctly, she then could apply the principle to all other sounds that required this distinctive feature.

One of the drawbacks of the distinctive feature approach is the plus-minus classification system. Since the act of articulation is a multi-positional, not a binary, function, many clinicians prefer the traditional three-part system of speech sound classification, namely, *place* and *manner* of articulation, and *voicing*.

Phonological Processes

Young children learning to speak use certain strategies, called **natural processes,** to simplify adult speech patterns. They seem to do this *naturally* (no one teaches them) because they have immature, and therefore limited, motor capabilities. Typically, children systematically (the simplifications are not random) alter mature speech models by deleting syllables and sounds or by substituting easier-to-produce sounds for more difficult ones. No doubt you have observed these two common natural processes: *deleting weak syllables* ('*nana* for *banana*) and *fronting* (*t*ake for *c*ake). A phonological process, then, is a way of describing how children attempt to duplicate adult speech. Here are only a few of the many other natural processes that have been identified (see Khan, 1982, for a description of sixteen natural processes).

> *Deletion Processes*
> Cluster reduction: [prɪŋ] for "spring"
> Stridency deletion: [tap] for "stop"
>
> *Substitution Processes*
> Stopping: [tup] for "soup"
> Gliding: [wæbɪt) for "rabbit"
>
> *Assimilation Processes*
> Alveolar assimilation: [dɔdi] for "doggie"
> Velar assimilation: [gɔgi] for "doggie"

A child who has the substitutions t/d, k/g, s/z, and f/v does not really have four errors but only one, the failure to recognize or produce the distinctive feature of *voicing*. As soon as he learns that some sounds must be voiced rather than unvoiced he may be able to produce all four of those sounds correctly.

Another phonological process often used by misarticulating children is *fronting*. They substitute t/k, d/g, and /n/ for /ŋ/, using consonants that require lifting the front of the tongue rather than the back.

Natural processes. Strategies used by children to simplify adult speech patterns.

Still another group of errors involving the s, z, f, v, /θ/ and /ʃ/ is due to the child's failure to recognize the distinctive feature of *continuancy*. All these sounds must be prolonged (continued) but the child does not recognize this distinctive feature and so says /tup/ for *soup*, /tɛbɛn/ for *seven* and /tu/ for *shoe*. She uses stop consonants to replace the continuants. The phonological process here is called *stopping*.

For reasons yet unknown, some children persist in using these simplification patterns long after they should have acquired more mature articulation (Shriberg, 1987). A few children have *deviant* rather than *delayed* phonology; they show idiosyncratic processes that are never found in normal phonological development (for example, the substitution of sibilant sounds such as s, z, etc. for stops such as t, d, etc.)

The speech pathologist's task is to analyze the child's defective speech and to reduce his sound errors to a small number of underlying patterns. Basically, this involves grouping the client's errors into clusters and then describing the general "rule" or "rules" by which he organizes his use of speech sounds. Here is an example of how a clinician wrote a rule for a child who deleted final stop phonemes (Emerick and Haynes, 1986, p. 180):

$$
\left.\begin{array}{l} p \\ b \\ t \\ d \\ k \\ g \end{array}\right\} \longrightarrow \phi \ / \ CV\_\_\# \qquad 80\text{–}100\%
$$

This rule says that the consonants p, b, t, d, k, and g are deleted in the context of the CVC word (for example, /mɪ/ for "mitt") when the target sound is at the end. The slash stands for "in the context of," the blank represents the location of the target sound, and # refers to a word boundary. Note that the percentage of occurrence is indicated after the rule.

Some diagnosticians use conventional articulation inventories to identify natural processes since apparently it doesn't matter how the sample is obtained. In addition, a number of manuals specifically designed for assessing articulation errors from a phonological process frame of reference are available.

We should note in closing this section that the complex tasks of examining linguistic characteristics and organizing the results thereof promises to become somewhat less tedious by virtue of computer-assisted analysis procedures. Several such software programs have been developed and continue to be refined (Bernthal and Bankson, 1993).

CORRECTING MISARTICULATIONS

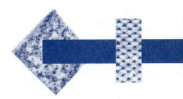

Once the speech pathologist has performed the diagnostic procedures described in the preceding section of this chapter, his next task is to design a tentative plan that takes into account the findings of that diagnosis. We use the word "tentative" because there will always be a need for revisions as the therapy proceeds. New information always comes in during the course of therapy and the clinician must always make adjustments to the treatment plan.

The Therapy Goals

Nevertheless, there are certain goals and subgoals that are to be found in all articulation therapy no matter how it is done or what strategies are used to enable it to be successful:

1. The client must become aware of the characteristics of the standard phonemes that serve as the targets of therapy and recognize how his misarticulations differ from those target sounds. Many, but not all, forms of treatment employ some *sensori-perceptual training* to assist a client in listening for his errors and comparing them with normal speech.
2. He must discover how to produce the standard phonemes at will. This second goal is termed *production* or *establishment* of the target sounds.
3. He must **stabilize** or strengthen the use of the standard phonemes in isolation (/sssss/), in syllables (/sa/, /isi/, /os/), and in words and phrases and sentences.
4. Finally, the client should be able to use the target sounds in spontaneous speech of all kinds and under all conditions. This latter objective is usually included under the terms *transfer, maintenance,* or *carryover.*

There are differing points of view concerning the most appropriate way in which to structure the learning and unlearning process that takes place in articulation therapy. Our clients learn in different ways. For some, the cognitive kind of learning (in which the clinician structures the training so that vital insights can be achieved) seems most useful. Other clients learn the standard speech sounds more readily when the learning process is highly structured as when operant conditioning procedures are employed. Clinicians, as well as clients, show preferences for one or another of these approaches and so they design the kind of therapy that suits their own needs and competence. We suspect that most speech pathologists are eclectic and will use whatever learning strategy seems most promising in terms of the client's personality, motivation, perceptiveness, and response to different kinds of trial therapy. Moreover, it is possible to use different kinds of learning procedures at different phases of the treatment. Often, for example, in training a child to produce a phoneme that he has never made correctly, we have used the cognitive approach, then shifted to operant conditioning when we wished to strengthen the new sound or to extinguish the habitual errors that he no longer needs to make.

Stabilization.
The process of making a response permanent and unfluctuating.

The Target Sounds.   If a client has only one misarticulated phoneme, it is, of course, the first target of therapy. However, most of our clients have more than one error, and so some decisions must be made. Few speech pathologists do what most parents do—try to correct all of the defective sounds at the same time. Instead, they decide to work on only one or a few of them with similar features (such as the cognates /s/ and /z/ or the /f/ and /v/ in which the manner of production is similar except for the feature of voicing). Many workers try to select a phoneme or phonemes that, if mastered, will facilitate generalized improvement to other sounds in the same class. Usually (1) they select as the first targets those phonemes that occasionally in certain phonetic contexts (as revealed by deep testing) are already produced correctly; (2) they choose phonemes whose coordinations are relatively simple (if a child has difficulty with the /r/, /l/, and /f/, they would begin with the /f/); or (3) they choose the sound that responds most readily to strong stimulation (if the child with /θ/ and /s/ errors can imitatively produce the /θ/ sound in isolation or a nonsense syllable but cannot make a good sibilant when imitating the clinician's /s/, that clinician would probably start therapy with the /θ/); or, (4) of a number of defective phonemes, they choose those that are acquired earlier by normal children over those that usually develop later (a misarticulated /k/ or /g/ sound would be worked with before an affricate such as the /ʤ/). The clinician has to use her own judgment as to the importance of these priorities and at times disregard them altogether if other critical factors are present.

> We worked with a little boy who had been teased unmercifully because he could not say his own name—Rodney. Although he had many other defective sounds that might have been easier to teach, that he could produce after stimulation, and use correctly in a few words, we chose instead to begin with the /r/. Once he had mastered it and was able to use it in his own name, the progress with all his other misarticulations was rapid. This illustrates again that motivation may be the most important factor of all in choosing the first target sounds.

Modes of Therapy

As we pointed out earlier, articulation therapy can take many forms. We have chosen to focus upon two prominent contemporary methods very briefly and then show how most clinicians combine many strategies in a traditional format of treatment.

The Behavior Modification Approach.   Many speech pathologists use operant conditioning procedures in their articulation therapy. Since we have presented the basic rationale for this approach in our chapter on language disorders, we shall not repeat this information here. However, we wish to emphasize that all the goals and activities described in this chapter may be programmed according to the methodology of operant conditioning.

Were you to observe a speech pathologist using the operant approach in helping a child to recognize the difference between the correct sound and its error, you might see him presenting paired sounds, syllables, or words and giving the child a marble for each time (or every three times) the child correctly identifies that they are the same or different and then later letting the child choose a small prize in exchange for those marbles. You would note that the speech pathologist has set up a hierarchy of discrimination tasks, beginning with the easy ones and then proceeding to those more difficult. He will establish **baselines** and then chart the child's progress as the criterion for each subsequent step is successfully accomplished. At times, when the task seems too difficult (e.g., in identifying the clinician's deliberate errors in conversational speech), the program will be revised or *branched* with additional substeps until the child can again be successful and get his reinforcing tokens. Occasionally, the clinician will use *prompts* (helpful comments or suggestions) to keep the child progressing. As the child's performance improves, the worker will gradually *fade out* her prompts and verbal modeling. At various times in therapy, the clinician will also *probe* (test performance in untreated situations, tasks) to determine if the client's improvement is generalizing.

Speech clinicians have been using similar techniques for years, but the programs used by the operant workers are much more systematized and objective. There is little doubt that behavior modification, with its emphasis on behavioral objectives and precision recording, has been of inestimable assistance to clinicians who must fulfill the accountability requirements in public schools and other work settings. Efficiency, however, may be achieved at the loss of effectiveness, to say nothing of the satisfaction for both the client and the worker.

> For these children, the efficient stimulus-response paradigms of behaviorism were not effective. The children did not like to "drill," no matter what the payoff. Moreover, the management structures were not all satisfying for the speech-language clinicians. (Shriberg and Kwiatkowski, 1982, p. 245)

There is no doubt that such programs can help a client identify the distinctive features of the correct phoneme and to recognize his errors. However, in contrast to its use in facilitating discrimination, the application of operant conditioning methods in helping a person acquire a new sound initially has been less successful. Although some individuals are able to produce the correct sound as soon as they can tell the difference between it and its error, this is not usually the situation. Far too many persons just cannot discover by themselves the necessary coordinations that will produce it. If a lateral lisper, for example, never emits a normal sibilant, it is obvious that we have nothing that can be reinforced. Punishing

Baseline.
An initial level of response prior to conditioning.

such a person for his errors usually just makes the matter worse. In such a situation, programs are designed that involve what is called *shaping*. A chain of target responses is set up, beginning with a sound the person can already produce, and then gradually progressing through a series of slight modifications that more and more resemble the standard sound. At each stage in the sequence, the patient is reinforced for successful production until that particular component sound in the chain is learned. Then this production is no longer reinforced and the client gets his reinforcement only when he varies his attempts enough to achieve the next transitional target sound. By working through this series of transitional sounds, the standard sound is finally acquired. We discuss and illustrate this shaping process later under the heading of "progressive approximation."

Linguistic Approaches.   Some speech pathologists set as their first targets not the learning of the correct forms of one or two phonemes, but instead the discrimination and production of distinctive features. These workers feel that the child either has not learned the rules that govern our phonology or has learned improper rules of his own. They, therefore, seek to help the child discover these rules, to recognize the distinctive features that he omits or replaces with others.

The basic point of view of these linguistically oriented clinicians is that the child does not need to learn how to make specific phonemes. The relevant unit of language, according to distinctive feature theory, is the feature or sound property. The proper focus for therapy, therefore, should be distinctive features, not phonemes. The assumption is that once he is trained to discriminate and produce appropriately the distinctive features he needs in order to speak correctly, all the misarticulations containing these feature errors will tend to be discarded. As McReynolds and Bennett (1972) long ago have stated and demonstrated, "If an error is a feature error, it should not be necessary to train the feature in all the phonemes in which it is relevant. The feature should generalize to other phonemes without specific training on each one" (p. 204).

But just how does the clinician administer the distinctive feature approach? McReynolds and Bennett (1972) describe their procedures as follows. First the child was taught to produce the desired feature in the initial (the beginning) position of a nonsense syllable. In these syllables the feature was discriminated and then produced through imitation. Stridency, for example, was taught on the /s/ phoneme in these syllables, then generalized to other strident phonemes. Contrasts between strident and nonstrident phonemes or productions of the same phoneme were made vivid by the clinician and taught to the child using the operant approach. Then the same procedure was used with the phoneme in the final position of nonsense syllables and words.

The *minimal-contrast* approach devised by Blache and Parsons (1980) commences on the word level. Since the function of speech sounds is to make words different, they reason, the treatment should focus on contrasts that signal changes in meaning. A child is shown that the minimal contrast of voicing, for example, in the words "bat" and "pat," distinguishes a wooden stick from an affectionate touch. Their program has four steps.

> First, the child must *understand* that two contrasting words differ in meaning. The child must have the concept behind a word pair.
>
> Second, the child should be able to *hear* that the two words are different. The clinician names pictures (pin-bin; peek-beak) and the child points to the items named.
>
> Third, the child must produce the words in response to the pictures or objects. In this step, the child now names one picture of the word pair. If the child makes an error, the worker may explain or show him how to produce the sound correctly.
>
> The last step involves using the words in communication situations outside of therapy.

The phonological approach stresses the *conceptual* (rather than the motor or production) aspects of speech sounds. By this we mean that the primary focus of therapy is to lead the child to see how word meaning is altered by sound contrasts. The youngster must come to realize that the word "cake" when uttered "take" (as in *fronting*) denotes something quite different.

Now we provide a final glimpse of phonological-based therapy by including a draft of a treatment plan prepared by a clinical supervisor for a team of student clinicians.

> Client: Alex McGuffie, age 5.3
> Sound errors: *t/s, d/z, p/f, b/v, t/θ,* and *d/ð*
> Phonological rule: *stopping*
> Target sounds: *f, v, s*
> Therapy procedures:
> 1. Auditory bombardment. At the beginning and end of each session, read lists of words containing the target sound to the child; use auditory amplification.
> 2. Establish meaningful minimal contrasts. Prepare lists of words that differ only by the target sounds, for example:
>
>   sip/tip   for *t/s*
>   see/tea
>
>   pat/fat   for *p/f*
>   pit/fit
>
> Then follow this training sequence:
>   a. Alex points to the picture of a word pair named by the clinician.
>   b. Alex repeats the target sound correctly in a word pair after the clinician models it.

      c. Alex names a picture without the clinician's model.

      d. Alex uses the correct production in a carrier phrase ("This is _____").

      e. Alex uses the correct production in a sentence modeled by the clinician.

      f. Alex uses the correct production in sentences of his own.

   3. You will want to review the treatment programs prepared by Monahan (1984; 1986) and Tyler, Edwards, and Saxman (1987) for additional information and procedures on conceptual training.

Our brief and oversimplified treatment of linguistic approaches to the correction of misarticulations cannot begin to do justice to these methodologies; so, again, we would urge our readers to explore other references (such as Bernthal and Bankson, 1993) that focus specifically and at length on this topic.

Traditional Therapy

Most speech pathologists do not confine themselves to either the operant or linguistic approaches we have described, although they may employ some of the procedures from each for special purposes in therapy. For example, they may use the distinctive feature approach when this seems appropriate to the discrimination difficulties of a child as he compares and contrasts the characteristics of the standard sound and its error. And again, they may use operant conditioning procedures only for strengthening and stabilizing a newly acquired standard phoneme. Or they may use neither. In the "traditional" approach to therapy, the speech clinician borrows and adapts procedures from a number of different methods to implement her objectives.

The hallmark of traditional articulation therapy lies in its sequencing of activities for (1) sensory-perceptual training, which concentrates on identifying the standard sound and discriminating it from its error through scanning and comparing; (2) varying and correcting the various productions of the sound until it is produced correctly; (3) strengthening and stabilizing the correct production; and finally, (4) transferring the new speech skill to everyday communication situations. This process is usually carried out first for the standard sound in isolation, then in the syllable, then in a word, and finally in sentences.

When the senior author first began to work with clients with articulation problems in the early 1930s, two main approaches were being used. In the first of these, the clinician, after some preliminary relaxation and breathing and tongue exercises, through diagrams and demonstration, provided a model and then demanded that the client say the word or phrase just as she did. That was all. A single word was presented by the clinician; the child tried to say it correctly through imitation. If he failed, the clinician said "no" and tried again. If he failed again, another word was attempted. The early texts were full of word lists to be used as drill material.

The other approach did not use tongue or breathing exercises but instead employed intensive stimulation with correct words produced by the clinician. A lisper for instance, might spend the whole session responding to the clinician's commands: "See, saw, so, sue. Say *see*. See, saw, so, sue. Say *so*." Once we watched a clinician bedevil a poor boy with this procedure for an hour and he never did say any of those four stimulus words correctly. A variant of this had the clinician produce and prolong the isolated /s/ sound using different degrees of loudness or duration and then asking the child to imitate her as she pronounced a word with a prolonged initial /s/ sound. These early techniques were so utterly boring and ineffective that in 1939 we devised the different approach now called *Traditional Articulation Therapy*, although at the time it seemed radical. Nevertheless, although it has changed over the years, as Secord (1989) has written, it has stood the test of time and is still more widely used than any other method.

This traditional approach is based on the belief that the client's articulation errors have become so fixed, reinforced, and automatized by the time he comes for help that not only does he not recognize them but also that he does not know how to produce the correct phonemes. Moreover, for the same reason, it seemed to be wiser to teach him first to make the new sound in isolation or in nonsense syllables rather than in words. Also, we recognized that once a client has been able to produce the correct sound, it would be weak and need to be strengthened if it were to win the competition with an error that has had a long history of usage. Finally, it seemed to us that instead of trying to correct all the errors at once we should concentrate our efforts on only one or two target sounds at a time. In selecting the target(s) we follow the guidelines already presented.

Operational Levels.   The mastering of a new sound so that it can be used in all types of speaking may be viewed in terms of four successive levels: (1) the isolated sound level, (2) the sound in a syllable, (3) the sound in a word, and (4) the sound in a meaningful sentence. This is the staircase our patients must climb. Once they have reached the top step of this staircase they find a wide platform on which they must explore the communicative, thinking, social control, and egocentric functions of speaking, using the newly mastered sound in each (see Figure 7-7).

With such a concept, it is possible for both clinician and client to know just where the latter is at each moment during therapy and to know what has been achieved and what remains to be accomplished.

At each level we use perceptual training to enable the child to identify, locate, and discriminate his error sounds from their targets. At each level we teach the client to produce the sound correctly, then to stabilize or strengthen it, and finally to use it in other contexts.

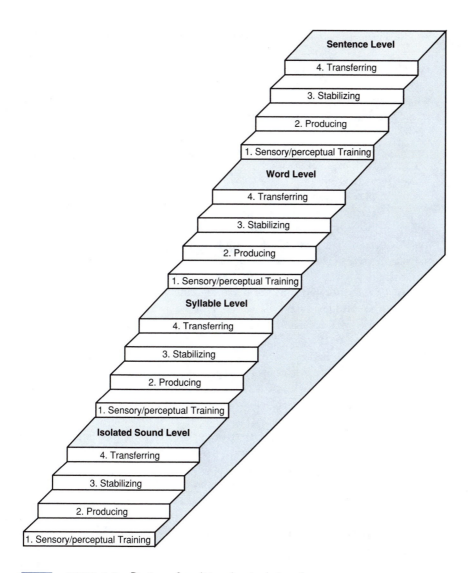

 FIGURE 7-7 Design of traditional articulation therapy

Why do we start by teaching the correct sound in isolation? For one thing, by doing this instead of teaching it in a word, we avoid the long history of usage that has so strongly reinforced the error. It's easier. Secondly, we must recognize that the production of that correct sound is our essential target.

The Focus of Therapy.   Since the essential error consists of a defective sound, it is upon this that we usually focus our therapy. Let us repeat: It is the *sound* that is in error. It is the misarticulated, nonstandard sound that spoils the syllable, spoils the word, spoils the sentence, and spoils whatever type of speech is being used. In whatever context it occurs, the acquisition and use of a standard sound must be our goal. The child's playmates say to him, "What's the matter with you? You talk funny. Say it this way!" and they provide him with an entire sentence to attempt. The child fails. Parents and teachers focus their therapy on the word level. "Don't say wabbit," they command. "Say rabbit!" The child fails again, or if, by chance, he does say it correctly, there is no transfer to any other /r/ word and there are thousands of /r/ words he must use.

You may wonder why it is necessary to progress from one level to another. The answer is that even after the client can produce the sound correctly in isolation we cannot expect him to be able to use it in syllables or words or sentences immediately. Only in rare instances does such generalization (transfer) occur and even then it is incomplete. Again we insist that the newly acquired standard sound needs to be strengthened before it can be incorporated into the person's communication.

Our second level is a syllabic one and we prefer to use the new sound in nonsense syllables instead of meaningful ones. Again they are easier to produce because the child has never used his error in saying them. Moreover, by using syllables, we can have the child practice his new sound in many different phonetic contexts, that is what he will have to do eventually. At this level, all types of syllables, (CV, VC, CVC) are used. By doing so, we make it easier for the client to master the next level, the use of the correct sound in words.

The clinician chooses the first target words with care and there are many factors to be considered. Familiar and often-used words may have their errors too thoroughly entrenched. On the other hand, if the child uses the correct sound in them, his improvement is more noticeable. Certain words will be easier to say correctly because of the influence of assimilation and coarticulation. Thus in treating a child with a frontal interdental lisp we would prefer the target word *soup,* /sup/, to *seed,* /sid/ because the /i/ vowel in the latter is made with the front of the tongue brought forward whereas in the /u/ vowel of /sup/ the back of the tongue is the part elevated.

Some generalization or transfer of the ability to produce the correct sound from one level to another does occur. Success in producing the isolated sound makes using it in nonsense syllable, and then in words, easier; and this transfer increases as therapy progresses. However, because the clinician cannot be certain that the transfer will be substantial, she usually trains her client at each of the levels. Only at the word level can she count on generalization being really effective. It appears as though once the child realizes that he can produce the correct new sound in certain words, he can do so on other words, too. This is fortunate because otherwise he would have to practice self-correction on each of the other words in his entire vocabulary. Similarly, the transfer of self-correction from single words to sentences rarely presents any real difficulty, because by this time he can recognize his errors and knows how to correct them. There will be occasional lapses but they the characteristics of mispronunciations rather than misarticulations. Eventually his errors will disappear.

Ear Training

Now that we have presented an overview of the course of traditional articulation therapy, let us describe the essence of the activities and goals for producing the isolated target sound.

Before we ever ask the child to attempt to make the target sound, we prepare her to do so by doing some intensive sensory-perceptual training. This consists of four major parts: (1) identifying the features of the target sound; (2) locating it when it occurs; (3) stimulating her strongly with it; and (4) discriminating how her error differs from the target sound. This first phase of therapy is commonly called *ear training.*

Identifying

Our goal here is to help the client recognize the essential characteristics of the isolated target sound—its auditory, visual, and movement features—when produced by the clinician. With small children it is often given an identity, even a name, the /s/ being called the "goose" or "snake" sound because of its hissing characteristics. Thus the clinician might give the child a picture of a goose or perhaps an actual rubber snake and have him use them to "scare her" every time he hears her produce a standard /s/, but not when she utters other isolated sounds or his error. With adults, of course, she would use more appropriate signalling devices. For both, she would demonstrate the way she produces a target sound such as the /s/, call attention to its high pitch, dental occlusion, and other features. This goal is easy to achieve but it is vitally important. It points out the bullseye that the client must shoot at.

Locating

It is especially important with children that they be able to recognize the target sound not only in isolation but in connected speech. This is not as easy as it may appear, because we do not listen to the sounds of our utterances. If we listen at all, we listen to the meanings we are trying to convey. The child, consumed by his need to listen for meanings, may hear the standard sounds flicker by, but he does not attend to them. Hidden as these sounds are in the fast torrent of speech, they have little stimulus value. Somehow we must make the characteristics of the sound vivid even in the fast flow of speech. Eventually he will have to recognize these tar-

Ear training.
Therapy devoted to self-hearing of speech deviations and standard utterance.

gets in his own sentences. To help him do so we first have him signal when they occur in the clinician's speech. We have been impressed by the ingenuity shown by clinicians as they invent appropriate signals that appeal to the child such as shooting a water pistol at the picture of a snake in the position of the letter S.

This perceptual training rarely presents any real difficulty but it is vitally important. If you have to hit a target you have to know where it is located.

Stimulating

In this phase of ear training, the clinician strongly stimulates the client with the target sound, flooding his ears with it. This is a new experience for the child. Before, he heard it only as it flits by; now he is bombarded by it. Many procedures are used to insure attentiveness. He may be asked to time with a stopwatch the varying durations of the sound presented by the clinician, for example, or to count the number of presentations, to indicate in that earphone of a binaural auditory trainer he is hearing the target sound, or to raise or lower his hand to represent its loudness changes.

Discriminating

Many children have difficulty in recognizing the differences between the features of the error sounds they produce and the features of the target sounds and so we try to help them do so as best we can. An experienced clinician trains herself to imitate the child's error very accurately. She tells him she has to learn to say it his way before asking him to say it her way. So they reverse roles and, for the moment, he becomes the teacher. Gradually, and after some deliberate failures she succeeds. Moreover, during this process, she points out features of the error, "Oh, I forgot to stick out my tongue like you do."

Samples or models of the child's error are compared with the standard sound using various techniques of presentation. We will provide a few illustrations.

The clinician, cupping her hands, stimulates the child with her duplication of his error in one ear and then with the target sound in the other ear. Then she asks him to point to the ear that heard the error—or the target sound. The clinician prolongs or repeats the target sound but inserts bits of the child's error and asks him to signal when they appear, or she makes a series of correct and error sounds, asking him to count only the errors.

Recalling, Perceiving, and Predicting Errors.   In this training in self-hearing, we operate in a time dimension. At first the child recognizes his errors only after they have occurred; next, when they are occurring; fi-

nally, he can predict them. The wise clinician understands this natural sequence of recognition and uses it. She signals her perception of the child's error at first only after an interval sufficiently long to let him listen to what his mouth has produced.

In the simultaneous perception of the error as opposed to this delayed perception, one very effective device is to have the clinician read or speak in unison with the child with her mouth to his ear. If at the moment he makes an error, she signals by making the correct sound very loudly, or by stopping her own speaking, or by some other stimulation, he will be brought to notice it instantly.

If the child is to learn to master his target sounds he must also learn to predict when they will occur. Even at this basic level where only the isolated sound is being presented, we start this prediction process. Clinician: "Watch my face and hold up the picture of the snake sound only if you think that's the one I'm going to say. Read my lips." She presents him with samples of the target sound and her imitation of his error.

This description of sensory-perceptual training may imply that it is difficult and time consuming. It is not. Many clinicians work on all four types of this training during a single therapy session (Figure 7-8). It constitutes the foundation the client needs.

Producing the New Sound in Isolation

When the clinician feels that the child is ready, she then seeks to evoke the new sound in isolation. Often, he will be able to imitate her model immediately because of the intensive sensory perceptual training he has experienced. Therefore, our first approach is termed auditory stimulation.

Auditory Stimulation.   This method relies upon simple imitation and demand. The clinician models the target sound and the child is asked to duplicate it. An example might run as follows.

> *Clinician:*   Now, Maria, I'm going to let you have your first
> chance to make the snake sound, *sss*. Remember not to
> make the windmill sound, *th-th*. This is the sound you
> are to make: *sss, sss, sssss*. Now you try it.

If the ear training has been adequate, this simple routine, in which the wrong sound is pronounced, identified, and rejected, then followed by the correct sound given several times, may bring a perfect production of the correct sound on the first attempt. Occasionally it will be necessary to repeat this routine several times before it works, and the child should be encouraged to take her time and to listen carefully both to the stimulation and to her response. She should be told that she has made an error or that she has almost said it correctly. She should then be encouraged to attempt it in a slightly different way the next time. No pressure should be brought

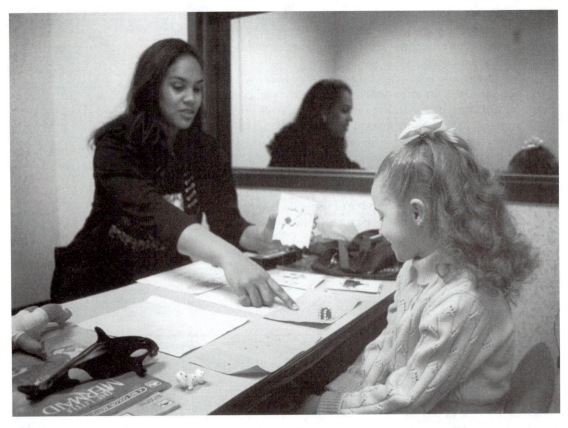

 FIGURE 7-8   Sensory-perceptual training combining auditory and visual stimuli (*Van Riper Clinic, Western Michigan University*)

to bear upon her; and a review of discrimination, stimulation, and identification techniques should preface the new attempt.

But this intensive stimulation does not always work. Some children, and some errors, require further measures before the isolated sounds can be produced consistently. Here are some of the other ways we teach them.

Varying and Correcting.   Whichever approach is used—and there are times when we must try one then another—the person must go through a process of varying his utterance. One of the basic problems confronting the clinician at this stage of treatment is to provoke such variation. Long-practiced habits are very resistant to change. Often before we can hope to get our client to have a fair chance of hitting his target, we must get him to try new postures, new attacks, new movement patterns. Variation must precede approximation. We must get our lisper to try and try again, but to try differently each time so that he comes closer and closer to producing the desired standard sound. Variation must precede approximation.

Progressive Approximation (Shaping).   The clinician joins the client and makes the same error the client makes. He then shows the client a series of transitional sounds each of which comes a bit closer to the standard sound until finally the standard sound is produced. Each little modification the client makes that comes a bit closer to the goal is rewarded. Those variations that move away from the target sound are ignored. Through this process, the *degree* of error is constantly determined, and new attempts are aimed at reducing the amount of deviation. The uniqueness of this approach is that it resembles the way in which infants seem to acquire normal articulation. They do not suddenly shift from saying *wabbit* to *rabbit;* instead they seem to proceed through a series of gradual and progressive approximations. This also is the process known to psychologists as *shaping*. Instead of asking the person to exchange a correct sound for his incorrect sound, we help him to shift gradually from where he is to where he has to go.

Progressive approximation is an excellent method for teaching a new sound. It permits reward for modification instead of reserving it for final attainment of the goal. It helps the identification of clinician and client. It reduces the task. If encourages variation. Even very resistant clients seem to move ahead under this regime.

Producing the Target Sound in Nonsense Syllables

Our next major step in therapy is to help our client to use the new sound in all phonetic contexts. This is very important since any sound changes slightly whenever it is preceded or followed by other sounds. The /s/ in the nonsense syllable *seeb,* for example, is acoustically higher in pitch than the /s/ in *soob.* Also the contour of the tongue varies a bit with differing phonetic contexts. Since we must be able to produce the new sound in all possible combinations, we must have some means of teaching these variations. The nonsense syllable provides us with such a vehicle.

There are three main types of nonsense syllables: CV (consonant-vowel syllables such as *la*), VC (vowel-consonant syllables such as *al*), and CVC (consonant-vowel-consonant combinations such as *kal* or *lod*). These syllables can be readily constructed by combining the new sound with common vowels and diphthongs. The first nonsense syllables to be practiced are those in which the transitional movements from consonant to vowel involve the fewest and simplest coordinations. For example, *ko* involves less radical transitional movements than does *kee*. The next nonsense syllables should be those that use the new sound in the final position (*ok*); and, finally, those in which the new sound is located in the medial position (*oko*) should be practiced. These nonsense syllables should be practiced thoroughly before familiar words are attempted.

Some speech pathologists prefer to start with this syllabic level—to teach *ree* and *ra* and *roo* rather than *rrr*, because they feel that the syllable is the basic unit of motor speech. They also point out that many sounds such as the plosives /k/ and /g/ can only be produced syllabically and that prolonging an isolated sound distorts its pattern in time and creates unnecessary difficulty in shifting from sounds into syllables and then into words. Why not begin immediately with the syllable and teach *la-lee-lie-lay-lo-loo* instead of the isolated *llll* sound? We will not argue the point with any real vigor, for we have often begun therapy with the syllable in certain cases where the person seemed to produce the sound more easily therein than in isolation. However, when therapy begins with the syllable, the clinician follows the same basic sequence we have outlined for the isolated sound.

Producing the Target Sound in Words

We are now ready to move onward to our third operational level—the word level. The new sound has been sufficiently strengthened so that it has a fair chance to hold its own in competition with the error if we can make sure that the odds are in its favor. We must remember that the client has used her old error in meaningful words thousands of times and that it would be unreasonable to expect her suddenly to be able to speak them correctly. We therefore need new techniques to ensure the successful incorporation of the newly acquired sound into words.

Selecting a Vocabulary.   We start, as you might expect, with simple words that have some relevance for the youngster. Here is a portion of a treatment plan for a ten-year-old boy that illustrates the way in which a clinician gradually increases vocabulary complexity when stabilizing at the word level.

> *Word Form.* (1) Start with one-syllable words with the target sound in the prevocalic position (*s*oup, *s*and, etc.). (2) Move to one-syllable words with the target sound in the postvocalic position (to*ss*, bu*s*, etc.). (3) Next, introduce words with the /s/ in two phoneme blends (*sl*am, *sp*in, etc.). (Note: Be sure to try *st* blends, such as *st*op, because when he anticipates making the /t/, he will pull his tongue tip back away from his teeth). (4) Then move to two-syllable words, three-syllable, and so on.

> *Word Content.* (1) Try to use words from the child's own vocabulary—use "rat*s*" or "*s*tinker" if these are words he uses. (2) Relate the vocabulary used to his interests—if he is a junior hockey player, include words like i*ce*, *s*kates, *s*tick. (3) Develop some word families—vocabulary relates to topics like food, television programs, hobbies.

Simultaneous Talking and Writing.   Simultaneous talking-and-writing techniques can be invaluable if used properly. The client should talk and write the first letter, the first syllable, and finally, the whole word. Thus, *s s s s s s s s s; s s si sick s si sick,* and so on. Later he can alternate the symbol and the word, and finally he can write only the symbol as he says the word.

We also ask our clients to draw on paper or trace in the air various figures. The client is trained to associate certain sounds with certain parts of the figures and then to trace continuously through the whole figure, thus producing a word.

Signaling Techniques.   This group of activities uses preparatory sets to integrate the sound or syllable into the words. Signaling can generate many key words. In this, the child prolongs or repeats the new sound and then, at a given signal, instantly says the prearranged vowel or the rest of the word. The child should be given a preparatory set to pronounce the rest of the word by preliminary signal practice. During this practice he waits with his eyes closed until he hears the sound signal that sets off the response. Thus, during the child's prolongation of *ssssss,* the clinician suddenly raps on the table, and the syllable *oup* is produced. With a preparatory set, the response is largely automatic and involuntary, and thus the new sound is integrated within the word as a whole. Often it is wise to require the child to say the word twice. Thus, *ssssss* (rap) *oup-soup.*

Producing the Target Sound in Sentences

When our client has shown that she can correctly produce the target sound in words, and correct herself when she makes the error in those words, we make its usage in sentences our primary goal. Those sentences should be meaningful. They should also vary in their purpose. They should make statements (declarative), ask questions (interrogative), and issue commands (imperative). When a lisping child discovers he can get the clinician to slap her own face when he says "/slæp jʊr fes/" but not "/θlæp jʊr feθ/" the experience will be highly motivating.

Even at this sentence level we employ the same identification, location, stimulation, and discrimination tactics we used in teaching the isolated target sound.

Transfer and Carryover

It is one thing to acquire the ability to use a new sound correctly in isolation, syllable, word, or sentence; it is another to be able to use it habitually and automatically. Somehow we must build in this person a control system that will continuously scan the utterance and notice and correct the errors automatically. No one can continually listen to the output of sound from his mouth. We need our ears to hear our thoughts and the thoughts of others. How can we automatize this corrective process? We have three main methods for doing so: (1) enlarging the therapy situation, (2) using the new sound in all types of speaking, and (3) emphasizing proprioceptive feedback.

Enlarging the Therapy Situation.　First, we must expand the therapy room to include the person's whole living space. He must be given experiences in scanning, comparing, and correcting in school, on the playground, on the job, and at home. Here are some of the ways we do this.

Speech Assignments.　Some typical speech assignments illustrating methods for getting the child to work on his errors in outside situations are the following.

> (1) Go downstairs and ask the janitor for a dust rag. Be sure to say *rag* with a good long *rrr.* (2) Say the word *rabbit* to three other children without letting them know that you are working on your speech. (3) Ask your father if you said any word wrong after you tell him what you did in school today.

The clinician should always make these assignments very definite and appropriate to the child's ability and environment. He should always ask for a report the next day. Such assignments frequently are the solution to any lack of motivation the child may have.

Checking Devices.　Checking devices are of great value when properly used. Typical checking devices are:

> (1) Having child carry card and crayon during social studies recitation, making a mark or writing the word whenever he makes an error. (2) Having some other child check errors in a similar fashion. (3) Having child transfer marbles from one pocket to another, one for each error. Many other devices may be invented, and they will bring the error to consciousness very rapidly.

Nucleus Situations.　Many parents make the mistake of correcting the child whenever he makes speech errors. It is unwise to set the speech standards too high. No one can watch himself all the time, and we all hate to be nagged. As a matter of fact, too much vigilance can produce such speech inhibitions that the speech work becomes thoroughly distasteful. Fluency disappears, and the speech becomes very halting and unpleasant. Then, too, the very anxiety lest error occur, when carried to the extreme, increases the number of slips and mistakes themselves.

Therefore, we recommend that parents and teachers concentrate their reminding and correcting upon a few common words and upon certain speech situations. Have a particular person picked out who is to serve as the speech situation where the child must use very careful speech. Use a specific speech situation, such as the dinner table, to serve as a nucleus of good speech. When errors occur in these nuclei situations, penalize them good-naturedly but emphatically. Freedom from errors will spread rapidly to other situations.

Negative Practice.   By negative practice we mean the deliberate and voluntary use of the incorrect sound or speech error. It may seem somewhat odd to advise clients to practice their errors, for we have always assumed that practice makes perfect, and certainly we do not want the student to become more perfect in the use of his errors. Nevertheless, when one seeks to break a habit that is rather unconscious (such as fingernail biting or the substitution of *sh* for *s*), much more rapid progress is made if the possessor of the habit will occasionally (and at appropriate times) use the error deliberately. The reasons for the effectiveness of this method are as follows. (1) The greatest strength of such a habit lies in the fact that the possessor is not aware of it every time it occurs. All habit reactions tend to become more or less unconscious, and certainly those involved in speech are of this type. Consciousness of the reaction must come before it can be eliminated. (2) Voluntary practice of the reaction makes it very vivid, thus increasing vigilance and contributing to the awareness of the cues that signal the approach of the reaction. (3) The voluntary practice of the error acts as a penalty.

Using the New Sound in All Types of Speaking.   In stabilizing and automatizing the new sound, we find it wise to provide systematic training that incorporates the new sound into real live message sending, social control, thinking, emotional, and self-expressive types of speaking. Again we must make deliberate nucleic implants of good speech in all these various functions. First in the therapy room, and then in all the person's living space, we must make sure that our client can use his new standard sounds in all the *kinds* of talking he must do. When the lisper commands his dog, he must say "Sit down!" When he responds affirmatively to a question he must say "Yes!" When he must mentally add four and three, he must think "seven," not "theven." In expressing his fear, he must say "I'm scared" not "thcared." He must be able to use good sibilants in his speech of self-display. Until certain correctly spoken sentences are used automatically in each of these forms of speaking, we cannot feel our task as a clinician is over.

Emphasizing Proprioceptive Feedback.   **Proprioceptive** feedback is a term that refers to the perception of contacts and movements and postures. If we place a finger on our lower lip, the felt contact is proprioceptive; if we cock our head to the left or move a foot, the sensa-

Proprioception. Sense information from muscles, joints, or tendons.

tions of posture and movement are proprioceptive. We know what has happened without seeing or hearing. In much the same way, we can know what is happening in our own speech even when we cannot hear ourselves speaking. It is quite possible to talk correctly in a boiler factory. We do not need self-hearing if our proprioceptive senses are operating well.

The most important automatic controls for monitoring articulation are proprioceptive. These controls see to it that we use the right movements, the right postures, the correct contacts. When the baby first learns to talk, self-hearing is most important. But after he begins to use language and to understand the meanings of others, self-hearing is given a less important role. Proprioception thus becomes much more important, so important, indeed, that obvious errors can persist for years without the person recognizing them auditorially. In articulation therapy, we must first reopen the self-hearing circuits and put more energy into them so that these errors can be distinguished. But we must not stop here. We must return to proprioceptive controls if the child is to use the new sound automatically. No one can listen to himself constantly.

Accordingly, in terminal therapy with a client with misarticulations, we teach him to use the new sound correctly by feel and touch alone. We put masking noise in his ears so he cannot rely on self-hearing. We ask him to speak in a soft whisper and in pantomime. All these activities decrease the monitoring of speech by self-hearing and emphasize its proprioceptive control. We have found these techniques invaluable in automatizing the new sound.

In Conclusion.   As we come to the end of this chapter we fear that you may be thinking that doing articulation therapy is both laborious and difficult. It really isn't if the client is a young child whose misarticulations have not become fixed through years of use. Most children respond readily and successfully to a systematic program. Once they have come to recognize the characteristics of the standard sound and its error and have been able to produce it in isolation or syllables, they move swiftly into normal utterance. We have had to describe many more techniques than those normally administered because there are always a few individuals whose problems are more severe. It's fun to work with all these children; it's very rewarding to see a troubled child untangle his tongue and life, to see him grow in self-esteem because he can now talk like other people. Our suggestions are not at all mysterious or difficult to administer. Many parents and teachers have been able to follow them once they found out from the speech pathologist what they were and why they made sense. Lost children should not have to try to find their way out of the swamp alone. They need a guide who has a map.

STUDY QUESTIONS

1. In simple terms, what is the difference between an articulation disorder and a phonological disorder? Into which of these categories does a "phonetic disorder" fall?
2. For what reasons may it not always be possible to label a child's speech difficulty simply as *either* an articulation disorder *or* a phonological disorder?
3. In what ways may dialect differences at times be mistakenly identified as articulation or phonological disorders? And how would you define the term *dialect,* anyway?
4. What are the three major ways in that speech sounds tend to be misarticulated? And what is the fourth but less common way?
5. With what types of speech sounds would you expect dental malocclusion to cause the greatest difficulties?
6. What is meant by "auditory discrimination" and why may this be of relevance in understanding a child's speech difficulty?
7. For what reasons does the clinician wish to explore the developmental history of a child who is having difficulty with the mastery of speech sounds?
8. Of what diagnostic significance is the *consistency* of a client's speech sound error(s)?
9. What types of observations and judgments must the clinician make in performing a linguistic analysis of a child's speech sound errors?
10. What steps and processes are involved in "traditional" therapy for articulation problems? What elements of traditional therapy may be equally useful in a linguistic approach?

REFERENCES

Battle, D. (1993). *Communication disorders in multicultural populations.* Stoneham, MA: Butterworth-Heinemann.

Bernthal, J., and Bankson, N. (1993). *Articulation and phonological disorders* (3rd ed.). Englewood Cliffs, NJ: Prentice Hall.

Blache, S., and Parsons, C. (1980). A linguistic approach to distinctive feature training. *Language, Speech and Hearing Services in Schools,* 11, 203–207.

Elbert, M., and Gierut, J. (1986) *Handbook of clinical phonology: Approaches to assessment and treatment.* San Diego, CA: College-Hill Press.

Emerick, L., and Haynes, W. (1986). *Diagnosis and evaluation in speech pathology* (3rd ed.). Englewood Cliffs, NJ: Prentice Hall.

Hodson, B., and Paden, E. (1983). *Targeting intelligible speech: A phonological approach to remediation.* San Diego, CA: College-Hill Press.

Iglesias, A., and Anderson, N. (1993). Dialectal variations. In J. Bernthal, and N. Bankson, *Articulation and phonological disorders* (3rd ed.). Englewood Cliffs, NJ: Prentice-Hall.

Khan, L. (1982). A review of 16 major phonological processes. *Language, Speech, and Hearing Services in Schools,* 13, 77–85.

Lowe, R. (1994). *Phonology: Assessment and intervention applications in speech pathology.* Baltimore: Williams & Wilkins.

McDonald, E. (1968). *A deep test of articulation.* Pittsburgh: Stanwix House.

McReynolds, L., and Bennett, S. (1972). Distinctive feature generalization in articulation training. *Journal of Speech and Hearing Disorders,* 37, 462–470.

Monahan, D. (1984) *Remediation of common phonological processes.* Tigard, OR: C. C. Publications.

Monahan, D. (1986). Remediation of common phonological processes: Four case studies. *Language, Speech and Hearing Services in Schools,* 17, 199–206.

Monnin, L. (1984). Speech sound discrimination testing and training. In H. Winitz (ed.), *Treating articulation disorders: For clinicians by clinicians.* Baltimore: University Park Press.

Morrison, J., and Shriberg, L. (1992). Articulation testing versus conversational speech sampling. *Journal of Speech and Hearing Research,* 35, 259–273.

Pollack, E., and Rees, N. (1972). Disorders of articulation: Some clinical applications of distinctive feature theory. *Journal of Speech and Hearing Disorders,* 37, 451–461.

Proctor, A. (1994). Phonology and cultural diversity. In R. Lowe, *Phonology: Assessment and intervention applications in speech pathology.* Baltimore: Williams & Wilkins.

Secord, W. (1989). The traditional approach to treatment. In N. Creaghead, P. Newman, and W. Secord, *Assessment and remediation of articulatory and phonological disorders.* Columbus, OH: Merrill.

Shriberg, L., and Kwiatkowski, J. (1982). Phonological disorders III: A procedure for assessing severity of involvement. *Journal of Speech and Hearing Disorders,* 47, 256–270.

Shriberg, L. (1987). A retrospective study of spontaneous generalization in speech-delayed children. *Language, Speech and Hearing Services in Schools,* 18, 144–157.

Stoel-Gammon, C., and Dunn, C. (1985). *Normal and disordered phonology in children.* Baltimore: University Park Press.

Taylor, O. (1994). Communication in a multicultural society. In F. Minifie, *Introduction to communication sciences and disorders.* San Diego, CA: Singular Publishing Group.

Tyler, A., Edwards, M. and Saxman, J. (1987). Clinical application of two phonologically based treatment procedures. *Journal of Speech and Hearing Disorders,* 52, 393–409.

Weiss, C., Gordon, M. and Lillywhite, H. (1987). *Clinical management of articulatory and phonologic disorders.* Baltimore: Williams and Wilkins.

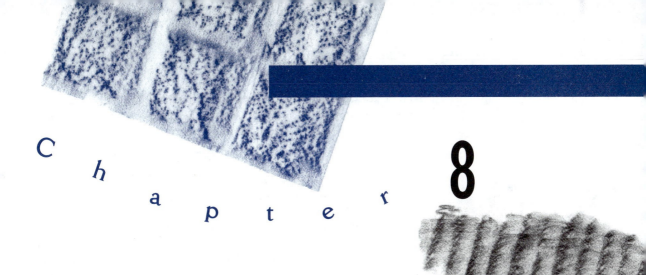

Chapter 8

Fluency Disorders

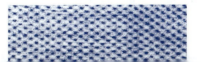

There are several disorders of fluency, stuttering and cluttering being the ones most frequently encountered by speech-language pathologists. Most of this chapter will be devoted to stuttering.

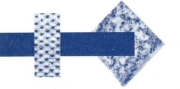

WHAT IS STUTTERING?

Curiously, major disagreements still exist concerning the very nature of stuttering itself. What is stuttering? A hundred wastebaskets could not hold all the articles and books that have sought to answer this question. Robert West, a founder of our professional association, once remarked: "Everyone knows what stuttering is—except the expert." Certainly the person who stutters knows, and so do his listeners.

All agree that the flow of speech is interrupted when one stutters. This is why it is called a disorder of fluency. The definition problem arises because all of us have interruptions in our fluency. No one is completely fluent all the time. Occasionally we all stumble, repeat, or hesitate, and our fluency breaks occur more often under communicative stress. But do we all stutter? The answer, of course, is no. What then constitute the essential differences between this so-called normal disfluency and the abnormal kind we call stuttering? Is it just a matter of degree or frequency? Again, we feel that the answer is no. The behaviors we label as stuttering are different.

Our own definition of stuttering goes like this: *Stuttering occurs when the forward flow of speech is interrupted abnormally by repetitions or prolongations of a sound, syllable, or articulatory posture, or by avoidance and struggle behaviors.* (The student should be advised that our definition is not universally accepted. Reference to other points of view will be found in the supplementary readings listed at the end of this chapter.)

The research shows rather conclusively that stutterers have more syllabic repetitions and sound prolongations than normal speakers. They have more syllabic repetitions per hundred words, and they have more of them per word. We examined one stutterer who repeated one syllable forty-three times on a single word. Normal speakers occasionally hang onto a sound or posture only briefly, but stutterers show a long duration on their prolongations. The senior author once had a silent prolongation on the posture of the first sound of the word "pass" that lasted 6 minutes by a schoolroom clock, although it was interrupted several times by the need for the intake of air for survival. Normal speakers do not have these experiences. There also seem to be differences in the form of the repetitions and prolongations that distinguish the stutterer from the normal speaker. When a normal speaker repeats a syllable (and he does so only rarely), he uses the correct vowel and repeats it at the regular tempo of his other syllables. He says "Sa-Saturday." The stutterer tends to say

"Suh-Suh-Sih-Suh-Suh-Seh-Sa-Saturday," and the variable repetitions occur irregularly and often with tension. Also the syllables in the stutterer seem to be arrested; they are terminated suddenly; the breath is interrupted. These phenomena do not seem to be characteristic of the few syllable repetitions shown by normal speakers. We say "few" because they are rare. When a normal speaker repeats, he tends to repeat words and phrases, not syllables or sounds. We do not consider the repetition of a word or phrase or the use of pauses, "um's" and "er's," or reformulations as abnormal. We even accept a few repetitions of a syllable. But when a sound or syllable is repeated not once or twice but many times, and when this behavior occurs too frequently, then we prick up our ears and say to ourselves that the speaker stutters. We tend to say the same thing when a sound is prolonged, as in this example: "I think that mm-mmmmmmmmmy mmmmmmmmm-mother wwwwwon't let me go." The tolerance for such prolongations of a sound seems to be much less than for repetitions of a sound or syllable. We have also used the word *posture*. Not all these repetitions and prolongations are vocalized. The stutterer often makes several silent mouth postures before the word is spoken, or he may assume a fixed position and struggle silently with it before blurting out what he wants to say. These fixed postures may be located anywhere in the speech structures. One stutterer may hold his breath with both true and false vocal cords closed tightly. Another may protrude his tongue or twist his lips to one side. Since these silent postures take time, they break up the normal time sequence of speech. Finally, we have included in our definition the terms "**avoidance**" and "struggle." Although most beginning stutterers show little struggle or avoidance, in the advanced stages of the disorder, these reactions may constitute the major part of the problem.

It is difficult to describe stuttering in words. One has to see it and hear it, and perhaps even feel it, to really understand what it is. However, we will present word pictures of just a few of the stutterers who have come to us for help.

> John was three and a half when his anxious mother brought him. "His stuttering is growing worse," she told us. "It happens more often and he repeats more than he did a month ago. His father is more concerned about it than I am, probably because he says he stuttered too as a child though he doesn't now."

> We took the boy into our playroom and procured a fairly good sample of his speech. Essentially, his stuttering consisted of repetitions of syllables, usually averaging about three of four per word. There were no signs of struggle or tension. He showed no awareness that they had occurred. He spoke easily and freely. However, most of his utterances had these easy repetitions in them, most often at the beginning of his sentences, but also on words within them. Only a few sentences were spoken completely fluently.

Avoidance.
A device such as the use of a synonym or circumlocution to escape from having to speak a word upon which stuttering is anticipated.

Eva was four years old and her parents said that she had been stuttering for about two years but that lately it had become much worse. Our examination revealed that she not only showed syllabic repetitions (which were irregular and accompanied by tension) but also she prolonged some of her continuant sounds ("Mmmmmmommy"). Several times she opened her mouth but seemed to be unable to produce any sound and once when this occurred, she began to cry. Some sentences were spoken entirely fluently.

Bob was a fourteen-year-old who had been stuttering for many years, almost since the beginning of speech, his parents reported. They said that recently he had shown a personality change, that previously he had been a happy, outgoing kid but now had begun to be withdrawn. His teachers had told them Bob refused to recite in school and was a loner. It was difficult to get an adequate sample but we did observe that he had long silent blocks with tremors of the lips and jaws and that he often jerked his head in an attempt to release them. At times, he exhaled and then squeaked out the word on the end of his breath. He averted his eyes when stuttering.

One of our most difficult stuttering clients, whom we shall call Bill, rarely showed any real overt stuttering because he was usually able to avoid doing so, yet we have rarely met a person so handicapped. A cum laude graduate from a small college, he was working as a common laborer for a construction company. The few blockings that he did have were silent prolongations of a consonantal posture. He would close his lips, for example, on a word beginning with /k/, /t/, or /m/ and go into a tremor of the tongue or lips. When this would happen, he would stop and either say "ah-ah-ah" interminably or repeat the preceding words or phrases. For example, he might say something like this: "My ah-ah-ah-um position" (He wanted to say "job" but feared he would block on it so he substituted a word he felt he could say) "My position with the building industry (He wanted to say construction company) doesn't shall we say ah-ah-ah-ah-pay very well." He often used these filler phrases to gain some time, hoping that his fear would diminish and he could speak the word or sound he feared so much. Bill's fears of sounds and words and speaking situations were incredibly intense. He reported instances in which he had given a false name so he wouldn't have to say his own. He never made a phone call because once a listener had hung up on him. He had crossed the street to avoid having to say hello to an approaching acquaintance. Bill had no friends and had never dated. About the only social conversation he had was with strangers at a bar, and that only when he was pretty drunk.

Our final example was also a severely handicapped but George was not an avoider but a battler. He fought his stuttering as he had fought his tormentors in his school days when they mocked him unmercifully. George was not afraid of speaking. Indeed, he talked a lot and refused to be interrupted. When he repeated syllables, his voice would go up in pitch like a siren. When he had a prolongation, he would try to force the word out explosively, sometimes almost shouting it. His face contorted with the effort and often he gasped in his effort to break out of his blockage. At times his whole body would thrash around so violently others had thought he was having an epileptic seizure. Not a pretty sight.

Of all the speech disorders, stuttering has been the one most studied, yet it continues to present problems that baffle clinicians and researchers. Over the years we have learned much about stuttering, but at the present time some of the pieces of its jigsaw puzzle are still missing. In this chapter we will show you what parts of the puzzle have been assembled and also the remaining gaps. Speech pathology is a new profession and stuttering is an ancient disorder. Much controversy exists about the nature of stuttering and its treatment, but there are also areas of agreement. We begin by presenting those facts about the disorder that are widely accepted.

Prevalence

Stuttering seems to occur in all cultures, as suggested by the following compilation (after Van Riper, 1982).

Words Referring to Stuttering

European
Finnish: ankyttää
German: stottern
French: begaiement
Portuguese: gagueira
Norwegian: stamning
Italian: balbuzie
Spanish: tartamundear
Yugoslav (Slovene): jeclijati
Latvian: stostisanas
Estonian: tölpkeel
Hungarian: dadogó
Czech: koktani
Russian: zaikatsia; zaikanie
Esperanto: babuti

Native American
Salish: sutsuts
Nanaimo: skeykulskwels
Tlahoose: ha'ak'ok
Haida: kilekwigu'ung
Chocktaw: isunash illi
Asage: the'-ce u-ba-ci-ge
Cherokee: a-da-nv-te-hi-lo-squi
Sioux: eye-hda-sna-sna; iyi-tag-tag
Eskimo: iptogetok

Pacific
Fiji: kaka
Hawaiian: uu uus

Asian
Tagalog: patalutal
Chinese (Cantonese): hau hick; kong'-tak-lak-kak
Japanese: domori; kitsuon
Vietnamese: su noi lap

Eastern
Persian: locknatezaban
Hebrew: gingeim
Arabic: fa faa; rattat
Hindi: khaha
Hindustani: larbaraha
Turkish: kekeke mek

African
Egyptian: tataha; tuhuhtuhuh
Ga: haamuala
Xhosa: ukuthititha
Luganda: okukunanagira
Ghana (Twi): howdodo
Nigeria (Ibo): nsu
Shangaan: manghanghamela
Somali: wùu haghaglayyá

We also know that stuttering has affected the human race since the earliest of times. The Chinese Laotze mentioned stuttering in a poem written 2500 years ago. Hieroglyphics for the word "nit nit" (stuttering) were found on clay tablets dated back to the twentieth century BC. In the *Bible,* Moses is said to have stuttered and had his brother Aaron read the tablets of the Ten Commandments he brought down from the mountain. We find this verse from the *Koran* that seems to corroborate the belief: "Moses said, My Lord, relieve my mind and ease my task for me, and loose the knot in my tongue that they may understand my saying." Demosthenes, who became the most famous orator of ancient Greece, was said to have conquered his impediment by putting pebbles in his mouth and leaden plates on his chest as he climbed a mountain or talked to the waves of the seashore.

Despite their stuttering, many individuals have become famous; we provide just a handful of their names: Virgil, Erasmus, King Charles the First of England who was cured by having his head cut off, King Edward VI who had to stutter to the entire world over the radio annually at Christmas, and Winston Churchill. Famous or infamous, rich or poor, we still find stutterers everywhere, and most of them are as still as possible, trying to hide their affliction.

Investigations of the prevalence of stuttering show that about one in every one hundred persons stutters. This means that in this country alone there are over two million stutterers. The percentage may be slightly less in undeveloped cultures where the pace of existence is not as frantic as our own, but there appear to be only relatively small variations in prevalence around the world.

The prevalence of stuttering seems to be lower among the hearing impaired (Montgomery and Fitch, 1988), and it is rarely found in the congenitally deaf (Van Riper, 1982). Among individuals with certain types of mental impairment the prevalence may be somewhat greater than in non-impaired populations.

About four times as many males stutter as do females. This sex ratio has been found in studies from many different countries. Why? We really do not know. We do know that boys mature later than girls and are slower in language development. Geschwind and Galaburda (1985) speculate that the known higher amounts of testosterone in boys may tend to make their speech coordinations break down more easily under environmental pressures. Kidd, Kidd, and Records (1978) attribute the difference to a sex-linked inherited predisposition to stutter. None of these explanations has won acceptance. All we know is that more boys than girls begin to stutter.

We now have enough research to be sure that children with relatives who stutter are more likely to develop the disorder than those without such a family history, but we also know that stutterers are also found in families where there is no such history. No gene for stuttering has as yet been discovered. Some have attributed this higher risk to a predisposition that is only fulfilled when certain environmental factors, such as stress, trigger its occurrence. Others have suggested that when parents stutter they may be overconcerned about the normal disfluencies of their children and worry about them or punish them until the child does react with struggle or avoidance. Still others feel that children with relatives who stutter acquire the disorder through imitation. This belief, once widely held, no longer seems credible, mainly because the symptoms of beginning stuttering are very different from those of the relative whom they are presumed to have imitated.

The Onset of Stuttering

It is generally agreed that most stuttering begins in early childhood, usually between the years of two and five. It can occur suddenly or gradually, usually the latter. By gradual onset we mean that periods of noticeable stuttering may be followed by periods of normal speech and also that its frequency and duration slowly (not suddenly) increase.

In its earliest forms the stuttering behaviors consist of excessive repetitions of a sound or syllable, or prolongations of a sound or articulatory posture that may be voiced or silent. The child says "/mɪmɪmɪlk/" or "/mmmmɪlk/," or forms his lips for the /m/ sound yet no sound is produced. All or any of these interrupt the forward flow of speech.

Again, usually though not always, these behaviors at first show little signs of tension or struggle and the child is seemingly unaware that he has produced them. There are no instances of avoiding speaking nor of avoiding certain words.

This description tells what usually happens when a child begins to stutter, but there are other children whose stuttering onset is very sudden and in whom awareness, struggle, and avoidance are present.

The risks of a child beginning to stutter after the age of six are very small but the onset of stuttering in adults has also been reported. Adult onset stuttering is rare but numerous studies show that it exists. A few of them report that they had stuttered in childhood and that the disorder reappeared in situations involving great communicative stress, but most develop their stuttering as a result of trauma involving brain damage due to strokes, accident, or diseases. Here is one account from the literature.

> She stuttered on 95 percent of the words she spoke, repeating initial consonants four to six times and medial consonants three to four times. The stuttering was not specific to any phoneme or group of phonemes. There was no adaptation effect. Whispering made no difference. She demonstrated marked effort in the production of speech but not poor eye contact, distracting sounds, or excessive body movement. (Nowack and Stone, 1987, pp. 142–143)

Another group of individuals who begin to stutter in adulthood develop the stuttering suddenly in situations involving great emotional stress. The stuttering seems to consist primarily of compulsive repetitions of syllables or whole words and the person shows little concern about them and little tension or avoidance are present.

Spontaneous Recovery.   Not all children who begin to stutter continue to do so. Indeed in many of them the stuttering behaviors disappear as mysteriously as they appeared. Precise figures of this spontaneous recovery are difficult to procure, but estimates range from about 40 to 80 percent. In short, there seems to be good evidence that even without therapy self-recovery occurs. Rarely, however, does this take place after puberty or after the child has become aware of his stuttering and has developed fears and avoidance and struggle. Unfortunately, some children do not "outgrow" their stuttering and as the years pass it can grow worse and worse.

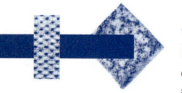

DEVELOPMENT OF THE DISORDER

One of the features of stuttering is that it tends to change with time. Usually beginning with brief repetitions or prolongations of a sound, posture, or syllable, it can grow in frequency and severity until the individual is almost incapacitated so far as communication is concerned. Bizarre facial jerks, gasps, even bodily contortions may appear as he struggles to release himself from his blockings. As a result, his inner world becomes one colored by anxiety, frustration, and shame.

One of our stuttering clients said this: "The worst about my stuttering is that I don't always stutter. If I would always do it on every word, maybe I could get used to it, like having a birthmarked face or a withered leg, but it comes and goes and I can never tell when I'll do it or when I won't." This inconsistency is one of the hallmarks of the disorder. All stutterers have some fluency and some have more than others.

Although different stuttering children may show different courses or tracks in their disorder's development, the one most frequently observed is as follows. First, the child shows an excessive number of simple repetitions of sounds or syllables uttered at the same tempo of his usual syllabic utterances. Then the repetitions per word increase and become swifter or irregular and the **schwa /ə/ vowel** appears in them. Next, prolongations of sounds occur and then silent articulatory postures, and then we find evidence of tension and tremors accompanying the repetitions and prolongations. Shortly after this, the child becomes aware of his fluency breaks and becomes frustrated. Then after this, the child begins to show signs of fearing to speak. He may leave the sentences unfinished, become unduly silent, refuse to answer, and may become withdrawn.

Schwa vowel.
The neutral vowel /ə/ as in the first phoneme in *above*.

When stuttering does occur he now tries to interrupt it by various devices or explosive struggle resulting in facial contortions, gasping, or tongue protrusions, thus increasing the abnormality.

Soon after this struggle appears, he begins to use avoidance devices, using synonyms for the words he fears, postponing the speech attempt by saying /ə/ repeatedly before attempting the feared word or sound, pretending to think or just refusing to talk.

At this advanced stage of development, he may also resort to various strategies for timing the speech attempt, such as tapping a finger or leg, using a head, finger, or leg, using a head jerk, or exhaling then squeaking out the word at the end of his breath. The varieties of these coping mechanisms are endless. Unfortunately, they soon become habitual parts of his stuttering.

Variability.   Confirmed stutterers show an almost bewildering variety of stuttering behaviors, though beginning stutterers do not. As the disorder grows in severity, different stutterers react differently to the interruptions in the flow of their speech.

There are literally thousands of possible reactions that can be used to escape, avoid, or disguise the inability to say a word fluently. We have seen identical twins who stuttered differently. Most adult stutterers pass through a whole series of different reaction patterns before they develop the final set that is as unique as their fingerprints. At four years of age, the stutterer may have only syllabic repetitions; at five, postural fixations. By his eleventh birthday he could be retching and gasping; by his sixteenth, his speech may also be punctuated by long pauses. When he becomes thirty, all of these behaviors may be in his stuttering repertoire, and there may also be some head jerks. But some of these behaviors may also be suddenly discarded or replaced by others less abnormal. We know one man, at the age of seventy, who stopped the struggling and avoiding of many years and began to stutter easily and with the syllabic repetition of his childhood. He told us he was too tired and too old to stutter so hard any longer.

At any age, a stutterer shows some variety in stuttering behavior. Those who are monosymptomatic are very rare. Most advanced stutterers have more than one behavior in their repertoire, and some have so many that at times of great stress they hardly know which one to use. Different kinds of behaviors may be used when stuttering on words beginning with vowel sounds than when stuttering on words beginning with stop consonants. A stutterer who used a nasal snorting noise to interrupt a long tremorous fixation on the first sound of the word "make" never showed this behavior when stuttering on the word "ache." Instead he had an intermittent vocal fry or a rise in pitch. One stutterer used a quick inhalatory vocalization to release himself from hypertensed laryngeal closures on voice CV or VC syllables, but never used it on syllables beginning with an unvoiced consonant. These different responses seem to have no reason for existing until we note that the nasal snort may at least initiate airflow, that vocal fry cannot be produced with true or ventricular vocal fold occlusion and so on. Many of the strange behaviors shown by stutterers seem to have some method in their madness when they are viewed as attempts to search for the integrations that will make the utterance of the word possible. If we look only at the variability itself, the picture is indeed confusing.

Thus far, we have been describing the development of the overt behaviors of stuttering, those that can be seen or heard. But there is also a similar course of development that is hidden from us, yet is vividly felt by the stutterer and often constitutes the major part of his problem. We refer, of course, to the emotional reactions the stutterer experiences.

Emotionally, the progression in severity usually follows this course: first, frustration and anger appear, then fear and anxiety, and then embarrassment, shame, and guilt. Each of these may lead to other reactions such as aggression, withdrawal, self-punishment, depression and the loss of self-esteem.

Because of the many rejections, mockery, or other penalties they receive when exhibiting their stuttering, confirmed stutterers feel not just embarrassment but intense feelings of guilt and shame. Until they begin to speak they look as normal as anyone else, but the moment they speak they feel they have committed a shameful act. One of them told us he felt as though he had been caught masturbating in public. Accordingly, they develop many behaviors that tend to disguise their stuttering. They learn to avoid speaking situations that they fear may reveal their disorder. They pretend to think. They may laugh inappropriately. They find ways of distracting their listeners. They may just stop talking altogether. There are literally thousands of these reactions, and all of them just contribute to their misery. In a verbal society such as ours it is tough to be a stutterer.

The Etiology (Causes) of Stuttering

Once again we regret to say that much controversy exists concerning the etiology of stuttering. Eventually we may know what the causes are, but at the present time we do not. An introductory text such as this should not lead the student deep into the jungle of hypotheses and theories about the origin of the disorder so we will content ourselves by presenting the three major ones, the *constitutional*, the *neurotic*, and the *maladaptive learning* theories.

Constitutional Theories.   These theories hold that stuttering has an organic basis, that stuttering is the outward symptom of some underlying bodily defect or malfunction. The ancients felt that an unruly tongue was at fault and the tongues of stutterers were slit to take care of the problem. Hippocrates, the father of medicine, attributed the disorder to blood full of black bile and recommended purges. Modern theorists are not so naive and tend to feel that the cause of stuttering resides in a malfunctioning nervous system.

But many of the constitutional theories of stuttering are more sophisticated. Let us look at just one of the most enduring—the cerebral dominance theory based on the concept of **dysphemia.** This word refers to an underlying neuromuscular condition that reflects itself peripherally in nervous impulses that are poorly timed in their arrival in the paired speech musculatures. It was felt to be an inherited problem or one due to a shift of handedness. At the present time few subscribe to the cerebral dominance theory in its original form, but the concept of dysphemia has been broadened to include a weakness or discoordination of the speech programming system.

The importance of the concept of dysphemia is that it explains the stutterer's speech interruptions in terms of a nervous system that breaks down *relatively easily* in its integration of the flow of nervous impulses to the paired peripheral muscles. In order to lift the jaw, for instance, nervous impulses must arrive simultaneously in the paired muscles of each side. In some stutterers these arrival times are disrupted; they are not synchronized. It is very difficult to lift a jaw or a wheelbarrow by one handle. The dysphemic individual is able to time his speech coordinations pretty well as long as the coordinating centers in the brain are not being bedeviled by emotional reactions and their backflow of visceral sensations. He can talk pretty well when calm and unexcited. But his thresholds of resistance to emotional disturbance are low. His coordinations break down under relatively little stress. We have all known pianists and golfers who could play excellently by themselves but whose coordinations were pitifully inadequate to the demands of concert or tournament pressures.

Although the constitutional theories have generated a tremendous amount of research, the findings are often confusing and contradictory. Nevertheless, belief in the presence of an organic factor in some stutterers stubbornly persists because of the disorder's tendency to run in families, as well as the sex ratio in favor of males, the tendency for some disfluent children to also show language disabilities, certain brainwave anomalies and coordination difficulties (Rastatter and Dell, 1987), and perhaps some organically determined perceptual differences that interfere with the monitoring of sequential speech (McKnight and Cullinan, 1987).

We may be on the threshold of a significant breakthrough in the prolonged search for the origins of stuttering. There is evidence that, in some cases, stutterers have difficulty coordinating airflow and voicing with articulation and resonance. Even their fluent speech shows tiny lags and asynchronies that are reflected in slower voice onset, longer transition times between phonemes, and asymmetry between lip and jaw movements. We remain optimistic that research is on the right track, but we are also cautious because it is so difficult to separate cause and effect in stut-

Dysphemia.
A poorly timed control mechanism for coordinating sequential utterance.

tering. It could be argued that some of the discoordination seen in the subjects is a *result,* not a cause, of abnormal disfluency. The discoordination observed might be a result of the excess muscular effort and emotional upheaval involved in chronic stuttering.

Stuttering as a Neurosis.   This point of view is held by many psychiatrists and some psychologists, perhaps because their clinical practice brings them, not the garden variety of stutterers, but those with deep-seated emotional problems. If you stuttered but were also deeply disturbed by emotional conflicts, to whom would you go for help—to a speech pathologist or a psychiatrist? In exploring *their* cases of stuttering, these workers therefore come to have a firm belief in the neurotic origin and character of the disorder. Stuttering behavior is viewed as the outward symptom of a basic inner conflict. In essence, the professional workers who hold these beliefs feel that stuttering is an outward manifestation of repressed desires to satisfy such inner needs as these; to satisfy anal or oral eroticism, to express hostility by attacking and smearing the listener, or to remain infantile.

We are pretty sure that some stutterers have this type of causation, but they are in the marked minority. In them the stuttering is symptomatic of a primary neurosis. But there are many more stutterers in whom the neurosis, if any, is secondary. By that we mean the individual becomes defensive, fearful, and hostile *because* he stutters—the speech abnormality provokes a negative emotional reaction. One of our former clients stated it succinctly: "I am bugged because my speech is plugged!"

Despite the distinct lack of scientific evidence that the majority of persons who stutter are different in any meaningful psychologic way from nonstutterers (see, for example, Bloodstein, 1995, pp. 211–237), personality and emotional breakdown theories of etiology remain a popular explanation among the general public.

Learning Theories

According to this point of view, stuttering has its origin in the early fumblings and hesitancies and interruptions that seem to be a natural and common phase of the speech learning process. Rather than a condition that the child *has,* stuttering is believed to be something he *does,* a form of maladaptive behavior that is somehow learned. We have already seen what a complicated business is this speaking we take so much for granted. We must master complicated muscular coordinations, use the right sounds, formulate our thoughts aloud, express the glandular squirting of our emotions, control others, and use it for the communication of messages. Let us survey some of the developmental explanations of stuttering.

According to Wendell Johnson, chief exponent of the *semantic theory,* stuttering begins, not in the child's mouth, but in the parent's ear. He lumped all types of repetitions and prolongations into the category of **nonfluencies,** which are quite normal reactions and common to all children. The difficulty, Johnson believed, arises when a parent hears these normal nonfluencies and reacts to them with anxiety and penalty. Johnson felt that even when the repetitions and prolongations are excessive, they are merely normal reactions to the abnormal conditions of communicative stress operating at the moment. He believed, therefore, that the source of the problem lies in parental misdiagnosis and misinterpretation, pointing out that when parents become anxious or punitive about normal hesitancies, the child, reflecting their attitudes, will begin to fear, avoid, or struggle to inhibit them.

According to the *frustration theory,* stuttering need not begin in the *parent's* ear; it may also begin in the ear of the *child*. The need to communicate a message, to verbalize one's thoughts, to control another person, to express emotion—these can be powerful drives. Besides, there are children whose appetites for speech for one reason or another are almost monstrous. They must be heard! When such speech-hungry children find these drives blocked by the repetitions and prolongations produced by listener loss or other fluency disruptors, they experience much frustration. The urge to consummate the response is blocked and impeded by the delay occasioned by the repetitions and prolongations. Interruptions frustrate, whether they come from others or from one's own mouth. Too many young stutterers we have studied do not appear to have the origin of their difficulty in parental mislabeling of normal nonfluencies to let us accept blindly Johnson's thesis. Some parents actually deny the existence of any problem. Usually, stuttering has had a gradual history of growth in frequency and severity before it ever gets labeled.

The *conflict reinforcement theory* suggests that speech disfluencies are the result of competitive and opposing urges to speak and not to speak. When these tendencies are about equal, oscillations and fixations in behavior occur. The conflicting urges may come from several sources. The child may want to speak but not know what to say or how to say it. He may need to speak at a time when he thinks his listener is not listening or does not want to hear him. He may have the urge to say something "evil" that may receive penalty. He may want to speak like big people, yet not have the fluency or articulatory skills to keep the flow going. He may have an urge to express himself at a time when he feels ambivalent. The lag of a clumsy tongue may oppose a strong need to talk quickly.

Sheehan explained stuttering in terms of conflicting roles, observing that the adult stutterer tends to vacillate between the roles of normal speaker and stutterer. Much of his speech is fluent; at times he can "pass" as a normal speaker. Only intermittently is he a deviant. When the stutterer uses different accents or plays a part as an actor, thereby escaping his usual roles, he may become very fluent. He has more difficulty talking to authority figures where he must reluctantly assume a subservient role and

Nonfluency.
Pause, hesitation, repetition, or other behavior that interrupts the normal flow of utterance.

much less trouble when speaking to someone of lesser status. When caught in false or conflicting roles, the ambivalence leads to hesitancy and stuttering.

The *operant conditioning view* of stuttering is sometimes called the *one-factor theory*. Proceeding from the observation that some repetitions are found in the speech of most speakers and that they occur more frequently in children and more frequently under communicative stress, there are those who seek to explain the nature of stuttering in terms of reinforcement alone. The repetitions are said to evoke desired parental attention or concern or to enable the child to escape listener loss. These desired listener reactions then reinforce the repetitive behavior, and so it tends to occur more frequently. Once stuttering has really taken hold, whatever the stutterer does to avoid or release himself from the habitual repetitions (which now have become unpleasant) will also be strongly reinforced, since the escape from fear or frustration is always rewarding.

Other writers find it very difficult to accept the view that the initial fluency breaks are operantly conditioned. The very consistency of the *core* behaviors of stuttering—the syllabic repetitions and fixations or prolongations—that are found in all stutterers and that in young children seem to constitute most of the abnormality seem to indicate that these are precipitated rather than learned. Accordingly, some have held that this core behavior occurs initially as a result of emotionally induced breakdown in coordination. Fluency failure then becomes classically conditioned through association of stimuli to negative emotionality. Advocates of this view agree with the operant conditioning writers that much of the struggle and avoidance behavior involve learned instrumental responses. By attributing the core behavior to classical conditioning and the avoidance and struggle responses to operant conditioning, they therefore support a *two-factor theory* of the nature of stuttering as a learned response.

What is a student to believe when so many different explanations exist? Our own resolution to this problem is an eclectic one. We feel that stuttering has many origins, many sources, and that the original causes are not nearly so important as the maintaining causes, once stuttering has started. We can find stutterers who partly fit any one of these various statements of theory and some stutterers who fit several. All stutterers are not cut from the same original cloth. It is important that we know these various explanations because the problems of some of the stutterers we meet can thereby be best understood. The river of stuttering does not flow out of only one lake.

Stuttering as a Self-Reinforcing Disorder

We have said that usually when stuttering develops into its final stage, little hope can be held that it will be "outgrown" or disappear. Even when the environment is changed so that it is permissive and free from fluency disrupters, the person continues to stutter. A few individuals are able to escape even after they enter this stage only because their morale is power-fully strengthened through other achievements. But usually, once fear and frustration, avoidance and escape, have shown themselves, the disorder becomes self-perpetuating.

There are several vicious circles, or rather spirals, that characterize the confirmed stutterer. The more he fears, the more he avoids certain words or situations, and with each avoidance his fears increase. Also, the more he struggles as he tries to escape from his communicative frustration, the more abnormal a picture he presents, and again, the more he stutters the more guilt he feels. Once caught in this trap—or whirlpool—stuttering seems to be able to maintain and to perpetuate itself with a tenacity that normal speakers find difficult to understand. Nevertheless, competent speech pathologists can do much to alleviate the difficulties of even the most severe stutterer and enable him to become reasonably fluent. They prefer, however, to work with the young child and his parents as soon as possible, knowing that if they can prevent the disorder from becoming self-reinforcing, the prognosis will be much more favorable and the stut-terer can be spared much distress.

Summary

Perhaps the best way we can summarize this material is to use the picture or map in Figure 8-1. Stuttering has three sources; the major one repre-sented by the largest, Lake Learning, into which the stream from Consti-tutional Reservoir flows. Neurosis Pond is also one of the sources of stuttering, but it is smaller. Its contribution to the flow also occurs further down the river's course. Stuttering can come from any of these three sources.

As the stream leaves Lake Learning, it flows slowly and many a child caught in its current may make it to shore by himself or with a bit of parental or therapeutic help. Some of them are cast up on Precarious Is-land and become fluent for a time, only to be swept away again by the swift-moving emotional currents from Neurosis Pond. The second stage in the development of stuttering is represented by Surprise Rapids, and the stutterer begins to know that he is in trouble. It isn't hard to rescue him, however, if you know how to do it.

Once he is swept over Frustration Falls, however, he takes a beating from the many rocks that churn the stream. Despite their random strug-gling, a few make it to shore even at this stage, the third, but they usually need an understanding therapist and cooperative parents to help them. The river flows even faster here, and soon it enters the Gorge of Fear. This is the worst stretch of the whole stream of stuttering, for below it lies the Whirlpool of Self-Reinforcement. Once the child is caught in its constant circling, there is little hope that he will ever make it to shore by himself.

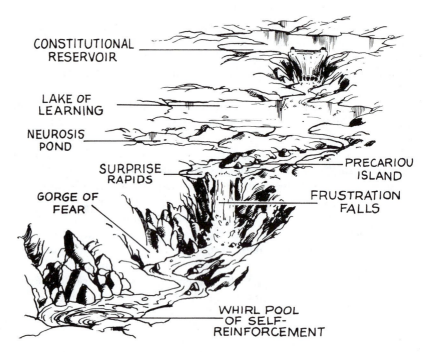

CONSTITUTIONAL RESERVOIR

LAKE OF LEARNING

NEUROSIS POND

SURPRISE RAPIDS

GORGE OF FEAR

PRECARIOU ISLAND

FRUSTRATION FALLS

WHIRL POOL OF SELF-REINFORCEMENT

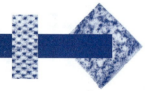

FIGURE 8-1
The origins and development of stuttering

Only an able and stout swimmer who knows not only this part, but all of the river of stuttering, can hope to save him. Where does the river end? King Charles the First knows.

THE TREATMENT OF STUTTERING

Our description of how we treat stuttering will be discussed in two sections because our aims and procedures for beginning stuttering differ from those for confirmed stuttering.

Treatment of Beginning Stuttering

Because therapy for confirmed or adult stuttering is difficult, time consuming, and often unsuccessful, many speech pathologists concentrate their efforts on prevention.[1] If the young child can be kept from developing situation and word fears and helped to withstand the communicative frustration, if he does not become ashamed or troubled by simple repetitions and prolongations, then his chance of becoming fluent is excellent. Therefore, our efforts are devoted mostly to reducing environmental penalties for stuttering, to building frustration tolerance, and to strengthening the fluent speech the child already has.

Assessment.   Before we can perform any therapy or parental counseling, we first must try to discern if in fact the child is stuttering. Two questions guide our evaluation: *How much* disfluency does he exhibit? What *type* of speech interruptions does he show? Generally, if a youngster has more than fifty speech breaks per thousand words—while talking in a free-play situation—then there is cause for concern. But it is more important to identify the type of disfluency he shows, for this will tell us how far the disorder has progressed. There is a hierarchy of danger signs (see Figure 8-2) in the development of stuttering, which ranges from rhythmic repetitions, to pitch rise (prolongations that end in an upward vocal shift), to avoidance behaviors. The higher a child is on this gauge, the more likely he is aware that talking is difficult. However, it is rather difficult to determine just how aware a child is of his speech disfluency. Children as young as three years have told us that they stutter and yet, upon gentle, indirect questioning, they were totally naïve and indifferent about their

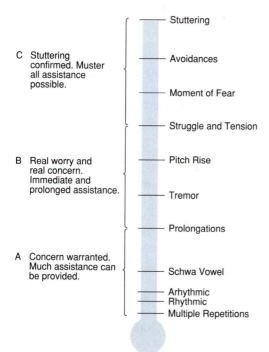

FIGURE 8-2   Danger signs leading to stuttering in young children (adapted from the Stuttering Foundation of America films on the prevention of stuttering)

speech interruptions. When in doubt about how far the disorder has progressed, it is better to err in the direction of treating the problem indirectly, with preventive therapy as outlined in the following discussion, rather than working directly with the child.

A complete assessment of a child beginning to stutter also includes an evaluation of his motor and auditory skills and the administration of a screening test of language abilities. Probably the most important aspect of the diagnostic process is an extensive interview with the child's parents. We want to know, among other things, their perception of the child and his speech problem, how they have tried to help him, and how the youngster has responded to their efforts.

Preventing and Reducing Negative Emotions.   One of the very first objectives in treatment of young children beginning to stutter is to eliminate or reduce PFAGH, the acronym representing the negative impact of penalty, frustration, anxiety, guilt, and hostility.

Penalty Reduction.   The stutterer's negative emotional states, as we have seen earlier, result from the rejecting and punishing reactions of his early listeners. Accordingly, much of the speech pathologist's time may be spent in counseling parents to help them understand that these vulnerable children need permissiveness rather than punishment and that it is unwise to make the child feel that he has done something wrong when he stutters. Sometimes when he quits getting punished for stuttering, he quits stuttering.

One of our young clients spoke the first word of almost every utterance with repetitions or prolongations. Often the repetitions would continue for several seconds. He would say, "Ca-ca-ca-ca-ca-ca-ca-ca-can I go now?" His frantic parents, who had been asking him to "Stop that!" or to "Stop and begin over again!" followed our advice and ceased these admonitions. The reduction of this penalty reduced the stuttering, but too much still remained. We then discovered that they were also breaking him of the habit of sucking his thumb. As soon as we persuaded them to stop their efforts in this regard, the child stopped stuttering completely.

Reducing Frustration.   Children in the early stage of the disorder usually experience little frustration so far as their stuttering is concerned. It comes in a bit later when the major reaction is the occasional expression of surprise and bewilderment, and the repetitions become faster, more irregular, and end in prolongations of a sound or posture. The child, without knowledge why, is beginning to sense that speaking is hard work at times, that it isn't easy. But the major frustrations come from other sources, from the daily business of living in a world geared to the needs of others as well as to one's own needs. One of the sad things about our culture is that the age of speech learning is made to coincide with the application of so many taboos. During the preschool years, there are so many things that a little child must learn he mustn't do. The frequency of usage of the word "No!" by mothers of children of this age is probably exceeded only by that of the expression, "Oh dear!" All children of this age hear a hundred "No's" each day of their lives, and some children hear more, or feel the sharp slap of a heavy hand on their bottoms. We do not wonder that the age of three is a negativistic age; the demands for conformity are especially heavy then. The child can't help feeling plenty of frustration.

In counseling our parents we must help them to understand the role of frustration in precipitating stuttering. We cannot ask them to stop being culture carriers. Their own needs for a peaceful, reasonably quiet, and orderly home life would then be frustrated. They know that each of us must learn to inhibit some of our infantile urges if we are to live in a civilized society. Are we then caught in a dilemma? On the one hand, to reduce the stuttering, we must reduce the frustration; on the other, if we do so, we create a continuing annoyance in the home that will provoke penalty outside the home if not within it.

The solution to the dilemma is simply to help the parents do two things: (1) *reduce* the number of the child's frustrating experiences and (2) *build up* his frustration tolerance. There is no need to eliminate all frustration; we merely need to decrease it. Indeed, since life is always bound to hold many frustrations in store, it is wise to help children learn to tolerate them.

Increasing Frustration Tolerance.   Many an adult should learn the lesson that it is possible to increase one's tolerance for frustration. The inappropriate infantile behavior shown by our frustrated friends (never ourselves!) is evidence that somewhere along the growth line, many of us fail to learn this lesson. Perhaps it is because we have never had the teacher we needed. There are two major ways in which we can build up frustration tolerance. One is through the empathic understanding of the needs of others; the second is through **desensitization** or adaptation. We shall not go into the first of these save to say that children should learn that parents have rights, too.

The second way in which to build frustration tolerance involves conditioning. It follows one method for breaking a horse. First you put a cloth on the horse's back, then later a sand bag, then a saddle, then a brave little boy, and then you can jump aboard. It takes time and patience and plenty of gentling and loving along the way, but some horses are taught to accept their riders this way. Through parental counseling and observation of the child, the major frustrating factors are defined. Then they are introduced into the child's life very gradually, but persistently, and only to the degree that he can tolerate them. The consequence is that the child will adapt and gradually be able to tolerate more and more frustration.

Desensitization. The toughening of a person to stress; increasing the person's ability to confront the problem with less anxiety, guilt, or hostility; a type of adaptation to stress therapy used for beginning stutterers.

Reducing Anxiety, Guilt, and Hostility.   We can reduce these reactions by reducing the penalties and frustrations that beget them. Second, outlets other than stuttering should be made available. Third, the beginning stutterer needs extra reassurance that he is loved and accepted. We have already considered the first of these three sources; now let us discuss the second.

We find many homes where the need to express one's feelings of anxiety, guilt, and hostility is neither understood nor accepted. If a child reveals that he is afraid of big dogs, thunderstorms, going to bed, or anything else, he is subjected to ridicule and "shamed out of his silly fears." His confessions of guilt and shame evoke a slap or a smile or parental embarrassment. His expressions of hostility are punished. He soon learns to keep them to himself. But we repress these emotional acids at our peril. They want out! And they always find a way. With the stutterer, that way is often stuttering.

These taboos against emotional release can be changed for some children by parental counseling, but some parents are themselves too inhibited or emotionally involved to make the necessary changes. And there are parents who do not cooperate, who cannot accept counseling. What do we do then?

Play Therapy.   We can offer the child an opportunity through play to release her forbidden feelings. We can provide her with at least one situation in which she finds a loved and loving adult who understands and accepts her feelings, who actually rewards their expression whether the child expresses them verbally or through acting out.

We have used play therapy with many of our young stutterers and not only with those in whom we suspect a primary neurosis. Where anxieties, guilts, and hostility play an important part in the child's stuttering problem and when their expression at home is denied or prevented by the parents, play therapy is absolutely essential. Not all young stutterers need it. There are some children who show no more than a normal amount of these feelings and in whose problems other factors are more important. With the neurotic stutterer it is the treatment of choice.

Creative Dramatics.   Another method for relieving the pressures of anxiety, guilt, and hostility so that they do not contribute to the stuttering problem is that of creative dramatics. In this activity, the children, guided by an imaginative adult leader, improvise a play, take the various parts, and invent their own dialogue. Children frequently select and play parts that provide for the expression of their more intense feelings.

We have found creative dramatics especially useful when much of the emotional conflict was due to sibling rivalry, fears of the local bully, or teasing by the child's playmates. In such instances, the child needs more than a permissive parent figure; he or she needs a permissive group.

Parental Counseling.   We have referred frequently to the counseling of parents in the reduction of all the factors that increase stuttering. Parents need education and information, but this is not all that counseling provides. They also need relief from their own anxieties, guilts, and hostilities. They need the opportunity to verbalize their own feelings in the presence of a permissive, understanding listener. They need to learn to view the stuttering child objectively. Jointly with the clinician, they must explore all his problems, not just his stuttering. In so doing, they often realize their own perfectionistic strivings, their own childhood conflicts, their own present acting out of relationships they had with their own parents long ago. There are many problems in counseling parents that produce difficulty. Some should be referred to the psychiatrist. With some, the conferences should be confined primarily to giving information. The depth of the counseling relationship should depend upon the clinician's own training and competence and on the severity of the interpersonal relationships which exist.

Reducing the Communicative Stress.   All stutterers at any stage show stuttering when they are bedeviled by the fluency-disrupting influences we now list. The beginning stutterer is especially vulnerable, and we have been able to cure more early stutterers by reducing the fluency disruptors in the speech environment than by any other means.

How to Prevent Hesitant Speech.   Hesitant speech (pauses, accessory vocalization, filibusters, abortive speech attempts) occurs as the result of two opposing forces. First, there must be a strong need to communicate; second, this urge must be blocked by some counterpressure. Some of the common counterpressures that oppose the desire for utterance are the following.

1. *Inability to find or remember the appropriate words.* "I'm thinking of-of-of-of-uh that fellow who-uh—oh yes, Aaronson. That's his name." This is the adult form. In a child it might occur as: "Mummy, there's a birdy out there in the . . . in the . . .uh . . . he's . . . uh . . . he . . . he . . . he wash his bottom in the dirt." Similar sources of hesitant speech are found in bilingual conflicts, where vocabulary is deficient; in aphasia; and under emotional speech exhibition, as when children forget their "pieces."
2. *Inability to pronounce or doubt of ability to articulate.* Adult form: "I can never say susstussusiss-stuh-stuhstiss—oh, you know what I mean, figures, statistics." The child's form could be illustrated by: "Mummy, we saw two poss-poss-uh-possumusses at the zoo. Huh? Yeah, two puh-pos-sums." Tongue-twisters, unfamiliar sounds or words, too fast a rate of utterance, and articulation disorders can produce these sources of speech hesitancy.

3. *Fear of the unpleasant consequence of the communication.* "Y-yes I-I-I-uh I t-took the mo-ney," "W-wi-will y-you marry m-me?" "Duh-don't s-s-spank me, Mum-mummy." Some of the conflict may be due to uncertainty as to whether the content of the communication is acceptable or not. Contradicting, confessing, asking favors, refusing requests, shocking, tentative vulgarity, fear of exposing social inadequacy, fear of social penalty in school recitations or recitals can produce this type of speech hesitancy.

4. *The communication itself is unpleasant, in that it recreates an unpleasant experience.* "I cu-cu-cut my f-f-finger . . . awful bi-big hole in it." "And then he said to me, 'You're f-f-fired'" The narration of injuries, injustices, penalties often produces speech hesitancy. Compulsory speech can also interrupt fluency.

5. *Presence, threat, or fear of interruption.* This is one of the most common of all the sources of speech hesitancy. Incomplete utterances are always frustrating, and the average speaker always tries to forestall or reject an approaching interruption. This he does by speeding up the rate, filling in the necessary pauses with repeated syllables or grunts or braying. This could be called "filibustering," since it is essentially a device to hold the floor.

6. *Loss of the listener's attention.* Communication involves both speaker and listener, and when the latter's attention wanders or is shifted to other concerns, a fundamental conflict occurs. ("Should I continue talking . . . even though she isn't listening? If I do, she'll miss what I just said . . . If I don't, I won't get it said. Probably never . . . Shall I? . . . Sha'n't I?") The speaker often resolves this conflict by repeating or hesitating until the speech is very productive of speech hesitancy. "Mummy, I-I-I want a . . . Mummy, I . . . M . . . Mumm . . . Mummy, I . . . I . . . I want a cookie." Disturbing noises, the loss of the listener's eye contact, and many other similar disturbances can produce this type of fluency interrupter.

We must remember that the beginning stutterer is still learning to talk. His speech is not stabilized. But the mere fact that he has some fluency, and all stutterers do, indicates that, with a little less pressure, stabilization may occur. If, through counseling the mother, and often by demonstrating better practices before her in play therapy, we can just ease his burden a little, the stuttering goes away. Often we are surprised to find how quickly these children respond to the reduction of any one of the precipitating factors. This is not so true of the children whose stuttering comes from constitutional or neurotic causes, but it is true of the large proportion of garden variety stutterers. And even the others are helped thereby.

Lowering the Standards of Fluency.   Communicative stress can also come from the need to talk like others do. If the parents or other children set standards of fluency far beyond the child's ability to imitate, he is almost certain to falter. Parents provide the models for all behavior whether they want to or not. It is not enough for parents to become better listeners; they must also provide models of fluency that are not too difficult for the child to follow. It is difficult for some parents to simplify their manner of talking to children, but most of them manage it once they understand why they should do so.

Reducing the Communicative Demands.   Parents frequently report that the young child has more stuttering when he first comes back from school or from playing with the other children. They think it is because of the excitement or some baleful influence of the teacher. The better explanation often is that this is the time that parents give the child a cross-examination. "What did you do at school today?" No child remembers. He did lots of things, but he didn't memorize them. One question follows another when all he wants is a cookie and to go out to play.

Removing the Stimulus Value of the Stuttering.   A final, but very important, component of communicative stress is the unfavorable attention given to the stuttering by the parents. They call attention to the repetitive speech. They tell the child to "stop it" or to "stop stuttering." We know of no quicker way to throw a child into more severe stuttering than by such suggestions. They should be terminated immediately. Other parents interrupt the child when he stutters and ask him to relax or to stop and think over what he is about to say. When we tell them not to do so, they protest and say, "But it really works. If we stop him and tell him to relax or to stop stuttering he does stop stuttering. Why shouldn't we do this?" Advice again is not enough. Parents must understand how stuttering develops, how frustration and fear are born. We do point out that the child is still continuing to stutter, and is probably getting invisibly worse, that the policies they are using are frustrating in themselves, and that they are training him to fear and avoid. We help them to see that they should reduce the stimulus value of stuttering, not make it more vivid.

Other parents do not nag their children when they hear them stuttering, but they respond to it by signals of alarm and distress, which are probably worse. They freeze in their conversational tracks. They hold their breath; they become jittery. Their faces suddenly become masks. Any little child will respond to such signals as though they were cannon shots. We must reduce these signals. They add too much to communicative stress.

Building Ego Strength

Ego strength is difficult to define, but we know when it's low and we know when it's high. It rises and falls in all of us depending upon our

Ego strength. Morale or self-confidence.

success-failure ratio, but its basic ingredients are love, faith, and opportunity. Some of our stuttering children are denied all three.

We have come to have a great respect for parents, once they realize that their child is in danger and know what to do. Some parents have to be taught to show their love. Some have to be shown how to put aside their own anxieties and to let the child run the risks of living in a dangerous world. Better to break a leg than break a spirit! We have found the overprotective parent to be one of our major problems in this regard. The child must have opportunity even to fail. Security does not come from success alone.

How do we build up ego strength, morale, self-confidence? It is difficult to generalize. Often the clinician must accept much of the responsibility for doing the job. We ourselves have done many things. We have taught a boy to box, another to swim, another to read, another to ride one of our horses. We once took a child to a cowboy movie every week for a whole semester.

> One little girl stutterer, the next to the youngest in a family of six girls, had failed to show any improvement in her stuttering for almost a year despite all our attempts to reduce the denominator of her own particular stuttering equation. Then one of our student clinicians bought her a puppy, and she stopped stuttering. I asked the clinician, a girl, why she had bought the puppy. "It was obvious," she answered. "I have been out to Nancy's home several times, and it was clear that she had no status whatsoever. She's shy and quiet, and the other girls dominate her completely. I felt that she ought to have something she could dominate or feel superior to, someone to whom she could talk and not be interrupted, something to love. I had a puppy once and I remember."

We aren't sure that her analysis was correct, but we are sure that the stuttering disappeared. And we are certain that self-confidence, morale, and ego strength can be increased with love, faith, and opportunity.

Increasing Fluency.   First, with the beginning stutterer, we should arrange things so that during the periods of more severe stuttering, he talks less. The converse is also true. Since early stuttering comes in waves, during the periods of excellent speech, the parents should provide him with every possible opportunity to exercise it. This simple policy has eliminated the disorder in many children.

Second, both in the play therapy sessions and in the home, self-talk should be encouraged. Parents should do it as they go about their ordinary activities, telling aloud what they are doing, perceiving, or feeling. In sessions with the clinician she should provide the same models of commentary. Only a few children stutter in their self-talk. It should be facilitated.

We also institute games that might be called "speech play." No attention to the stuttering, of course, should be involved. The child should only know that he and the clinician or parent are having verbal fun. Some of these games involve speaking in unison, or echoing, or speech accompanied by rhythmic activities, or talking very slowly and lazily. There are variations of these activities, but the purpose of all of them is to increase the experience of fluency.

Desensitization Therapy.   Any fluency under any conditions is to be sought, but fluency under conditions of communicative stress is especially to be prized. Most beginning stutterers respond favorably to a coordinated program of the type we have described, but there are some who become worse as the environmental pressures are removed, and there are many whose parents and teachers cannot be persuaded to change their unfortunate policies. What can we do with these children? Give up the case and blame the failure on the child's peculiar constitution or the parent's guilt? No, there is another alternative, if we can toughen the child, build up his tolerance to stress, and create calluses against the hecklings, rejections, or impatience.

This is what the speech clinician does. He first establishes a social relationship with the child in which the latter does not realize that he is doing any speech therapy. They may be setting up a toy railroad on the floor or participating in any other similar activity. The speech clinician then works to achieve a basal fluency level on the part of the child. This usually consists of simple statements of fact, requests, observations, and so forth. The clinician, as he works, thinks aloud in snatches of self-talk, commenting on his activity. Soon the child will begin to do the same, and by appropriately altering the communicative conditions, and his own manner, the clinician gets the child to speak with complete fluency. In the young stutterer, this is not too difficult. Then, once the basal fluency level has been *felt* by the child, the clinician begins gradually to inject into the situation increasing amounts of those factors that tend to precipitate repetitions and nonfluency in that particular child. He may, for instance, begin gradually to hurry him, faster and faster. *But,* and this is vitally important, the clinician stops putting on the pressure and returns to the basal fluency level as soon as he sees the first sign of *impending* nonfluency.

As soon as the clinician returns to the basal fluency level, he again begins slowly to turn up the heat, to hurry the child a little faster, to avert his gaze more often, or whatever he happens to be trying to toughen the child against. Then an interesting thing occurs. The child can take more pressure the second time than he could the first. But again, the first signs of approaching stuttering appear, and again the clinician goes down to the original basal fluency level. It should be made clear that throughout this training, the child never does stutter, if the clinician has been skillful. What he feels, probably, is that he is being fluent under pressure. Fluency becomes associated with the feeling of being hurried. The effects of this toughening to stress are not confined to the speech sessions. The child seems to be able to stay fluent even when his father keeps interrupting him.

Prognosis.   If we can locate the child soon enough and initiate the type of therapy outlined earlier, the chances of a favorable outcome are excellent. Children in the early stages of the disorder usually seem to present no great difficulty if systematic treatment can be administered. For these children it seems as though all that is needed is the reduction of one or two of the factors that are precipitating the speech hesitancy so that self-healing, can take place.

Treatment for Confirmed Stuttering

At the present time there is no one form of treatment for confirmed stuttering that has gained general acceptance by all speech pathologists. Some of them, relatively few, use only psychotherapy, hoping that psychological counseling will lead to the lessening of the negative emotions that created or continue to play a part in maintaining the disorder. Another group of workers concentrate their efforts on conditioning the stutterer not to stutter. A third group, using what has been termed traditional therapy, trains the stutterer to respond without struggling or avoidance to his fear or experience of being blocked, that is, to learn to stutter easily and fluently. One interesting perspective on the evolution of stuttering management theory has been well synthesized by Prins (1995). Since many approaches have some successes and some failures, students should be wary of the many claims of cure or improvement from some ostensibly "new" treatment for stuttering. Confirmed stuttering is a tough nut to crack. It is very easy to get even a very severe stutterer to be fluent for a short time, but keeping him that way is an entirely different matter.

Let us now take a look at these three major ways of treating stuttering.

Psychotherapy.   There is some psychotherapy inherent in all forms of stuttering therapy because the close relationship between the clinician and his client provides an opportunity for the ventilation of emotion and an opportunity in a permissive setting to explore new ways of coping with stress. Most speech pathologists confine themselves to providing this supportive relationship and refer their stutterers elsewhere when they discover deep-seated emotional conflicts that are not speech-related. Some stutterers, mainly the affluent, are referred to psychiatrists; others to psychologists or to counseling centers. Speech pathologists need enough background in psychotherapy to be able to make the proper referrals.

With a highly permissive clinician, the stutterer verbalizes his feelings and perceptions at deeper and deeper levels and, on the basis of the insights so achieved, becomes able to accept and change himself.

We wish to emphasize, however, that most stutterers, despite the constant emotional stress under which they live, are pretty normal individuals. Most of the research has shown that they are no more neurotic or psychotic than fluent speakers. Their anxieties, guilt, and frustrations seem to be the result of their stuttering, not the cause of it, and once they become fluent, their emotional upheavals usually disappear. Deep psychotherapy is for the relatively rare stutterer whose stuttering stems from and is maintained by basic emotional conflicts.

The Fluent Speech Approach

The second major form of treatment currently being used for the confirmed stutterer in this country is based upon the belief (or supposition) that the stutterer's fluent speech can be strengthened sufficiently to enable him to withstand any threat of stuttering. Zero stuttering is the goal, certainly one to be desired if it is possible to attain. There are many variants of this kind of stuttering therapy, but all of them use some technique to produce some nonstuttered speech, and then some program is administered to reinforce and maintain the precarious fluency evoked in the therapy room. All the ancient techniques, such as rate control by metronome or delayed feedback, relaxation, unison speaking or **shadowing (echoing)**, speaking while sighing or using passive breath control, various forms of suggesting (including hypnosis), rewarding fluent speech and punishing stuttering, prolongation of the vowels or syllables, and many others are still being used despite their long history of failure.

Why does this situation exist? The first reason is that most stutterers can be made temporarily fluent by any of these procedures; the second is that they are relatively easy for the clinician to administer. We repeat: All stutterers can speak fluently under special conditions and not one of them stutters on every word or every sentence every time he speaks. He can speak normally when he is unafraid or calm or relaxed or when he feels confident and assured or has faith in the clinician's presumed competence. His stuttering also tends to disappear if he is asked to speak in a way that is markedly different from his usual manner, such as using a falsetto, drawling his words at a very slow rate, using a singsong kind of utterance, adopting a dialect, or making the voice very nasal and so on. By concentrating on any of these strange ways of talking, the stutterer temporarily can distract himself from the fears of words and sounds that usually precipitate his stuttering, and, for a short time, become fluent. Unfortunately, these strange ways of speaking prevent stuttering only as long as they are novel. When they become habitual they lose their distractive value and back come the fears and the stuttering. Most speech pathologists are aware of this situation, but many of them (especially the advocates of operant conditioning) feel that no matter how the first fluency is obtained, it can be reinforced sufficiently and any stuttering pun-

Shadowing.
Echo speech.

Echo speech.
A technique in which the patient is trained to repeat instantly what he or she is hearing, following almost simultaneously the utterance of another person. Also called "shadowing."

ished contingently, so that the person will be able eventually to speak normally. When relapses occur, as they tend to do no matter how the stutterer is treated, booster sessions are provided for those who return for further help. Many, alas, do not return.

There are many different forms of the fluency-inducing approach to the treatment of stuttering. All of them seek, as we have said, to "establish" fluency in a clinical setting and then, using carefully programmed small steps, transfer the new speaking skills to conversational situations. In almost every instance, advocates of the "don't stutter" approach use some variation of behavior modification, usually featuring either classical or operant conditioning.

The Modification of Stuttering Approach

The third way of treating a confirmed stutterer seeks to make her fluent by training her to stutter without struggle or avoidance. Believing that most of the stutterer's abnormality and communicative deviance consist of learned responses to the threat or experience of breaks in the speech flow, many speech pathologists seek to reverse the vicious developmental spiral and to teach the stutterer to stutter as easily and as effortlessly as she did when the disorder first began. Even the most severe stutterer will occasionally exhibit some of these easy early stutterings, and if her characteristic stuttering behaviors can be modified and shaped to resemble them, most of her abnormality will disappear. Certainly, she will not get many penalties or feel much frustration if all that she shows are a few easy syllabic repetitions or a slight lagging prolongation of a sound. In short, the speech pathologist does not penalize stuttering or try to get the stutterer to avoid it. Instead, he encourages that stutterer to stutter if he must but in a new and different way, one that will not interfere with his communication.

What usually happens is that the amount as well as the severity of stuttering dramatically decreases once the stutterer finds he can cope with his fears or his feeling of being blocked, once he discovers that he is no longer helpless, that he can be fluent even though he does stutter. Advocates of this approach believe that only a few advanced or confirmed stutterers can ever be made permanently fluent by strengthening their normal speech or by punishing their stutterings or by merely undergoing psychotherapy. They believe that the stutterer needs to know what to do when he fears he may stutter or finds himself doing so.

We now describe the third approach in some detail since it is the kind of therapy that these authors have found most successful. In many ways it is eclectic, combining psychotherapy, classical and operant conditioning, and insightful therapies. Its major focus is on the stutterer's fears and frustrations and the avoidance and struggle behaviors they generate. In this approach the stutterer is encouraged to seek out stuttering rather than avoid it or try to talk without stuttering.

And he is trained to modify that stuttering so that, if it does occur, little abnormality will be exhibited. In other words, we try to shape the stuttering into a more fluent form.

The stutterer already knows how to speak normally, but he does not know what to do when he fears or finds himself stuttering. We simply teach him better ways of coping. The stutterer's fluency increases because once he stops being terrified of stuttering or ashamed of it and once he finds that he can stutter easily and effortlessly, the number of his stutterings decreases in both frequency and severity. Advocates of this approach feel that psychotherapy alone ignores the abnormal speech behaviors that constitute the essence of the disorder. They also feel that trying to extinguish the stutterer's fears by classical conditioning or merely strengthening the fluent speech or punishing the stuttering usually results in relapse and eventual failure. They believe that merely experiencing the *absence* of fear or having a period of fluency does not solve the stutterer's problem. He has had many such experiences before. What he needs are new and better ways of coping with fear and stuttering when they beset him.

To understand how the speech pathologist of this persuasion goes about the task of making the confirmed stutterer fluent you should know something of the program's sequence (see Figure 8-3). We have coined an acronym, MIDVAS, to help you remember. Each separate letter of this word refers to the goal of a particular phase of therapy, and they follow the order of the letters of the word. *M* is for motivation; *I* is for identification; *D* for desensitization; *V* for variation; *A* for approximation; and *S* for stabilization. This is the sequence of our therapy. We structure our therapy plan so that each new phase has a special emphasis, but all preceding goals are continued. New experiences are added but the old are reviewed. It is cumulative therapy. For convenience of exposition, we describe the treatment as though it were being administered to severe adult stutterers. Modifications must of course be made for young children or for the very mild stutterer, as well as for the special needs of any given individual. All stutterers present special problems. All need special treatment, but there still are general principles and practices that help all of them.

The First Phase of Therapy: Motivation.   One who has not worked much with confirmed stutterers would expect to have little trouble motivating them to do the things necessary to find relief. Certainly, the interruption to communication, the social implications and deprivations, and the struggling and the fear are unpleasant. Why then do we find so much resistance? We think there are two answers. First, it is always difficult to confront one's abnormality, to expose it enough to modify it, and this resistance is found in healing all emotional ills. Second, the fact of the stutterer's fluency when alone or in nonstressful situations makes him feel that no major overhaul is needed. But deep in his bones he knows he has a tough job to do, that the seizurelike behavior and the panic of his fears

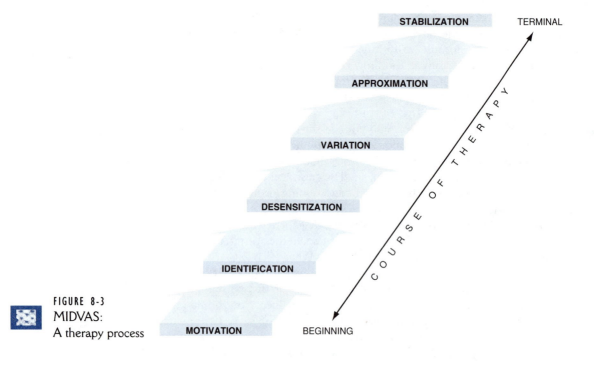

STABILIZATION   TERMINAL

APPROXIMATION

VARIATION

DESENSITIZATION

COURSE OF THERAPY

IDENTIFICATION

FIGURE 8-3
MIDVAS:
A therapy process   MOTIVATION   BEGINNING

are not going to yield to any waving of a savior's hands; yet it is only human to hope for easy miracles. We keep in our desk a little bottle of pink aspirin with a label reading, "One of these will cure stuttering forever." In an early session, we always hand a new stutterer the bottle. He always grins and hands it back. We have never had one so much as open it in thirty years. They know.

When the confirmed stutterer first comes for therapy, he usually speaks with great difficulty; and we have found it wise to begin by defining our role, not as a teacher or preacher or medicine man, but as a guide and companion on a joint quest. We do this in the initial interview, explaining why we ask the questions we do, and sharing with him the implications of his answers. When he stutters, we provide a running commentary of our own objective evaluations of his behavior. When he avoids, or postpones, a speech attempt on a feared word, or when he uses some trick to start his utterance or disguise the stuttering that occurs, we recognize and identify what he has done with complete acceptance. Suddenly he finds not only a permissive listener but one who understands. This is one of the crucial experiences in all successful therapy.

Another crucial experience that the stutterer should have as soon as possible is that of observing her clinician actually *sharing* her abnormality. We do this by attempting to duplicate her moments of stuttering. The stutterer can be asked to teach the clinician how to replicate her blocks so that she may better understand the scope of her problem. By pantomiming what she is doing as she is doing it, we become a human mirror for her. This interaction not only helps to produce a close relationship between the stutterer and the clinician, but it also partially extinguishes some of the persisting evil effects of old traumatic wounds.

Another important experience occurs when the clinician reveals that she is interested and desires to share not only the outward behavior of the stutterer but also to understand his *inner feelings*. We find it wise to begin with the feelings created by the immediate moment of stuttering. A few stutterers are able, with skillful counseling, to express these feelings, but most are not. The stuttering itself interferes with expression. We therefore verbalize the stutterer's feelings for him. We do this tentatively and ask for corrections and additions.

The stutterer soon comes to feel that this person is a competent guide who seems to know one way out of the swamp. Let us outline how we help him to come to this conclusion.

First, we try to provide some person whom he can see or hear who has been able to conquer his stuttering problem. We also have the tales of many others on tape, and we use videotapes and films for the same purpose.

Next, we try to help the stutterer realize that he possesses in his own present speech both a certain amount of fluency and also, what is more important, a certain amount of stuttering that does not interrupt communication unduly or show much abnormality. This latter item is of utmost importance. All stutterers have some moments of stuttering that are unforced and unaccompanied by struggle or avoidance. We point these out when they occur and often make a tape in which many samples of these fluent stutterings are combined. We ask the stutterer to listen to this tape frequently. Also in our pantomimic sharing of his stuttering, we often repeat again and again these fluent stutterings so that he can see them, and we ask him to repeat them also. We point up this easy, fluent sort of stuttering as a goal object. Even a rat runs a difficult maze better when he has a taste or smell of the cheese to be found at the end of that maze.

It is possible to help the stutterer to have another very important experience: *The realization that it is possible to stutter in many different ways and that some ways may be better than others.* We make it possible for him to observe and duplicate the kinds of stuttering shown by other stutterers and ask him to experiment a bit in modifying his own. This is another of the crucial experiences that are the mile markers on the road to freedom. There are many of them.

It is also necessary that a clear picture of the course of therapy be given to the stutterer. He needs some kind of a map before he becomes willing to undertake a journey, even though he now knows he has a guide. We have found it useful to give him some understanding. This first phase of therapy requires the imparting of information. The stutterer is usually as ignorant of the nature of his disorder as he is of the behavior he uses so compulsively. He needs to know something of the causes of stuttering and the way in which it develops, and we also help him to find information about the way in which stuttering has been treated in the past as well as how it is being treated by other clinicians. We do not believe in blind therapy. We want him to know where he's going, where he is, and what he has to do. We find that we get a better motivated client this way.

The Second Phase of Therapy: Identification.   As soon as possible we move directly into the second phase of our therapy, in which the basic goal is the identification and evaluation of the various factors in the client's *personal* stuttering equation. There is no emphasis on trying to speak more fluently. Just the converse. The stutterer is to seek out stuttering experiences and to analyze the behavior and identify the forces that created it. This is the period of self-study, of self-exploration. (Note that this goal structuring increases the approach and decreases the avoidance vectors in the **approach-avoidance** conflicts.) The objective observation of the stuttering behavior gets down to what the semanticists might call "first-order facts." The more the stutterer stutters, the more opportunity he has to make his observations. The clinician shares and rewards these discoveries.

The first targets for identification are the core stuttering elements—the repetitions and prolongations—and then the escape and struggle behaviors. Here is how we introduced the task to one client.

> In this session we want to start getting acquainted with what you do when you stutter. We need to move from the general feeling you have of "being stuck" to some very specific descriptions; we will be making an inventory of your stuttering pattern. Before you can alter your reactions to the anticipation or presence of speech breaks, you need to know very precisely what those reactions are. We will use a mirror so we can see it, listen to it on a recorder, and use our fingertips to search for areas of tension. I know this is not easy work—it will be stiff and uncomfortable at first to confront the old out-of-control behaviors.

Approach-avoidance. Refers to conflicts produced when the person is beset by two opposing drives to do or not do something.

Many times during these identification sessions we have had stutterers literally yelp out loud in self-discovery when they suddenly realize how much they are fighting themselves, how much they are holding back while trying to go ahead as they try to talk. These moments of self-discovery are very important.

One of the unique features of this type of therapy is the use of the speech assignment. In addition to the stutterer's own attempts in self-therapy, certain required activities and experiences are devised by the clinician to provide guidelines and models for what the client should be doing himself. Some stutterers need few of these; others need many; but the emphasis is always on self-therapy. The devising of self-assignments is constantly and vividly rewarded. Reporting the experiences and *feelings* evoked by these experiences is a very necessary part of the clinical routine. This may be done orally either in private sessions with the clinician or in group sessions with other stutterers, or the reports may be written in certain instances.

Many **secondary stutterers** have become a bit paranoid about the reactions of listeners to their stuttering. Even when no overt rejection is evidenced, they think the listener is merely covering up a punitive or embarrassed reaction. It is vitally necessary that they do some reality testing. Some assignments which could begin this testing might run like this.

> Keep track of the number of listeners who frown or show objective signs of impatience when you stutter. What proportion do not? Get a sample of ten strangers with whom you stuttered obviously to determine the proportion.

> How many store clerks did you talk to before you found one who showed signs of mirth or mocking when you stuttered? Try a minimum of five.

> If possible, ask one of your friends how he really feels when you stutter to him. Ask him to tell you the truth. Report what he said and whether you think he was being honest.

These assignments happen to revolve about the speech disorder itself, but we wish to make clear that we explore all penalties, not just those evoked by stuttering. Punishment of any kind seems to add an increment of stuttering. The client becomes aware of sources of rejection other than his stuttering. In this phase of therapy, we make no attempts to eliminate the behavior that provokes the penalty but merely to explore and to define it, and often the stutterer starts making some changes anyway. The emphasis at this phase of therapy is merely to *identify* those penalties which contribute to stuttering.

In exploring *frustration* the stutterer compiles an account of the frustrations characteristic of his present situation and also a history of those of the past. He also thereby becomes aware of basic drives and needs other than to speak fluently. Many stutterers become so focused on stuttering that other major problems are completely disregarded, even though they contribute to the disorder and may be more easily rectified. In the identification phase of therapy, the whole target, not just the bull's-eye of stuttering, comes into view.

Secondary stuttering. Refers to the advanced forms of stuttering in which awareness, fear, avoidance, and struggle are shown.

Now we confront the stuttering directly. In this phase of treatment, the stutterer explores and identifies the types of communicative stress to which he is most vulnerable. Again he is *seeking* speaking experiences instead of avoiding them, which is healthy in itself and a reversal of old practices. Here are two typical assignments.

1. Which of these two audience reactions seems to produce more stutterings: (a) interruption by having the listener finish what you are trying to say, or (b) having him look away when you're stuttering? Collect two experiences of each kind and report.

2. Read a passage aloud to some other stutterer very swiftly; then another of equal length at a normal rate; then another at a normal rate; and finally a fourth at a fast rate. Using hand counter, have him count how many blocks you have under fast and ordinary speaking rates, averaging the two trials for each. How much of a factor is speed in producing more stuttering? Report your findings.

In exploring *situation fears,* the stutterer should not only identify those of the present and the past but also attempt to assess their intensity. He should also try to discover what he specifically dreads. Many very important insights come from this sort of investigation. He may even find that he doesn't know what he is afraid of. The stutterer should also study the relationship between situation fears and the amount of actual stuttering that does occur. He may find that the correlation is not as high as he thinks it is. We find that experiences of this sort are very salutary because they weaken the *fear of fear.*

Word fears include not only fears of specific words but also the phonetic fears of sounds. It might be objected that by focusing the stutterer's attention on them, we only make them that much worse. All we can say in this regard is that any increment of this sort is negligible. They already have their full strength based upon a thousand memories. Stutterers also fear these phonetic fears; they attempt to distract themselves from them, to repress them, to escape from them. We have found it healing to look them directly in the face.

We also feel it very important for the stutterer to study his own variable feelings of self-worth. As we have said, stutterers are focused so much on their stuttering that they fail to see their other difficulties. In much the same fashion they are also unable to evaluate with any objectivity the other assets they possess. In this phase of the treatment they learn objectivity, and it is important that they apply it to the favorable factors as well as to the unfavorable ones.

Only his stuttering seems to have stimulus value for the stutterer; the quite evident amount of fluency he also possesses does not. At this stage he has become morbidly conscious only of his abnormality, not of his normality. Also, most confirmed stutterers have an exaggerated concept of what constitutes normal fluency. They do not realize that normal speak-

ers are also nonfluent, at times of stress very nonfluent. This area must also
be investigated.

1. On what percentage of words do you really stutter? Make tape
   recordings of yourself (a) reading to another person, (b) explaining
   something to a friend, and (c) making phone calls. Count the words
   spoken and the stutterings, and find out how fluent you are in each.
2. Listen to the conversations of other people, and be able to show us
   all the different kinds of nonfluencies they demonstrated.

In this section describing the *identification* phase of the therapy we
have tried to show how we help the stutterer recognize the scope of his
problem as expressed in terms of the various factors that make his stuttering better or worse. We would like to re-emphasize here that this exploratory phase by itself often produces immediate decreases both in the
amount of stuttering and in the intensity of the fear and avoidance. As in
motivation, identification experiences will continue throughout therapy.
We find, however, that we have more success when we stress it early in the
treatment.

The Third Phase of Therapy: Desensitization.

The third major
phase in the treatment of confirmed stuttering we have termed desensitization because our major goal in this part of the therapy is to toughen our
client to those factors that normally increase the frequency and the severity of his stuttering. In this phase, we are raising the thresholds of breakdown. It is very necessary that the stutterer understand why this is being
done. But there are immediate rewards from desensitization. He will soon
learn that as he becomes more hardened, he stutters less and suffers less.
As he becomes tougher, he finds that penalties do not throw him so
quickly; that frustration has a less evil effect; that he can tolerate more anxiety, guilt, and hostility than he could before; that communicative disruption and fear do not precipitate stuttering as frequently as once they did.
And the morale factor rises, as any soldier knows, when he has learned
what he can endure.

It is obvious that this phase of therapy takes some skill and empathy
on the clinician's part. He must not overload. Indeed, often the clinician must keep the client from overloading himself. But there must always be present the faith that comes from realizing the enormous
potentials that all humans seem to possess, and the support which only
a loved and respected clinician can give. Evidence must be provided that
the clinician can also share these experiences, can also bear the stress, can
also suffer but endure. Often he must become the receptacle for the hostile attacks that result from the hurt the stutterer experiences when he
tries and fails.

Assignments are given that provide opportunities for desensitization
to occur. Again, the stutterer is prevailed upon to construct his own

assignments and to bring to the clinician for sharing and analysis all the trophies and the failures which result. Group therapy provides an excellent situation for sharing these accounts, and the stutterers vie with each other and support each other. Also, as they often do assignments together, a sense of comradeship is established, which relieves the feeling of isolation so many stutterers know so well.

Usually, we begin fairly gradually to introduce the stress challenges, and the clinician sets models for the client to follow. We have found it wise to enter a store or similar speaking situation and to fake a very long stuttering block in the presence of the stutterer or stutterers. And we show we are not upset, that we remember exactly what the clerk did and how he reacted. We also verbalize our own feelings honestly. And then we do it again. We have found this often to be another crucial experience in the stutterer's life. The fact that another human being, a normal speaker perhaps, would be able to undergo such an experience and remain well integrated and relatively unperturbed, seems to impress the stutterer greatly. After a few of these demonstrations, he is willing to try himself.

Assignments must be so structured that an objective report can be produced. They must provide enough stress to permit desensitization to occur. For any given case, their difficulty must be so tailored that more success than failure ensues, but failure is not to be avoided entirely. Indeed, in the sharing period with the clinician or other stutterers, often the failures when expressed and accepted do more good than even the successes. But there must be clinician approval and reward for meeting these challenges. And constantly we must emphasize the basic purpose these desensitization experiences are designed to fulfill: the building of a thicker hide on the stutterer's sensitive soul.

The Fourth Phase of Therapy: Variation.   It is not enough to motivate, to identify, and desensitize, although these bring reductions in the frequency and severity of stuttering. In this new phase of therapy we begin to change, to modify the reactions to the factors that determine stuttering. Our purpose is to break up the stereotype of the stutterer's responses, to attach new responses to the old cues. Much of the strength of habitual compulsive reactions lies in their stereotype, in the consistency of their patterning. Varying them weakens them. Until new responses are made available, the stutterer has no choice except to yield to the old ones. We must help her to know that she has this choice. We cannot persuade her through intellectual argument. Only by behaving differently can she know that it is possible to behave differently.

This variation phase of treatment is usually short in duration because it passes directly into the next one of approximation, in which we seek to help the stutterer learn not just *new* responses to old pressures, but *good* responses. By "good" we mean only that new responses can be learned that will facilitate fluency rather than reduce it. We must help her learn new responses that do not continually reinforce her stuttering as her old responses do. But before these new ways of behaving can be learned, the old ways must be weakened. Variation must precede approximation. The stutterer must realize that she has a choice of responses before she can pick out and master a better one.

Again we seek to provide for the stutterer experiences in which this learning may occur and to motivate her to seek such experiences herself. Here are just a few examples.

> On every other word on which you stutter, be sure to stutter repetitively but slowly on the first syllable. Do this to three listeners.

> Ordinarily you walk around the block several times before entering a store to ask for something. Today, ask questions in three stores, but stand absolutely still looking in the display window for as long as it would take you to walk around that block. Then go in and ask for it. Report your introspections.

> Get a companion and hunt for the noisiest places you can find. Try not to speak more loudly to your friend but speak more slowly and distinctly.

> You say you find yourself worrying vaguely about everything and find it hard to get to sleep. Tonight, assign yourself to worry on purpose and do so aloud in self-talk just before you hop into bed. Worry aloud about everything you can possibly think of.

> Whenever a listener interrupts you or finishes a word on which you are stuttering, say to him, "Don't interrupt me. I have a hard enough time talking anyway."

As we write this chapter we are constantly aware of the inadequacy of our presentation of such assignments in reflecting what actually occurs in therapy. These assignments by themselves have no value. Only when shared with the clinician and when feelings are expressed and when rewards are appropriately timed, do the experiences they evoke have potency in modifying the attitudes and outward behavior of the stutterer. It would be easier and perhaps safer to resort to statements of vague general principles, but students seem to profit more from specific examples. So be it!

The Fifth Phase of Therapy: Approximation.

Once the stutterer has learned that his habitual reactions to the factors that make stuttering worse can be varied, we try to help him learn *new responses that will diminish that stuttering.* We now seek not just different responses but the best responses, those which tend to extinguish stuttering rather than reinforce it. Why do we call this phase the approximation phase? Because we feel that new responses are acquired, not by sudden exchange, but by gradual modification. You just don't stop stuttering severely and suddenly begin to stutter easily. By approximation we mean the progressive modification of behavior toward a goal response.

The basic goal, then, of this phase of therapy is to learn how to stutter and to respond to stress in such a fashion that the disorder will not be reinforced. The clinician's responsibility is to see that rewards are felt whenever the stutterer moves closer to this goal. Approval is contingent upon *progress,* not merely upon performance. Happily, the relief from communicative abnormality seems to follow the same course, and provides even more powerful reinforcement. The goal is getting nearer now.

In our discussion of this phase of therapy, we will confine ourselves to the exposition of what we do with the fears and experiences of stuttering itself. It must be remembered, however, that the characteristic responses to penalty, frustration, and all the other disturbing factors must also be modified in the direction of nonreinforcement of the stuttering.

One of the best ways we have discovered to help the stutterer learn an easier, nonreinforcing kind of stuttering is to do it with him. He watches us and hears us as we join him in his stuttering, duplicating the first of his behavior, but then we ease out of the tremors, cease the struggling, and smoothly finish the word. Often at first, the contrast between his continued struggles and our smooth utterance tends to shock him, but gradually he begins to follow our lead and to stutter as we do. He finds us sharing his initial behavior but then diverging. We make the changes gradually, at first setting models of minor changes that he may be able to follow, and rewarding them when they appear. Once he can make these minor changes (e.g., stuttering with his eyes open rather than closed), he gets no more approval until a further change occurs (e.g., lips are loosened from their tensed closure), and so on. We move only as far as the client is ready and able to go in any given session.

As soon as any change in the stuttering behavior has been learned, the stutterer is encouraged to use it in **cancellation** (Figure 8-4). By this term we mean that the stutterer stops as soon as a stuttered word has finally been uttered; pauses; and then says it again, this time using the modification he has learned in unison stuttering with his clinician. He still stutters this second time, faking, if he must, a duplication of the same stuttering he has just experienced; but now he modifies it in accordance with the new behavior he has learned. Then he finishes his sentence. Communication stops once he stutters, and it continues only after he has used a better stuttering response. This is also powerfully reinforcing.

Pull-out (Figure 8-4) is an awkward term, stemming from the stutterers' own language usage, referring to the moment of stuttering itself and what the stutterer does to escape from his oscillations or fixations. Evil pull-outs are the jerks, the sudden exhaling of all available air. These only increase the penalty and all other factors that make for more stuttering in the future. There are better ways of terminating these fixations and oscillations, and once these new ways have been learned in unison speaking with the clinician, and practiced frequently in cancellations in all types of speaking situations, the stutterer should begin to incorporate them within the original moment of stuttering itself.

Cancellation.
The voluntary repetition of a word on which stuttering has occurred.

Pull-out.
The voluntary release from a stuttering block.

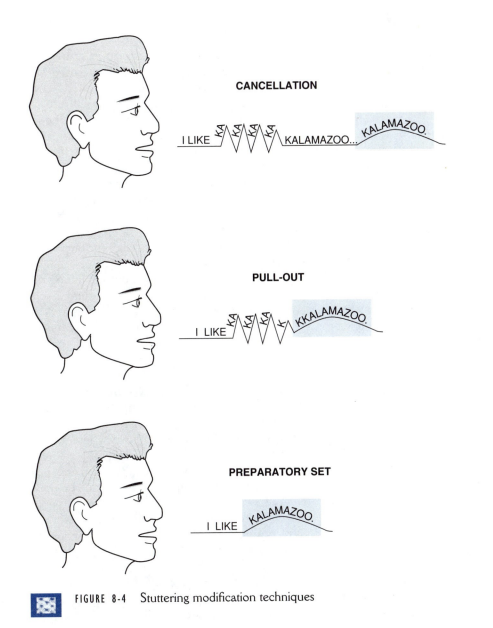

CANCELLATION

I LIKE KA KA KA KA KALAMAZOO... KALAMAZOO.

PULL-OUT

I LIKE KA KA KA K KKALAMAZOO.

PREPARATORY SET

I LIKE KALAMAZOO.

FIGURE 8-4   Stuttering modification techniques

Our next step is to move into the period of anticipation, into what has been called the "prespasm period." Usually, in response to word or phonetic fears, the stutterer actually makes little covert rehearsals of the stuttering abnormality he expects. These *preparatory sets* (Figure 8-4) to stutter often determine the kind and length of abnormality that result. Therefore, once the stutterer has shown that he can incorporate change not only in cancellation but also during the actual stuttering behavior, he is challenged to incorporate it within his anticipatory rehearsals, to plan to stutter this new way. Often we can help him by rehearsing for him and by getting him to duplicate our model before he attempts the word he has indicated he will stutter upon. Again, we reward the successes and disregard the failures.

As each new modification of stuttering is learned and starts up the series of experiences in cancellation, pull-outs, and preparatory sets, new modifications are being born, either with the help of the clinician through unison stuttering or through self-discoveries. With each new change comes a decrease in the severity and often in the frequency of stuttering as well. Fears of words, then of situations, lose their intensity. The stutterer's self-confidence begins to grow with each new achievement. The fluency factor grows larger. He becomes able to tolerate more communicative stress. It is also interesting to watch how he applies the same therapeutic principles to his other inadequate behaviors.

We cannot end this section on approximation without reminding the student that most of the progress made must be due to the stutterer's solo efforts. Many speech assignments are devised to provide the necessary opportunities for progressively modifying the stuttering behavior under stress. But this is how we begin.

The Final Phase of Therapy: Stabilization.   For lack of a clear-cut *stabilization* program, many stutterers have experienced frequent relapses and despair. It is not enough to bring the stutterer to the point where he is fluent, where he can speak with little struggle or fear. We must stabilize his new behavior, his new resistance to stress, his new integration. Anxiety-conditioned responses are very difficult to extinguish entirely. New adjustments must be made, new responsibilities undertaken now that the stuttering excuse is no longer valid. Terminal therapy must be done carefully. It must be done well.

Often stuttering seems to go out the same door it entered. More of the easy and unconscious repetitions and prolongations appear; periods of fairly frequent small stutterings alternate with periods of very good fluency. Sudden bursts of fear and even avoidance occur. Under moments of extreme stress an occasional severe blocking may be evident. It is important that the stutterer understand this and accept it as part of his problem. Often the clinician must be available for the verbalization of these traumatic episodes and receive the confession of avoidance and compulsive behaviors with accepting reassurance and remedial measures.

Even when the stuttering disappears, there remain gaps in the flow of speech where the stuttering formerly occurred. These people have had so little experience in smooth-flowing speech that some training is needed to provide it. One of the best ways we have found to do this is through echo speech or shadowing, in which the stutterer, while watching TV or observing some fluent speaker, follows in pantomime the speech that is being produced, saying it silently as it is being spoken aloud. Often we train the stutterer to repeat whole sentences exactly as the speaker spoke them. We also ask him to cancel whole sentences of his own in which gaps or hesitancies appeared so that they can be made to flow more smoothly. At the same time we also show him that even excellent speakers have some nonfluencies and that these are different from the residual breaks that come from a long history of broken speech.

We also train our stutterers to fake easy repetitive or prolonged stutterings, to put these into their fluent speech casually in certain situations every day. We ask them, too, to demonstrate an occasional faking of a short block of the old variety and then to follow it with a cancellation. Occasionally it is wise to fake a pull-out or some of the modifications of postures and tremors so that these basic skills may remain fresh for use in emergencies. Most stutterers dislike doing these things, and they will not do them unless the activities form a basic part of the stabilization phase of treatment.

The practice of taking an honest daily inventory must be encouraged. In this phase of treatment, we help the stutterer to learn to survey his own personal stuttering equation, to assess the variations in strength of the various factors, and to be honest in his evaluations. Here the accepting attitudes of an understanding clinician are most essential.

In this final phase of active therapy, we work especially hard to help the stutterer learn to maintain his new methods of fluent stuttering and fluent speaking in the face of pressures of all kinds. When he first comes to us, the stutterer has but two choices: to stutter on the feared words or to avoid them. We now have given him a third choice, the ability to stutter in a relatively fluent and unabnormal fashion. It is necessary not only to stabilize his new behavior of this third choice under conditions of stress but also to give him a fourth choice—to resist stuttering.

In helping the stutterer to resist communicative stresses of all kinds and yet maintain his new ways of short, easy stuttering, we deliberately create conditions in which the pressures to stutter in the old way are strong, and then the stutterer does his utmost to resist them. We seek out and enter the feared situations of the past; we look for more and more difficult situations. By programming this stress so that the stutterer is largely (not always) able to beat it and yet can stutter easily when he does stutter, we enable him to strengthen the new behavioral responses.

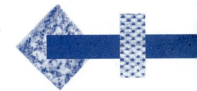

TREATMENT OF THE CHILD WHO HAS BECOME AWARE OF STUTTERING

Unfortunately, far too many children who begin to stutter do become aware of their disorder. From the rejecting reactions of their listeners or from their frustrations in not being able to communicate effectively, they come to recognize that there is something unacceptable in the way they talk. This is one of the real danger signs and it is marked by the beginnings of struggle. Every speech pathologist hates to see the appearance of facial contortions, pitch rises or tensions, and tremors in the speech musculatures of a young stutterer for they signal the beginning of the vicious spiral of self-reinforcement. Even though there is yet no evidence of fear, shame, or avoidance, the morbid growth of severe stuttering has begun. Fortunately, if the proper measures are taken at this critical period, that morbid growth can be reversed.

The treatment of children in this stage follows much the same course as that used in the treatment of beginning stuttering. We must increase the essential emotional security, remove the environmental pressures that tend to disrupt speech, and increase the amount of fluent speech that he experiences. Every effort should be made to prevent traumatic experiences with other children or adults who might tend to penalize or label the disorders. By creating a permissive environment in which the nonfluency has little unpleasantness, much can be done to help the child regain his former automaticity of repetition. The wise parent will find ways of distracting the child so that the struggling will not be remembered with any vividness. Some parents have increased their own nonfluency, reacting to it with casualness and noncommittal acceptance. One of them used to pretend to stutter a little now and then, commenting, "I sure got tangled up on that, didn't I? What I meant to say was . . ." It is also wise to provide plenty of opportunity for release psychotherapy, for ventilation of the frustration. Let these children show their anger. Help them discharge it.

If teasing has reared its ugly head and the child does come home crying or unpleasantly puzzled by the rejecting behavior of his playmates, the situation should be faced rather than avoided. Here is a mother's report.

> Jack came home today at recess. He was crying and upset because some of the other kindergarten children had called him "stutter-box." And they had mocked him and laughed at him. He asked me what was stutter-box and for a moment I was completely panicky, though I hope I hid the feelings from him. I comforted him, and then told him that everybody, including big people, sometimes got tangled up in their mouths when they tried to talk too fast or were mixed up about what they wanted to say. Stutter-box was just a way of kidding another person about getting tangled up in talking. I told him to listen for the same thing in the other kids and to tease them back. Later on that day he caught me once and called me a stutter-box. We laughed over it and I think he's forgotten all about it today. I hope I did right. I just didn't know what to do.

Many parents have been told so often that they should always ignore the stuttering that they continue to do so even when it sticks out like a second nose. This is very unwise. When the child is struggling with his stuttering, when he is obviously reacting to it, no good is obtained by pretending that it doesn't exist. There is a time for ignoring it, for distracting the child's attention from it, but there also comes a time when we must confront it and share the child's problem with him. Otherwise, he will feel that his behavior is shameful, unspeakably evil. He will feel that his parents cannot bear even to mention it. This is the road to fear and avoidance. It is a dangerous road to travel alone and in the dark.

Desensitization

The desensitization therapy used with these stutterers varies in one respect from that used earlier. We do not use complete fluency as our basal level from which we start and to which we return after gradually increasing the stress. Instead, it is wiser to use the first appearance of tension in the repetitions or postural fixations as the cue to return to the basal level. As in early stuttering, we try to harden the child to the factors that precipitate his nonfluency, but in this third stage of stuttering we keep putting on the stress (the interruptions, impatience, hurry, etc.), even though the repetitions begin to appear. But we stop short and return to our basal fluency level just before the tension, forcing, or tremors show themselves. By this technique, it is possible to bring the child back to a condition where there may be many of the primary symptoms, but little or no struggle reactions.

Direct Therapy.   Depending upon how far the child has entered this stage of frustration and struggle, there comes a moment when direct confrontation of the stuttering is necessary. There comes a time when the child needs some adult to show him that he need not struggle, that it is better to let his speech bounce and prolong easily, that this way "the words come out faster and easier."

This new direct attack on the problem should be done by the professional speech pathologist, but we have found it wise to do it in the presence of the parents so that they can feel the objective attitude employed and observe what we do. Here is a glimpse from the transcript of one such session (Figure 8-5).

Clinician:	I understand that you've been having a lot of trouble talking lately, Peter.
Peter:	Yea, I, I, I, I've been sssss . . . stutt . . . stuttering, *(The boy squeezed his eyes shut and fast tremors appeared on his tightly closed lips. The word finally emerged after a surge of tension and a head jerk.)* I've been stuttering bad.
Clinician:	So I see. Let's try to help you. I know what you're doing wrong. You're fighting yourself. You're pushing too hard. Let me show you how you just stuttered and then show you how to do it easy. *(Clinician demonstrates.)*
Peter:	Oh!
Clinician:	Now I'm going to ask you a question, and if you stutter while answering it, I'll join you but show you how to let

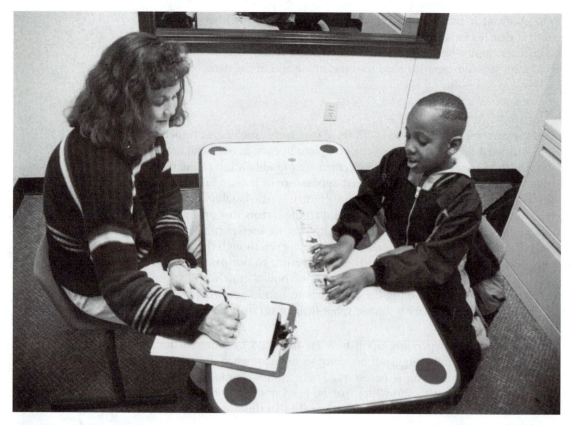

 FIGURE 8-5   Direct stuttering therapy with young child *(Van Riper Clinic, Western Michigan University)*

	it come out easy. OK? All right, how close is the nearest drugstore to your house?
Peter:	It's over on the next b . . . b . . . bbbbbbblock. *(While the boy is struggling, the clinician first duplicates what he is doing, and then slowly slides out of the fixation without tension. The child hears him, opens his eyes to watch him, and an expression of surprise is seen on the child's face.)*
Clinician:	Yea, I told you I was going to stutter right along with you, but you'll have to watch me if you're to learn how to let the words come out easy. Let's try another. If I went through the front door of your house, how would I find your room?
Peter:	YYYYYYYYYYYYou'd . . .*(The child joined the clinician in his grin.)* Yyyou'd have to gggggggo upstairs.

Clinician: That second time you didn't push it so hard, did you.
Good. You went like this . . . *(Clinician demonstrates.).*
Look, you've got to learn how to stutter my way, nice
and easy, either like th-th-th-this or like th . . . is. *(Clinician prolongs the sound easily and without effort.)* Now
let's play a speech game of follow the leader. You be my
echo and say just what I say and stutter just like I do.
Sometimes I'll stutter your way and sometimes my way,
the better way, the way you've got to learn to do it.

The session continued along this line and, before the end of the half-
hour, Peter was beginning to cease his struggling. It took four more meetings before he really learned how to stutter easily, but the parents reported
a marked reduction not only in the severity of his stuttering, but in its frequency as well. We saw him again after four months and the only stuttering behavior he showed was that of the first stage. Within a year it was
gone. Children learn quickly and forget their troubles quickly.

Fortunately, in these younger children, the disorder is not yet deeply
rooted. They unlearn more easily. Once they give you their trust and love,
they will follow your demonstrations and directions most willingly. We almost always use play therapy along with speech work to relieve the pressures. We provide situations in which there is little communicative stress.
We do desensitization therapy often, as though the child were still in the
earlier stages of the disorder. We give him many experiences in being
completely fluent through the use of echoing, unison speaking, rhythmic
talking, and relaxation. We combine fluency building with language
development activities. We do our utmost to build his ego strength in
every possible way. We use no speech assignments but, through parental
counseling and home and school visits, we gradually incorporate his new
ways of talking into his entire living space. We can help these children.

In concluding this section we urge the student to do what she can to
make the lot of the stutterers she meets a less miserable one. What they need
most is understanding and hope, and surely by now you have the information to provide both. No one needs to go through life with a tangled tongue.

CLUTTERING

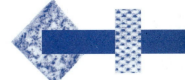

Another disorder of fluency is called *cluttering.* It is well named because
the speech of the clutterer is so disorganized he often cannot be understood. Moreover, the words are uttered very rapidly. They tumble from
his mouth pell mell. Phrases are left uncompleted. Frequent repetitions or
omissions mainly of whole words or part phrases occur and often are so
slurred they contribute to the jumble. The speech flow is jerky, not con-

tinuous; it comes in spurts. Listening to a severe clutterer for any length of time is sheer torture.

And yet the clutterer can speak perfectly if he speaks more slowly and carefully. He can—but he won't be able to sustain that normal utterance very long. Very soon he will be speaking rapidly again compulsively and almost incoherently.

One other feature of the disorder is that the clutterer seems completely unaware of his deviancy. If others fail to understand him, he feels it's their fault, not his. Rarely do clutterers refer themselves for therapy. They come to the clinician reluctantly only because an employer or lover insists. They are difficult to motivate. Stulli said the only way to treat a clutterer was to beat him with a stick.

The disability associated with cluttering is rarely confined to speech. The individual who clutters usually also has reading disabilities, difficulties in writing, spelling, grammar, word-finding, and activities involving the finer coordinations. Her brain waves may be atypical. Although cluttering is often found in children with Down's syndrome, most clutterers are of normal intelligence, though they sometimes do not sound as though they were. Because their perceptual processes seem to be speeded up as abnormally as their motor processes, they often have listening problems and fail to understand what is said to them. They listen in snatches just as they speak in spurts.

Let us now tackle the problem of distinguishing between cluttering and stuttering. It is a diagnostic problem of some importance because the treatment of cluttering differs widely from that of stuttering. We have listed below some contrasting features that may help in making the diagnosis. We should acknowledge, however, that both disorders can be present in a single individual. Thus there are stutterer-clutterers, clutterer-stutterers, and pure clutterers.

Cluttering	Stuttering
Very rapid speech (spurts)	Usually slower, halting
Unaware of disability	Highly aware of disorder
No fears of words	Fears of words, sounds, and speaking situations
No embarrassment	Frustration, guilt, avoidance, struggle
No avoidance	
Disorganized sentence structure	
Repetitions of whole words and phrases	Repetitions and prolongations of syllables, sounds, or vocal postures
Articulatory errors, slurring, omissions, distortions	No articulation difficulties
High variability in cluttering behaviors	Consistent behaviors in stuttering
Grammatical errors	Few grammatical errors
Lack of motivation	Usually motivated

Treatment

The clinician's first and unfortunately most difficult task is to convince the clutterer that he has unacceptable speech. We have already stated that the clutterer is oblivious to his abnormal utterance. If we confront him with some tape-recorded samples of his rapid disorganized speech he will say the recorder is faulty. We always insert some of our own or other's speech to counter this reaction. Clutterers hate to be recorded and often become very angry when forced to listen to the the flood of their pell mell, disorganized, and confusing messages. Often they cannot understand what they have said on the recording.

We have found it wise sometimes to omit the audio recording and to record our first interview on videotape. Only after several information and desensitization sessions do we let him see and hear himself. Then calmly and patiently we analyze the deviant behaviors, often asking the client to repeat and echo them. We may have him transcribe the garbled utterance into written script. We may ask him to say the same thing but more carefully. Our purpose in these activities is to get the clutterer to be willing to identify the target of therapy.

Our next major goal attacks the *tachylalia*, the abnormally accelerated pace of his utterance. Again this poses real difficulties. Clutterers seem to have a different perception of time than we do. Their speech motors race; so do their perceptual processes. Many of them have complained that others speak unbearably slowly and that is why they find it hard to listen. The clinician's speech rate, though quite normal, may sound labored and slow to the cluttering client. He tries to guess what is being said and then gets keyed up and frustrated when he guesses wrong. So he just lets his words come out willy nilly and uncontrolled. He rides a runaway horse.

Since the clutterer can speak perfectly well when he speaks slowly, one might think that merely being instructed to do so would solve his problem. But you'll find he cannot tolerate the slower rate very long. We must increase that tolerance. Some procedures for achieving this goal are as follows:

Have the clutterer signal when he hears the clinician using rate surges or bursts of very rapid speech, then signal when he hears them in his own speech.

Practice cluttering behaviors deliberately (negative practice).

Insert pauses in his speech at appropriate times and prolong them. Adequate pausing will slow down the clutterer's speech more than any amount of exhortation to talk slowly. (Let us say here that we never ask him to speak more slowly—just more carefully.)

Have the clutterer echo or shadow your utterances when spoken at different tempos. Insist upon fidelity in his echoing and, after first using swift models, finally have him repeat after you at a normal rate of utterance.

Record his speech when urged to speak faster and faster, then have him listen to it as it breaks down.

Have him tap out the words of a forthcoming utterance before he says it. Similarly have him pantomime or whisper what he intends to say before he says it.

The use of mirrors, and audio and video recorders is almost mandatory when working with these clients, because they almost seem to have disassociated themselves from their speech. They must repeatedly see and hear themselves producing the garbled utterance before they will attempt to change it.

Once the clutterer has achieved some success in speaking carefully, we have him memorize and recreate various passages—especially jokes, which require a lot of verbal discipline. We have him paraphrase selections from books or TV news programs. We have even had clutterers do mental multiplications aloud, not silently, to help them discipline their thinking processes. We have them role-play job interviews or asking a girl for a date.

The clinician who works with clutterers (Daly, 1993, and Weiss, 1964, offer additional suggestions) must set realistic goals. Few clutterers if any ever become cluttering-free in all speaking situations. We seek mainly to give them controls so they can speak carefully and without undue abnormality.

STUDY QUESTIONS

1. What is the definition of stuttering, according to Van Riper and Erickson?
2. What is the rate of prevalence of stuttering in this country, how does this differ between males and females, and at what age levels does stuttering typically begin?
3. Describe the most common stages through which a child passes during the development of a stuttering problem.
4. *Constitutional* theories differ in what ways from *neurosis* and *learning* theories regarding the etiology of stuttering?
5. What is the basic theme of Wendell Johnson's *semantic* theory of stuttering onset?
6. How would you respond to the well-meaning pediatrician who reassures the mother of a four-year-old beginning stutterer that she should "just ignore your son's stuttering and he will outgrow it within a few years"?
7. What "danger signs" tell us that a child's nonfluency has reached a point where assistance is definitely needed?

8. Knowing some of the "common counterpressures" that can cause a child's speech to be hesitant, what suggestions can you make to the parents of a beginning stutterer to reduce such pressures?

9. Describe the basic process of *desensitization therapy* as it should be used with the child who stutters.

10. What has MIDVAS to do with helping the confirmed stutterer to become fluent?

11. What features differentiate cluttering from stuttering?

12. For what particular reason(s) may therapy sometimes be more difficult for cluttering than for stuttering?

ENDNOTES

[1]Two films, *Identifying the Danger Signs* and *Family Counseling,* dealing with the problems of beginning stuttering and its prevention may be rented or purchased from the Stuttering Foundation of America, P.O. Box 11749, Memphis, TN 38111–0749 (1–800–992–9392).

REFERENCES

Bloodstein, O. (1995). *A handbook on stuttering.* San Diego, CA: Singular Publishing Group.

Daly, D. (1993). Cluttering: Another fluency syndrome. In R. Curlee (ed.), *Stuttering and related disorders of fluency,* New York: Thieme Medical Publishers.

Geschwind, N., and Galaburda, A. (1985). Cerebral lateralization: Biological mechanisms, associations, and pathology. *Archives of Neurology, 4,* 429–459.

Kidd, K., Kidd, J., and Records, M., (1978). The possible causes of the sex ratio in stuttering and its implications. *Journal of Fluency Disorders, 3,* 18–23.

McKnight, R., and Cullinan, W. (1987). Subgroups of stuttering children: Speech and voice reaction times, segmental duration, and naming latencies. *Journal of Fluency Disorders, 12,* 217–233.

Montgomery, B., and Fitch, J. (1988). The prevalence of stuttering in the hearing impaired school-age population. *Journal of Speech and Hearing Disorders, 53,* 131–135.

Nowack, W., and Stone, R. (1987). Acquired stuttering and bilateral cerebral disease. *Journal of Fluency Disorders, 12,* 141–146.

Prins, D. (1995). Modifying stuttering—the stutterer's reactive behavior: Perspectives on past, present, and future. In R. Curlee and G. Siegel (eds.), *Nature and treatment of stuttering: New directions* (rev. ed.). San Diego, CA: Singular Publishing Group.

Rastatter, M., and Dell, C. (1987). Reaction times of moderate and severe stutterers to monaural verbal stimuli: Some implications for neurolinguistic organization. *Journal of Speech and Hearing Research, 30,* 21–27.

Van Riper, C. (1982). *The nature of stuttering.* Englewood Cliffs, NJ: Prentice Hall.

Weiss, D. (1964). *Cluttering.* Englewood Cliffs, NJ: Prentice Hall.

SUPPLEMENTARY READINGS

Freund, H. (1966). *Psychopathology and the problem of stuttering*. Springfield, IL: Charles C. Thomas.

Guitar, B., and Peters, T. (1989). *An integrated approach to the treatment of stuttering*. Baltimore: Williams and Wilkins.

Johnson, W. (1961). *Stuttering and what you can do about it*. Minneapolis, MN: University of Minnesota Press.

Luterman, D. (1991). *Counseling the communicatively disordered and their families* (2nd ed.). Austin, TX: Pro-Ed.

Myers, F., and St. Louis, K. (eds.). (1992). *Cluttering: A clinical perspective*. Leicester, England: Wurr Publishers.

Sheehan, J. (1970). *Stuttering: Research and therapy*. New York: Harper & Row.

Van Riper, C. (1973). *The treatment of stuttering*. Englewood Cliffs, NJ: Prentice Hall.

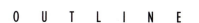

Chapter 9

Voice Disorders

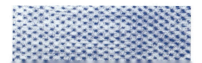

Problems with phonation, as illustrated by the following comments from a 50-year-old businessman with only rather mild symptoms of spasmodic dysphonia, can have profound effects on our lives.

> I just don't participate in anything like I used to. You begin to be antisocial, or at least that's how you feel. I'm at a meeting and someone stands up to make a point, and I think, "I could have said that and maybe even said it more convincingly," but I never do speak publicly anymore. And when someone does hear me speak and asks what's wrong with my voice, I just say that I've got a little sore throat today. It's better than trying to explain the whole problem to them.

> Even on days when my voice seems better, I'm always worried about when it will break down. I know that worrying about it makes me more tense and probably will cause my throat to tighten, but there's no way *not* to be worried. In my business, customers can really be turned off if I don't sound calm and collected and completely objective. Sometimes, when my voice is really bad, it sounds to people on the telephone like I'm about to cry. It has to leave them bewildered, and I can't blame them if I lose their business to a competitor.

The human voice is a remarkable instrument. A speaker can evoke a wide range of emotions and mental images by slight changes of vocal timbre, loudness, or subtle nuances in inflection. Furthermore, a person's voice is a sensitive barometer of his physical and emotional health. To paraphrase Luchsinger and Arnold's artful metaphor (1965, p. 147), "If it is true that the eyes are the mirror of the soul, then surely the voice is its loud-speaker." Since it is the spokesman for the personality, each individual's voice is unique; it is so distinct, in fact, that graphic representations of speech, called voiceprints, identify a person even more reliably than do fingerprints. Recording devices and security systems are available which can be activated only by the spoken command of one individual. Not only can we recognize other people by their unique vocal, quality, but we monitor our awareness of self in part by the distinct and constant character of our own voice. Quite literally, our voice is us. Perhaps this is why some clients with voice disorders are so resistant to therapy—altering one's voice implies a major change in self-identity.

While less frequently found than those of articulation,[1] the disorders of voice can be truly handicapping despite the fact that our culture tends to be more tolerant of vocal deviations than those of language or fluency or articulation. Perhaps this is because intelligible communication is still possible when the voice is harsh or nasal or unduly highpitched or of low intensity. Although a hoarse voice may not be aesthetically pleasing to listen to, we can still readily understand the speaker's message. Perhaps we may be more tolerant of phonatory deviations because there are so many of them within the normal range. There is no single standard of **pitch,** intensity, or quality.

Like noses, voices have to be quite prominent in their abnormality before they are noticed. Parents and teachers become concerned when a child's

Pitch.
The perceptual correlate of fundamental frequency.

language, phonemes, or fluency are different from those of other children, but unless the child's voice is grossly conspicuous and unpleasant they feel no need to seek help. Nor, for that matter, do many persons who themselves should be getting professional voice therapy. The reason for this is that we listen to what we say—to the message we seek to impart—rather than to how we say it. You doubtless were surprised or even shocked when you first heard yourself on a tape recording. Although that recorded voice sounded strange to you, it is the voice that others hear. Other voices on the same tape probably sounded quite familiar. The discrepancy is due partly to the fact that we sense our own vocal tones through bone and tissue conduction as well as from airborne sound and also because the sound field is different (our ears being behind our mouths but in front of the mouths of others).

All about us are voices that could be improved, made more pleasant and efficient. And there are some so markedly unpleasant or peculiar that they are advised to seek help. The singing teacher gets some of these, the speech teacher gets another group, the physician sees the pathological ones, and the speech pathologist is usually called upon last. Some of them will be among the most fascinating of all his clients. Often the most challenging of all the speech disorders, those of voice may reflect not only organic pathology but emotional and even vocational problems. A hoarse voice, for example, may be the first sign of laryngeal cancer in a client who has long disregarded the Surgeon General's warning printed on his packs of cigarettes. Or it may result from habitually speaking at a pitch level too close to the bottom of his pitch range because, as with one of our clients (a very short, essentially effeminate fellow), he wanted to sound strong and manly. Or perhaps that strained hoarse voice results from communicating in the presence of very loud masking noise. This happened to a foreman in a factory after he worked in a roaring, banging environment for many months. Voice disorders arise from many different conditions.

Since the human voice varies in pitch, loudness, and quality, the disorders of voice reflect these three features either separately or in combination (Figure 9-1). And although many useful systems exist for classifying dysphonias (see, for example, Aronson, 1990, or Colton and Casper, 1990), for this introductory text we shall use these simpler features.

Loudness.
The perceptual correlate of intensity or amplitude.

Aphonia.
Loss of voice; without phonation.

DISORDERS OF LOUDNESS

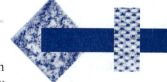

There are three major disorders of **loudness** in which the basic problem is the inability to produce any voice at all or to be able to phonate loudly enough to be understood. The term **aphonia** is used to refer to the complete loss of voice. A person whose larynx has been removed because of cancer always becomes completely aphonic, but some persons with a perfectly intact larynx may also show a complete or partial loss of voice. They

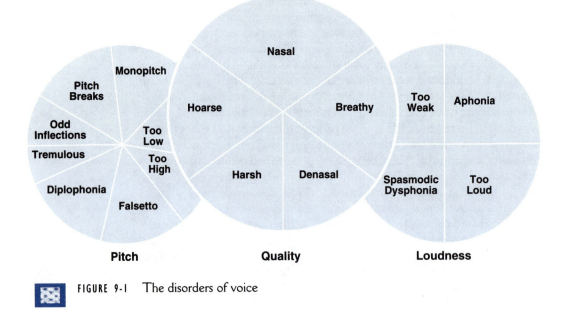

FIGURE 9-1   The disorders of voice

are those with *hysterical aphonia* or *dysphonia* and those with *spastic* or *spasmodic dysphonia*. Besides those two disorders of vocal intensity, there is a third, *phonasthenia*, which refers to a voice which is so soft and weak that intelligibility is impaired. One final disorder of vocal intensity, talking too loudly for the communicative circumstances, is also seen in the clinic, sometimes in association with a sensorineural hearing loss.

Hysterical Aphonia

This disorder, the loss of voice due to emotional stress, usually begins suddenly. The person may begin to talk, then suddenly find himself unable to finish a sentence with any phonation. One of our cases went to bed, quite happily, he told us later, and arose to find himself unable to speak aloud. A schoolteacher lost her voice in the middle of an explanation of a geometry problem. A preacher who had just conducted the opening exercises and participated in the singing was unable to produce even a squeak of sound when he started his sermon. A housewife about to give her mate a good calling down for coming in late at night found herself unable to say anything except in a whisper. A lieutenant in the jungle of Vietnam started to give the order to his men to enter a particularly dangerous thicket and found that he was not even able to whisper the command, that his mouth moved but no sound came out. Many hysterical aphonias arise from laryngitis or colds, the illness creating the necessary explanation for voice failure, though the real reasons lie deep in basic emotional conflicts. Clinical psychologists classify functional aphonia as a conversion disorder, a neurosis in which anxiety is converted into a physical symptom—blindness, deafness, paralysis, loss of voice. Despite the absence of physical abnormality, the afflicted person is not being devious; he genuinely believes he cannot see, hear, walk, or speak. Notice in the following illustration that the client's aphonia is not a problem, but rather it is a *solution* to a problem.

> Larry Synder, a twenty-seven-year-old enlisted man, was referred to the speech clinic by a psychiatrist at the K. I. Sawyer Air Force base. The physician's report stated:
>
> Airman First Class Synder experienced sudden onset of aphonia one month after reassignment as chief clerk. Our examination showed no pathology of the larynx; however, a slight reddening of the vocal folds was noted. The patient reports frequent upper respiratory infections and allergies of an indeterminate nature.
>
> In a low whisper, the client told us this revealing account of the circumstances leading up to his loss of voice:
>
> I joined the Air Force when I graduated from high school, and it's been my home for the past nine years. I really like it. I never have to worry about what to wear, where to get a meal, or a place to sleep. The service really takes care of you. And my job—I was a clerk—was super. But when they made me chief, I didn't think I could handle it. I don't like telling others what to do, especially new recruits who don't seem to care about their job. Now I guess they will have to reassign me—too bad.
>
> Throughout this recital, we were struck by the client's passiveness, his seeming indifference to the sudden loss of voice. There was no forcing or struggle to regain phonation, and his constant sad-sweet smile seemed incongruous in relation to the severity of the presenting disorder.

The medical reports on these clients usually state that no laryngeal pathology is present or that in attempted phonation the vocal folds are bowed. Occasionally the laryngologist will say that although the vocal folds are easily abducted (moved apart), they do not meet in the midline when the patient attempts to produce voice for speech, although they do so in coughing or clearing the throat. Indeed, many of the more naïve hysterical aphonics can hum or sing without difficulty. These features indicate that the disorder is not of organic origin. We do not find persons with a true laryngeal pathology who cannot produce at least a whisper or airflow during attempted phonation.

Many of our clients—most of whom have been female—were emotionally immature, suggestible persons who had an exaggerated need for approval. Typically, they found it difficult to express their feelings, particularly negative emotions, in an open manner. For some of them, aphonia provided an escape from an acutely stressful situation; for others, the loss of voice served as a revenge ("See what you have done to me!") or a sure way to prevent the utterance of the unutterable. Despite the dramatic symptom, however, the majority of our hysterically aphonic clients are not acutely disturbed psychiatrically.

Treatment of Hysterical Aphonia.

Since this type of aphonia must be viewed symptomatically as a protective device to cope with real or imagined difficulties that have become intolerable, some psychotherapy is often necessary; and the speech clinician may need to refer the patient to a psychiatrist or clinical psychologist and work closely with them. Quite often, especially in recent years, psychotherapists refer the case back to us, indicating that they prefer to undertake counseling after the person's voice is restored.[2]

There are some cases whose loss of voice persists even after the conflict situation has been resolved; and these provide some of the most sudden and dramatic cures known to speech pathology. At times even in a single session we have been able to help them "find" their voices again and to leave us talking as well as they ever had. When recurrences and relapses occur (and they do not always take place), we can be pretty sure that deeper psychotherapy or environmental change will be required. The largest number of our own clients with hysterical aphonia have been schoolteachers who just needed a rest from their duties. They often come to us in March when summer vacation seems too far away, and they cannot bear to cope with their schoolrooms another moment. The speech therapy gains time, and the speech clinician provides understanding and hope; often this is all that is required.

Since the person is convinced that his or her problem is organic, it is unwise for the clinician to peremptorily challenge this belief by pointing out that nothing is physically wrong with his or her larynx. It is best to lead into the issue of emotional causation by gradually providing more and more information.

If the client has had his or her unconscious profit from the aphonic symptom and is ready to get rid of it because it is a nuisance, we usually can find some way to restore phonation through massage or kneading of the laryngeal region; sighing, singing, or humming; the prolonged clearing of the throat; or through the use of the *vocal fry*. We have found these approaches generally useful in working with many kinds of voice disorders. One of the favorable prognostic signs when the voice does come back is the ability to produce it without tension. If the voice is strained or forced, our experience is that relapse is likely.

Adduct.
To move toward the midline.

Spasmodic Dysphonia (SD)

In this disorder, we have a mixture of aphonia and a strained, tense voice. In severe **adductor** SD the person labors hard to squeeze out some intermittent voice. It sounds like the strained voice of someone performing tremendous strenuous muscular effort and trying to speak at the same time. The mountain labors and produces a mouse of sound. At times there are facial contortions almost as in the severe stutterer. More rarely, SD occurs in an **abductor** form with attendant intermittent breathiness and aphonia. Fear of speaking is present, but usually not fear of words. This is also to be found in the cerebral palsied and some other types of central nervous system disease.

Spasmodic dysphonia seems to be slightly more prevalent in females than in males; the disorder typically starts in the fourth or fifth decade of life, although our clients have been as young as twelve and as old as eighty years. It may begin quite suddenly, but here is a case illustration in which the disorder progressed slowly and more typically over a span of six months.

> Shortly after starting her part-time job as a receptionist-secretary for a urologist, Emma noted a slight tightening in her throat and that her voice was tired at the end of the day. She attributed this to her working conditions: In order to ensure confidentiality in the crowded waiting room, she leaned over her typewriter and talked to each new patient in a low-pitched whisper. She dosed herself with cough medicine, chewed throat lozenges, but the problem persisted. And got steadily worse. By the time a laryngeal examination was performed—the physician found no **lesion** or other physical abnormalities—she spoke with a "staccato, jerky, squeezed, effortful, hoarse, or groaning voice."
>
> Our diagnostic evaluation revealed several features that are often associated with spastic dysphonia: extreme hyperadduction of the vocal folds when trying to phonate; larynx pulled up high in the throat; glottal fry; and jerky respiratory movements of the upper thorax. The client's stressful life circumstances dominated her conversation during the initial interview and in subsequent therapy sessions. Here is a portion of her story.
>
> I thought that when I went to work my husband and four teenaged sons would offer to help out at home. Far from it! I'm still chief clerk and bottle washer. And my boys are just like their Dad—they drop clothes all over and depend on me to remember where everything is in the house. Oh, my elderly father also lives with us and he comes in and out of senile episodes. Last week he got up early to prepare the family breakfast, which was nice, but he built a fire—with kindling and paper—on top of the electric range! I like going to work, but there is stress there, too. The phone is ringing constantly, I have bills and letters to type, and I must sign in each new patient and list his presenting complaint. How can you talk about VD or a vasectomy in a confidential manner with a waiting room full of other patients listening?
>
> There was more to Emma's tale of woe, but you get the picture of a middle-aged woman overwhelmed by responsibilities. Strangely, and rather typically, she never expressed her anger openly to her family. Although she wanted to scream, "I'm mad as hell and I'm not going to take it any more," she was afraid that others would stop loving her. Subsequent at-

Abduct.
To move away from the midline.

Lesion.
A wound; injured tissue.

tempts at voice therapy, later combined with psychological counseling through the university women's center, were not successful.

Long regarded as a psychiatric problem resistant to treatment either by psychotherapy or voice therapy, spasmodic dysphonia is currently a topic of considerable interest among clinicians and researchers. In recent years substantial progress has been realized in the success with which symptoms of SD—particularly SD of the adductor variety—have been relieved, at least temporarily, through medical intervention (see list of suggested supplementary readings).

Surgical sectioning of one **recurrent laryngeal nerve (RLN),** with resultant unilateral paralysis, has been demonstrated with many patients to result in a dramatic and immediate resolution of adductor spasm of the larynx, although some patients have been reported to experience a return of symptoms—some to a level of severity greater even than that characterizing their pretreatment condition—with the passage of time. The probability of relapse, however, appears to be reduced in patients whose surgery is accompanied systematically by voice therapy. RLN sectioning, however, also has resulted in excessive breathiness in some patients.

More recently, based upon evidence that SD can reflect the operation of a focal laryngeal dystonia, botulinum toxin (Botox) has been used to treat the disorder. Injections of laryngeal musculature (typically the thyroarytenoid, either uni- or bilaterally) with small quantities of Botox (intended to weaken rather than to paralyze the injected muscle) have resulted in elimination or reduction of adductor spasm in the vast majority of SD patients receiving this treatment, although maintenance of freedom from spasm requires periodic reinjection at intervals of two to four months. In the use of Botox, too, it has been observed that the efficacy of treatments, including the uneventful management of transient dysphagic side effects, may be enhanced if patients receive at least brief periods of voice therapy. As in the case of RLN surgery, some patients present with excessive breathiness following Botox injection (presumably reflecting "overdosage").

Spasmodic dysphonia of the abductor type, seen far less frequently, has been treated with Botox injections into the posterior cricoarytenoid (PCA) muscle—with encouraging but more equivocal results.

In any event, it must be noted that the long-term (and even short-term) effects of Botox injections, including diffusion, distant spread, and possible aspiration (in the case of PCA injection) are not yet fully understood.

Infrequently, but not to be discounted, there have been reports of patients whose spasmodic dysphonia has been alleviated through voice therapy alone. Moreover, there has been at least one instance of apparent permanent resolution of SD following a single Botox treatment. In both instances it has been presumed that the SD symptoms were of **psychogenic** etiology or/and that patients have learned to "mask" the symptoms by adopting compensatory laryngeal control strategies.

Recurrent laryngeal nerve (RLN).
Branch of the vagus nerve that innervates all but one of the intrinsic muscles of the larynx; also called the *inferior laryngeal nerve.*

Psychogenic.
Caused by underlying psychological or personality factors.

Although studies of SD, particularly of SD and Botox treatment, are being conducted in many centers, there clearly are many questions that must be addressed regarding the disorder and its responsiveness to current intervention strategies.

Weak Voices

The old term, phonasthenia, refers to the voice that is too little and too weak to carry the normal burdens of communication. Voices that are not loud enough for efficient communication are fairly common, but they seldom are referred to the speech pathologist. Imitation, overcompensation for conductive hearing loss, and feelings of inadequacy leading to retreat reactions account for most of them. Many pathological reasons for such disorders are common, but they are frequently accompanied by breathiness, huskiness, or hoarseness or other symptoms sufficiently evident to necessitate the services of the physician, who should rightfully take care of them.

> One individual with a history of prolonged laryngitis, but with a clean bill of health from the physician, claimed that she was afraid to talk loudly because of the pain she had experienced in the past. Something seemed to stop her whenever she decided to talk a little louder. She constantly fingered her throat. She declared that she was losing all her self-respect by worrying about her inability to speak as loudly as she could. Use of a masking noise during one of her conferences demonstrated to her that she could speak loudly without discomfort. Under strong clinical pressure, she did make the attempt, but the inhibition was automatic.

When we speak we expose ourselves, and the louder we do it, the greater that exposure is. The insecure, withdrawn person finds even ordinary levels of intensity almost unbearably revealing. His very nature resists the display of self. Usually he has good reasons for his inhibited utterance, although they may remain hidden until counseling makes them bearable and manageable. An emotionally healthy person enjoys a certain amount of display speech. One who is not finds it traumatic. And once again, we find that even when psychotherapy is successful, often there is need for voice therapy to enable the person to use an adequate vocal intensity.

Where there is no organic pathology such as **vocal nodules,** paralysis, or contact ulcers, we can assume that the person does possess an adequate voice. Our task is to help him find it. Often we discover that emotional insecurity lies at the bottom of the problem, and we must provide opportunities for exploration and release of these feelings. These people often are fearful of establishing close relationships, and their barely audible voices reflect this fear. A warm, permissive clinician can make the vocal therapy itself a means of creating at least one non-threatening relationship. Often the speech therapy is less important than the client's testing of the clinician's acceptance, but we use the vocal exercises as the pathway to re-

Vocal nodules.
Small callus-like protuberances on medial edge of vocal folds, usually bilateral; caused by misuse and abuse of the voice.

assurance. By extending the therapy to other communicative situations, the person comes to find that the world may not be as threatening as he had supposed.

But there are often habits involved too. Whatever the original cause of the weak voice, these people often show inefficient forms of breathing when speaking. They may habitually exhale much of the inhaled air prior to vocalization (air wastage), or make a series of small inhalations rather than one large one (staircase breathing), or speak on the very end of the exhaled breath, or speak while the chest is expanding (**opposition breathing**). A certain amount of air pressure is needed for adequate phonation, and these methods of speech breathing make it difficult to speak loudly enough for communication. We seldom need to teach the person how to breathe; but there are times when we have to teach him to stop breathing in an abnormal way. Once he knows what he is doing incorrectly and recognizes the moments of normal breathing that he shows occasionally, the normal patterns will return.

Often, the problem may consist of the use of improper pitch levels. The person who speaks at the very bottom, or very top, of his pitch range, for any reason, cannot have normal vocal intensity. We may therefore have to change the habitual pitch. We have had clients referred to us as having weak voices who merely were fearful that if they spoke in their usual way, they would have pitch breaks upward into the falsetto. With these, it was necessary to work on pitch control and to ignore the intensity. Generally, intensity becomes louder as the pitch rises. By prolonging tones and then introducing rhythmic pulses of pitch rises that go higher and higher, the intensity of the pulses becomes louder and louder.

Some of these cases are difficult to hear merely because they speak with their mouths almost shut—because they do not articulate with any energy. Putting a stopper in any horn diminishes the loudness of its tones. We teach these people to uncork their mouth openings. Also, by making the plosives distinctly or by stressing the fricative consonants, we can compensate for the lack of vocal intensity. Many of the bad habits of utterance are due to excessive tension in the mouth, tongue, or throat; and by relaxing these focal points of tension, the voice becomes freer and louder. One of the common areas of excessive muscular contraction is the region just above the larynx. The larynx is often raised almost into the position for swallowing. When a person habitually assumes this abnormal posture prior to vocalization, it is difficult to produce a normal voice no matter what effort is expended. Again, we must identify this abnormal behavior and bring it up to consciousness so that it can be brought under voluntary control and eliminated. Voice should not be squeezed out. It needs an open, relaxed, natural channel. At times we have these persons talk while chewing to discover the normal function. Some of our voice clients have forgotten how to produce voice normally. We must show them.

Opposition breathing. Breathing in which the thorax (chest) and diaphragm work oppositely against each other in providing breath support for voice.

A few of our voice clients, especially those who have some paralysis of the vocal folds, need more energy rather than less, and they need it in the right places. Certain pushing exercises with the arms or legs, or sudden contractions of the fist may aid if they are accompanied by phonation.

Excessive Loudness

Only rarely have we seen for treatment clients who talk excessively loudly (a seldom-used term for an overloud voice is *macrophonia*). As in the case of weak voices, inappropriate vocal loudness can have organic or functional causes.

In certain types of hearing loss, an individual will raise his voice in order to hear himself. Persons with cerebral palsy or Gilles de la Tourette's syndrome may emit inappropriate bursts of loud speech.

Most of the bombastic voices we hear, though, are due to functional rather than physical causes. Some persons, probably only a small minority, display their large egos by a loud mouth. Individuals who work in noisy environments or whose occupation (military, teaching, preaching) requires prolonged loud talking may acquire habits of vocal intensity that are inappropriate.

Prolonged loud talking, particularly in combination with improper breath support and body tension, can cause structural damage to the vocal folds. Children seem to be especially vulnerable to laryngeal pathology from vocal abuse, but unfortunately the speech pathologist does not become involved until parents and teachers are alarmed by the youngsters' chronic hoarseness. Unless bad vocal habits are eliminated or reduced markedly, thickening of the vocal folds, vocal nodules, or polyps may occur. The wisest course of action is a program of vocal re-education, a comprehensive plan to reduce loud talking, minimize prolonged use of the voice, and teach easy initiation of phonation. To accomplish a re-education program, clinicians employ a variety of activities. Here is a brief description of how a student speech clinician helped a nine-year-old junior hockey enthusiast to monitor his constant shouting:

> A large "shouting graph" was prepared and decorated with a picture of a famous hockey player. Enlisting the assistance of one of the client's teammates, I asked them to obtain a baseline measurement of the total number of shouts observed during a one-hour hockey practice. The two boys were then asked to tally the total number of episodes of vocal abuse each day for the next two weeks (see Figure 9-2). Note the decline in the shouting episodes over the initial period—charting the maladaptive behavior apparently increased the child's vigilance and helped him to monitor its occurrence.

Some clinicians use voice-activated devices that light up when a child's speech exceeds a designated intensity, thus providing instant feedback and

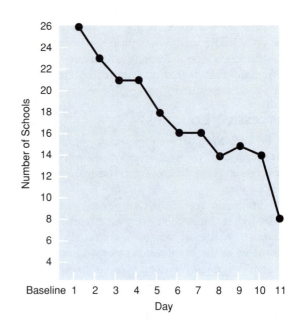

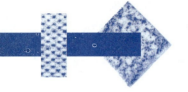 FIGURE 9-2 Shouting graph

enhancing awareness of inappropriate loudness. The VisiPitch and the IBM Speech Viewer also are useful for this purpose.

PITCH DISORDERS

Thus far we have been describing those voice disorders in which the basic problem is one of loudness or intensity. We must remember, however, that there are two other main aspects of voice that may also be deviant—*pitch* and *quality*. Indeed, the professional speech pathologist knows that except for aphonia (in which no voice is present), the majority of his voice clients tend to show abnormality in all three features, although one is usually most prominent in its deviation. Moreover, he knows, too, that by changing the pitch level, changes in loudness or vocal quality can often be achieved, and often by altering the intensity, or the vocal quality, pitch levels can become more normal. Therefore, when he examines a client with a voice problem he surveys all three aspects of the voice—the intensity, pitch, and quality—and seeks to determine how they may be related.

Suppose, however, that the speech pathologist recognizes immediately that the most noticeable deviation is one of pitch. He then asks himself some diagnostic questions: Is the habitual pitch level too high or too low for the client's age and sex? Is it appropriate relative to the client's total pitch range? Is this client speaking in almost a monotone? Do the pitch breaks resemble those of the adolescent male when his voice is changing? Is he speaking with the falsetto? Is the voice tremulous in its pitch? Is the deviation primarily one of stereotyped or peculiar inflections? Is he using two pitches (diplophonia) at the same time? Are there times or conditions when the client's pitch levels are within the normal range?

Habitual Pitch Levels

The concept of a habitual pitch level must be clearly understood. Except in the case of monotones, it does not refer to a certain fixed pitch upon which all speech is phonated. It represents an average or **median** pitch about which the other pitches used in speech tend to cluster. For example, in the utterance of the sentence, "Alice was sitting on the back of the white swan," the fundamental pitch of each vowel in any of the words may differ somewhat from that of the others. Moreover, certain vowels are inflected—that is, they are phonated with a continuous pitch change that may rise, fall, or do both. Of course, each inflection has an average pitch by which it may be measured, if the extent of the variation is also considered. If all the pitches and pitch variations are measured and their durations are taken into account in the speaking of the preceding illustration, we shall find that they cluster about a certain average pitch, which may be termed the "key" at which the speaker phonated that sentence. It should be understood, of course, that different pitch levels will be used under different communicative conditions. Nevertheless, each voice can be said to have a habitual pitch range in which most of the communication is phonated.

The pitch of the normal human voice presents many mysteries and much research needs to be done before we can hope to understand its abnormalities.

Almost anyone can raise or lower the pitch of his or her voice at will, and yet the adjustments are all involuntary. The individual does not know how he or she does it, nor can we give instructions how to alter his or her pitch level. But we do know that the *size* of the vocal folds (their length and mass), the *tension* they are under, and, to some extent, the *volume* of *subglottal air* determines a person's habitual or modal pitch level. The average fundamental frequency of adult male voices is approximately 128 Hz; for adult females it is 220 Hz. For a frame of reference about frequencies, musical notes, and sounds that resemble pitch levels of human voices, consult Table 9.1.

Many of our clients with voice problems have tried to use a pitch level that was too high or too low for their particular mechanism. In therapy we help them to find their *optimum* or natural pitch where they may phonate most efficiently. For most persons, this **optimal pitch level** is located four or five notes above the lowest tone they can produce comfortably.

We know that the voice of a young child is high pitched when compared with that of the adult and that in old age it sometimes tends to creep

Median.
Midline, in the middle.

Optimal pitch level.
The relatively narrow range of pitches, toward the low end of an individual's vocal pitch range, within which the individual may phonate most efficiently and effortlessly.

TABLE 9.1 Fundamental frequency (F_n), musical notes, and common environmental sounds

Frequency (cps)	Piano/Musical Scale		Sounds Like
1,024	C_6		Emergency warning tone: radio, television
—	—		
—	—		
—	—		
—	—		
512	C_5		
—	—		
—	—		
480 infant cry	B_4		Flute
—	—		
—	—		
—	—		
300 child, age 7			
—	—		
—	—		
256	C_4	Do	
—	B	Ti	
—			
220 average F_0; adult females			
			Truck air horn
—	A	La	
—	G	Sol	
	F	Fa	
	E	Mi	
	D	Re	
128 average F_0; adult males	C_3	Do	Fog horn
—	—		
—	—		
—	—		
100			Horn on large boat

back again to higher levels. We know that the major pitch changes occur at puberty, the bottom of the girl's pitch range descending from one to three tones. Boys' voices usually drop a full **octave,** and there is a less marked but noticeable loss at the upper end of the pitch range. Usually, but depending upon the onset of sexual changes, the voice changes occur in boys between the ages of thirteen and fifteen, with the girls showing the same basic changes a year earlier. Occasionally, the change of voice has been known to occur very suddenly (usually when puberty comes late), but most frequently it takes from three to six months on the average.

Why do some people fail to use the normal pitch change? There are several reasons besides delayed sexual development. Some clients have voices that are high pitched primarily because of infantile personalities, because they cannot or prefer not to grow up. This case study may help to make the point:

> Charles Juliff was first referred to the public school speech clinician for his articulation difficulty at the age of twelve. He substituted *w* for *r* and *l, t* for *k,* and *d* for *g.* He had a marked **interdental** lisp. He sucked his thumb and cried easily. He preferred the company of very young children and still played with dolls at home. He was rejected and despised by boys of his own age and bore the nickname of "Sister." He was an only child, pampered and babied and overprotected by an anxious mother. Although intelligent, he had failed the third grade twice. He was absent from school a good share of the time for chronic headaches and stomach upsets. The articulation defects were very resistant to therapy, and the child was not cooperative. Consequently, he was dismissed from speech therapy classes and referred to the school psychologist, who was unable to solve the home problem because of the mother's attitudes.
>
> At seventeen he was again referred to speech therapy, this time at a college clinic. No articulation defects were present, but the voice was very high pitched, rather nasally, whiny, and weak in intensity. The secondary sex characteristics were present, and he was quite fat. The personality was still infantile.

In such cases psychotherapy is the indicated treatment, although vocal training may be used along with it, either to make the psychotherapy more palatable or to help the person to make changes in the habitual pitch as he comes to accept and solve his psychological problem.

Similarly, an abnormally low-pitched voice appears deviant and can cause the person much distress. Although a few of our clients with this problem have been adult women who have passed through their menopause and have taken medication containing hormones (testosterone compounds) that produced a *virilization* ("maleness") of the voice, we also have had a few young female college students with deep bass voices. They were almost afraid to open their mouths, afraid to talk for fear of the listener reactions, which had often traumatized them. A low-pitched voice

Octave.
Unit of measurement of frequency intervals; doubling or halving a fundamental frequency raises or lowers the sound by one octave; on the equal tempered music scale, one octave is equal to six tones or twelve semitones.

Interdental.
Between the teeth. An interdental lisp would show itself in the substitution of the *th* for the *s* as in *thoup* for *soup.*

may have organic (paralysis, hypothyroidism, chronic **edema,** growths on the vocal folds) or functional causes.

There is much that we still do not know about why we habitually use the pitch levels that we prefer. The voice of authority in this country is pitched deeply; in Japan, it is very high. Do soprano mothers and tenor fathers beget children with pitch levels higher than their playmates? Certainly, we find a few clients with very tiny laryngeal cartilages who speak far above the normal range, but most persons with pitch disorders have normal larynges (plural for larynx). Why do the deaf tend to have high-pitched voices? Again we do not really know. Speech pathology is full of unknowns.

Monopitch

We have never seen a client whose voice could be viewed as strictly mono-pitched, although we have known many whose voices were highly mo-notonous. All of them were capable of some pitch change, and all of them had some inflection. The key characteristic was the narrow range of in-flection and pitch change, often no more than one or two **semitones.** Also, these individuals often substitute a change in intensity for the pitch change, and this creates the impression of deviancy. Many persons whose voices strike us as entirely lacking in inflection are merely those with stereotyped inflections. These are the ones whose voices fall after every pause, comma, or period. There is deadly monotony, to be sure, but no monopitch. Nevertheless, these restricted, lifeless voices are miserable to listen to, and they interfere with communication by sheer lack of variety.

The causes of monopitch are (1) emotional conflicts, (2) lack of physical vitality, (3) hearing loss, and (4) the use of habitual pitch levels too near the top or bottom of the pitch range. The role of emotional causation in producing the monotonous voice has been described by various authors and researchers. A review of the literature indicates that individuals who are in states of depression and schizophrenics tend to show this type of voice. We have also found it in paranoid or suspicious individuals or those who are barely able to keep their emotions under control, as a defensive mechanism to prevent others from knowing how they feel.

Undernourished, sick, or fatigued persons also tend to show little range of pitch or inflection. They seem to have insufficient energy available for the normal melody of speech. Those who are very hard of hearing also present the picture of monotonous voice, although careful scrutiny often reveals certain stereotyped inflections, most of which are alike and yet unlike those of the normally hearing person. Finally, when the habitual pitch for any reason is either too near the ceiling or floor of the pitch range, we find a tendency toward monopitch. We need voice room to maneuver. If we cannot go downward, we do not go upward.

Edema.
Swelling caused by accumulation of serous fluid.

Semitone.
A half-tone, a half-step on the musical scale.

Pitch Breaks

Most of us tend to think of the change of voice as occurring abruptly when it does occur, and "pitch breaks" have been the subject for a good deal of humor in our culture. Indeed, some children, boys and girls alike, do have these sudden shifts of pitch as characteristic of the period of voice change; and also, some children as young as seven and eight can show similar sudden shifts. We also are prone to think of the pitch changes as always shifting toward the higher notes, but breaks can be downward as well.

The majority of the pitch breaks that do occur are generally an octave in extent in most children. They occur involuntarily, very suddenly, and the child seems to have little control over them, reacting at first with great surprise. The upward pitch breaks of boys start when the word spoken is pitched below the habitual pitch of the moment. It often seems as though, in the attempt to return to the level they feel most natural, they overshoot their mark. In a few children the experience is so traumatic that they resort to a guarded monotone and develop a very restricted range.

The cause of the pubertal pitch changes is not entirely understood, although we do know that profound alterations in the organs of voice occur at the time. The male larynx grows much larger, and the vocal folds grow longer and rather suddenly; the female larynx increases more in height than in width, and the vocal folds seem to thicken. The male vocal folds lengthen about 1 centimeter, the female's only a third as much. At the same time, the child is growing swiftly in skeletal development. The neck becomes longer, and the larynx takes up a lower location relative to the opening into the mouth. The chest expands greatly, and perhaps one of the causes of voice breaks is the greater air pressure that suddenly becomes available. The following case may be illustrative.

> One of our cases was a boy who had been delayed markedly in physical growth until his sixteenth birthday, at which time a great spurt of development occurred. He grew 6 inches in three months and his voice seemed uncontrollable as far as pitch was concerned, so much so that he developed a marked fear of speaking. Speech therapy was ineffective until he was taught by the speech therapist to fixate his chest and to use abdominal breathing as exclusively as possible. Immediately the pitch breaks disappeared, and the technique tided him over the next six months, at which time he returned to his normal thoracic breathing pattern without difficulty.

Too high a pitch in some individuals, either male or female, may be the result of failure to make the necessary transition to the adult voice. The social penalties upon the male with a voice pitched too high are severe in our culture. Indeed, an old name for this voice problem was the **"eunuchoid voice."** The penalties upon the female are less severe. Nevertheless, the high-pitched voice is rarely much of an asset. We have seen some near tragedies resulting from the disorder. Personalities have been

Eunuchoid voice.
A very high-pitched voice similar to that of a castrated male adult.

warped by social rejection; vocational progress has been blocked; self-doubts have impaired the person's ability to cope with the demands of existence. There is nothing humorous about a high-pitched voice.

The Falsetto

All of us have the capacity for speaking in a falsetto voice even if we cannot yodel, but there are some individuals who use it involuntarily. It involves a different way of using the vocal folds. The falsetto register constitutes an entirely different mode of vibration. In normal phonation the entire shelf of muscular tissue vibrates whereas in the falsetto only the thin ligaments do. This condition is produced by stretching the vocal ligaments, and at the same time, relaxing the muscles within the folds.

The falsetto voice is usually located beyond the upper limits of the normal pitch range. The causes of the habitual falsetto voice appear to consist of emotional factors (1) as a protest against sexual or social maturity, (2) as a defense against pitch breaks, and (3) as a method for preventing the hoarse or husky voice. In some cases a falsetto voice may be producible even when laryngeal paralysis is present. The emotional causation presents a problem in counseling and psychotherapy in some cases and professional help may be needed.

> R. James S. III came to us with a very high-pitched falsetto whose only inflection was at the end of his phrases and sentences. He was a fat boy at eighteen, and he was a boy rather than a youth. His divorced mother had spoiled and babied him for years, and he was almost totally unable to cope with his freshman year in the university. She phoned him every evening and wrote to him every day. He refused to eat in the dormitory, he wept easily and frequently and also in a falsetto. We recorded his voice, played it back to him, and then referred him to a psychiatrist. He dropped out of school and we lost track of him for a year. When he returned, he told us that he had continued his psychotherapy, had cut his ties with his mother, and was working as a janitor. His psychiatrist reported that he was now ready for voice therapy. Within a single week he found his deep bass voice. It was one of the easiest bits of therapy we have ever had. Had we attempted earlier to work with Bob, as he had finally come to call himself, we are sure we would have been unsuccessful.

This case points up another significant bit of information. Abnormal voices can persist of their own momentum and habituation long after the original cause has ceased to exist. They perpetuate themselves by the reinforcement they get from successful consummation of communication.

Other Pitch Disorders

Muscular dystrophy.
A disease characterized by progressive deterioration in muscle functioning and also by withering of the muscles.

The tremulous voice may be due to paralysis, **muscular dystrophy,** or other similar neurological disorders. It may also be due to cerebral palsy on the one hand, or to fearfulness on the other. Referral to medical or psychological services is indicated. Females or children with very low-pitched voices should be referred to a physician before undertaking speech therapy; often glandular and hormonal problems are present. Stereotyped inflections may be due to foreign language influence, to psychological conflicts, or to hearing loss.

The most common cause of *diplophonia*, a rare disorder in which the person produces two distinct pitches at the same time, is unilateral vocal fold paralysis.

Treatment of Pitch Disorders

When the problem consists of an habitual pitch that is abnormally high or abnormally low, the clinician's basic task is to discover ways of helping his case produce a more optimal pitch level. First, there must be some confrontation through tape recording, an experience that often shocks the client terrifically, for she has not really recognized before how her voice sounds to others.

Our next task is to help the person vary her pitch levels, to explore the range of pitches of which she is capable but has not discovered. The pitch of the voice usually varies with the intensity. By increasing the loudness, the tone will usually be made to rise in pitch. Even high-pitched falsettos will shift downward if a tone is first initiated very loudly, then gradually softened as it is prolonged. Pitch rises when the laryngeal musculature is tensed, and we can use this feature in therapy. Tension in almost any part of the body seems to be reflected and finds some focus in the larynx. By asking the person to pull upward on the seat of her chair, or to push down on the table, we can increase the tension of the vocal folds and perhaps raise the pitch of a sustained tone. This works best if the effort is applied in pulses. Conversely, if we wish to lower a pitch, we can begin by using strong muscular contractions and let go jerkily in a series of relaxations.

The self-perception of pitch is still mysterious. We still do not know why some individuals with excellent hearing seem to be unable to match a given pitch or to locate their own voices on a scale. They sing off key and do not know it. However, there seems to be some evidence that pitch perception is tied in somehow with body postures and **kinesthesia.** Even little children who have never seen a musical scale lift their heads and rise on tiptoe when they reach for a high note. When we try to sing very low, we tuck our chins in, lowering our heads. At any rate, we have found that by having the client follow our head or arm body movements as we show her how her pitches are rising or failing or being sustained, we can improve his faulty pitch placement.

Another approach frequently employed uses the vocalized sigh or yawn to produce the desired pitch. These sighs and yawns must be accompanied by decreasing intensity and relaxation in order to be most

Kinesthesia. The perception of muscular contraction or movement.

effective. Still another makes use of the grunts and noises symbolic of relief or feeding. Clearing the throat may also be used to provide a lower pitch.

An example of some actual therapy that produced a change from a high falsetto into normal male phonation within a single hour may now be given, although it should be understood that further work was necessary to stabilize the new voice thereby obtained.

> T. J. was a nineteen-year-old boy with a high-pitched monotonal falsetto that was inconsistent in that occasionally nonfalsetto tones were heard, although they, too, were spoken at the same high level. After the usual ear training in identifying the problem, we had a session in which we demonstrated the following kinds of phonation and asked him to join us and to duplicate what we heard. (1) We asked him to do some vocalized donkey breathing, alternately on inhalation and on exhalation, and very rhythmically. As we produced the model, we occasionally changed the pitch of the exhaled sound. Several of his tones were very good. (2) We asked him to retract his head as far as he could, then to bring it forward until it dropped down on his chest, producing a long sigh as he did so. We showed him and first did what he did so far as sound was concerned, then gradually let our own pitch fall as the sigh ended. He followed us and ended with a weak, breathy, but very low tone. (3) We showed him some stretching and yawning and asked him to join us, saying "Awwwww" in the middle of the yawn. (4) We placed some tissue paper over a comb and asked him to buzz it, using a prolonged *z* sound with his lips against the paper. The tone we used was of low pitch, and so was his. We then asked him to say *zzzeezzz* and *zzzooozzz* and then *zzzzoooooo* as he buzzed the comb. This failed, for he used a falsetto buzz. (5) We asked him to duplicate a vocalized clearing of the throat as he held his fingers to his ears. It was very low pitched and without any falsetto. (6) We than taught him the clicking vocal fry until he could sustain it for several seconds, then had him open and shut his jaws and lips during the fry phonation. In this activity we heard normal phonation along with the vocal fry. (7) We demonstrated head and jaw shaking from side to side while we produced various vowels of different pitches. (8) As he duplicated our model by head and jaw shaking in unison with us, we slowly said, "I am using my real voice," and he echoed it in the new low pitch. (9) We played back the recording of his voice to him, called it quits for that session, asked him not to speak very much until we saw him again, and made an appointment to do so.

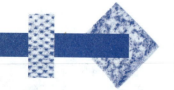

DISORDERS OF VOCAL QUALITY

Disorders of vocal quality are the most frequent type of voice problem. Although the terminology is notoriously ambiguous, quality generally refers to the smoothness or clarity of the phonated tone, another aspect of quality is resonance, the selective amplification of the glottal tone in the cavities above the larynx. We divide disorders of quality into two main categories: *disorders of resonance,* hypernasality, and denasality and *disorders of laryngeal tone,* breathiness, harshness, and hoarseness.

Nasality

The most common disorder of resonance is hypernasality, a condition involving abnormal mixing of oral and nasal resonance. Hyponasality, usually called denasality, results from a lack of nasal resonance on the consonant sounds /m/, /n/, and /ŋ/.

Hypernasality. Nasal resonance occurs primarily because the back door to the nose fails to close sufficiently (Figure 9-3). The contraction of the soft palate and pharyngeal muscles that elevate, spread, and squeeze the rear opening to the nasal passages may be said to constitute that door. Research has shown that the closure need not be complete on all sounds to prevent hypernasality, but there are definite limits to the amount of opening permitted. Influenced by the abnormal flow of air through the nasal cavity, the vocal folds may also behave differently in hypernasality. Certain organic conditions reflect themselves in excessive nasality because they make it difficult to close this valve like mechanism sufficiently. The person with an unrepaired cleft palate shows hypernasality; so does the person

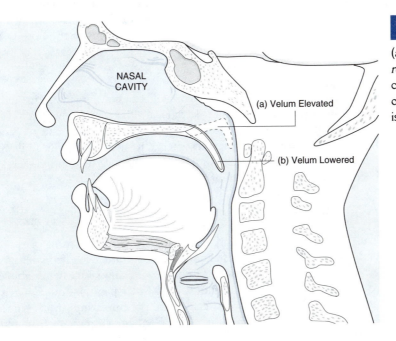

NASAL
CAVITY

(a) Velum Elevated

(b) Velum Lowered

FIGURE 9-3
Hypernasality: (a) During *normal resonation* the velum is closed; (b) nasality occurs when the velum is lowered.

whose soft palate has been paralyzed or made sluggish by other disease. Investigations have also revealed that hypernasality tends to occur after the adenoids have been removed, a process that leaves a relatively larger channel than had previously existed, due to the adenoid mass.

Hypernasality, when excessive, creates a voice quality that most listeners find unpleasant. It has some virtue in enabling the speaker to get his message across in the presence of masking noise, for it carries piercingly. Auctioneers and barkers at carnival sideshows find it useful, if not ornamental.

Assimilation Nasality.

Hypernasality may be general and exist on most of the vowels and voiced consonant sounds, or it may be restricted only to the sounds which precede or follow the nasal consonants /m/, /n/, and /ŋ/. This latter type is termed *assimilation* nasality. Many speakers of general American English show some assimilation nasality in such a sentence as "Any man can make money." This is because of the need for alternate openings and closings of the velopharyngeal opening. In the word *man* the passageway to the nose must be, open on the *m*, closed on the *a*, and opened again on the *n*. It's easier just to leave the space open. Also, even on a word such as *and*, we tend to prepare for the *n* opening while we're still saying the *a*, and this may cause a premature lowering of the soft palate, thereby producing the sound nasally. The assimilation may thus be either forward or backward. Hypernasality of either type seems to be more likely to occur on certain sounds than on others. High back vowels such as /u/ and /o/ may show less hypernasality than the lower front vowels. The consonants /z/ and /v/ tend to show more hypernasality on them than do the other consonants. It is possible to have much hypernasality without ever having any airflow coming out of the nose because it is the resonation of the sound, not the airflow, that creates the unpleasant voice quality. The louder the voice, the more prominent the hypernasality appears.

There are other causes for hypernasality besides organic. Through imitation and identification, children can learn the excessively nasal voices of their parents or associates. Low vitality and fatigue also tend to produce more of the problem, for it takes energy to make the swift adjustments needed. Finally, whining children and adults have whining voices; complaint prefers the trombone of the nose.

Denasality

This is the voice of the head cold, of the hay fever victim, of the child with enlarged adenoids. The nasal passages are occluded, perhaps by growths within the nostrils, by congestion in the nasal cavities above the roof of the mouth, or by adenoids in the rear passageways. Often some of the nasal consonants are affected, the person saying "Mby syduhzziz are killig mbe." The voice sounds are dulled and congested. Listeners de-

Assimilation.
A change in the characteristic of a speech sound due to the influence of adjacent sounds. In assimilation nasality, voiced sounds followed or preceded by a nasal consonant tend to be excessively nasalized.

sire to clear their own throats or to flee. Again, as we have found before, denasal voices may be maintained long after the cause has ceased to exist, but the basic treatment of denasality usually is medical or surgical in nature.

The Breathy Voice

This disorder often coexists with other problems. It may show itself in intermittent aphonia, in instances of weak intensity, and in conjunction with the hoarse voice. Its major characteristic, as the name implies, is an excessive output of airflow along with phonation. Breathy voices are not whispered, but they are aspirate in quality. Phonation is present, but the rush of air is obvious. At times, the huskiness accompanies the tone; at other times the constricted hissing of the air precedes or follows the tone. There is air wastage. Because of the air leakage and the asymmetrical movements of the vocal folds, a noise component is generated and accompanies the glottal tone. When the breathy voice is subjected to acoustic analysis, the turbulence is apparent as a "broad-band noise superimposed on the periodic vocal tone" (Zemlin, 1981, p. 222). Figure 9-4 illustrates spectograms of normal and several abnormal voice qualities.

In some cases, a sort of gasping series of short inhalations throughout the person's speech produces the impression of huskiness. When this occurs, the phrases are short and choppy, and the rhythm of utterance is disturbed. From this description it is obvious that there are different types of breathy voices, but all have in common the imperfect adduction of the vocal folds during the closed phase of the phonatory cycle.

 FIGURE 9-4 Spectrograms of various vocal qualities (from W. Zemlin, 1981, used by permission)

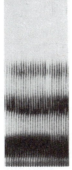 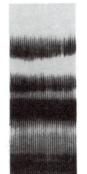 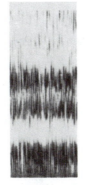 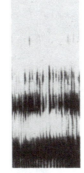 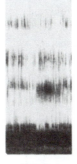

Normal   Nasal   Breathy   Harsh   Hoarse

Causes. The causes of the breathy voice may be either organic or functional. A paralyzed vocal cord may fail to join its twin at the midline for part of its length, thus leaving a gap through which the airflow may leak. Certain diseases may inflame or swell the membranes of the vocal cords so that they vibrate inefficiently. Excessive strain may make them weak—as it does any muscle when overloaded too long. Whenever you meet such a disorder, you should first make sure that the person hasn't just been yelling too long at a football game or has a bad cold, and then, if the condition has persisted or is getting worse, the person should be immediately referred to a physician.

In Figure 9-5 we present illustrations of some of the organic conditions that can lead to weak, breathy voices. Some persons abuse their voices so much that they develop these pathologies. Vocal nodules—tiny cornlike growths of the edges of the vocal cords—may prevent complete closure; they are usually found on the anterior portion of the cords. The laryngeal polyp, if it is large enough, not only produces weak and breathy phonation but also a fluttering, tremulous pitch. Usually benign, it can be removed by surgery. Contact ulcers are often the result of vocal abuse and strain, but gastric reflux also is a causal factor. To aid in their healing, physicians may prescribe silence, but unless the person is trained by the speech pathologist in better ways of producing voice, they tend to recur.

There are also other causes. We have known individuals whose breathy voices were being produced and maintained solely by improper habits of vocal attack. They always began voicing with a preliminary exhalation of air. We had to teach them to start speaking without this preparatory windup. Some persons use a breathy voice because of the fear of being heard or exposed. And a few of them employ it deliberately.

FIGURE 9-5
Three organic causes of laryngeal tone disorders (vocal folds are seen from above as during a laryngoscopic examination)

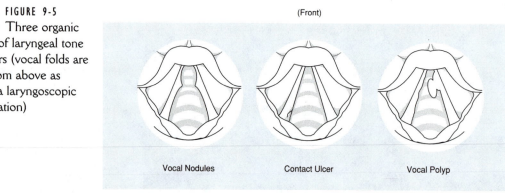

(Front)

Vocal Nodules   Contact Ulcer   Vocal Polyp

(Back)

The Harsh or Strident Voice

There are voices that are so rasping and piercing that they repel listeners. One characteristic of these voices is the presence of what is called the "vocal fry," because, perhaps, it sounds like the sizzling of bacon in the frying pan. As we said earlier, it is hard to describe but fairly easy to produce. By opening your mouth and making a tickerlike, crackling sort of sound, you can produce it and even slow it down until the separate clicks can be distinguished. When this vocal fry is fast, however, and accompanied by great tension, we have the basic quality of the strident or harsh voice. It is often accompanied by strain localized about the larynx, and often this structure is pulled up almost to the position used in swallowing. If you will place the tip of a finger against your Adam's or Eve's apple and produce a very harsh voice, you will know what we mean. In some instances, persons who have harsh voices are attempting to phonate at a pitch level that is too high (shrill) or, more often in men, too low (gutteral) for their particular structure.

Along with these features we also find the presence of what is called the "hard attack." Normally, the vocal folds should be brought together almost simultaneously with the pulse of air pressure. In the aspirate or soft attack, as we have already seen, the vocal folds close *after* the air has begun to flow. In the hard attack, the folds are closed and held tightly prior to the breath pulse. To break them open and start them vibrating from this tight position requires extra effort. If you will squeeze and hold your vocal folds tightly closed and suddenly utter a vowel, you will hear the little strained click that indicates the hard attack. It is not a good way to produce voice; vocal nodules or contact ulcers may result from the strain.

The usual causes of the harsh voice are imitation, personality problems involving hostility and aggression, the need to make oneself heard in the presence of masking noise, and the use of improper pitch levels. We need not belabor the obviousness of the first two of these causes, but some comment on the others is necessary. Strident voices seem to be able to make themselves heard more easily than normal voices, even though the effect is often unpleasant. In this regard they are somewhat like hypernasality. They're harsh but you can hear them. Those of us whose professions demand constant speaking in noisy situations often develop them, and sound more aggressive than we are. One of the nicest persons we have ever known was a lady who was in charge of the woman's swimming classes at our university, and she sounded like a witch until she developed vocal nodules and had to have voice therapy as well as a change of jobs. The only way she had found to pierce the echoing noise of splashing, squealing girls was to scream at them harshly. One of our cases was a foreman in a noisy factory whose harsh straining voice finally gave out due to the formation of contact ulcers near the back ends of his vocal folds.

The Hoarse Voice

Perceptually, the hoarse voice may be said to be a combination of the breathy and the harsh voice quality disorders. In it you can hear the air wastage and also the straining vocal fry of the strident voice. Research has shown that a hoarse or rough voice quality reflects irregularities in how the vocal folds move during phonation. Since the folds do not close and open smoothly or evenly, the glottal wave is distorted by perturbations. The physical correlates of these irregularities are **jitter,** the extent of variations in the fundamental frequency, and **shimmer,** the magnitude of intensity variations.

When voices suddenly become hoarse, we look for evidence of overuse or abuse. Most of us have become hoarse from too much yelling at one time or another—but not from praying. Usually with rest the hoarseness disappears. You've got to stop calling the pigs from the back forty. The same situation occurs as the result of a severe cold or laryngitis. Vocal nodules and polyps (see Figure 9-6) also are associated with hoarseness. But we wish to sound a strong note of warning about hoarseness. When it persists long after the abuse or laryngitis has disappeared, and there seems to be no apparent reason for its continuance, referral to a laryngologist should be made. Cancer of the larynx often shows its ugly head first in this form. Hoarseness is also a warning sign of **papilloma,** a benign tumor that grows in the throats of some young children.

A hoarse voice may also be produced through ventricular phonation. By this term we refer to the vibration of the false vocal folds that lie above the true ones. It is uncommon but we have found it in some few clients, nearly always when the true vocal folds are impaired.

Treatment of Voice Quality Disorders

Speech pathologists who have watched professional singers working hour upon hour to perfect their tone, practicing scales, spending long hours with their voice teacher sometimes envy that teacher. To find the same devotion in a person with a voice disorder is unusual. Even when the person has a falsetto or a husky voice due to severe vocal nodules, it is difficult to get him to work hard enough to hope for a favorable result. The reason for this state of affairs seems to lie in the relative lack of attention we pay to our voices. In the expression of emotion, we are more concerned with the cargo of anger rather than the voice vehicle that carries it. In most communicative interchanges, the basic message is carried by the articulation rather than the tones; and unless the voice is so weak that it cannot be heard, the fulfillment of communication may reward unpleasant voices as well as good ones.

Identification of the Problem.   One of best ways we have found for helping these clients is to have them hear their own voices on tape record-

Jitter.
Small perturbations/irregularities in the fundamental frequency of a voice; excessive jitter may be perceived as vocal "roughness."

Shimmer.
Small variation in vocal intensity from cycle to cycle.

Papilloma.
Benign wart-like growth that can occur in the larynx; may create breathing difficulty as well as dysphonia.

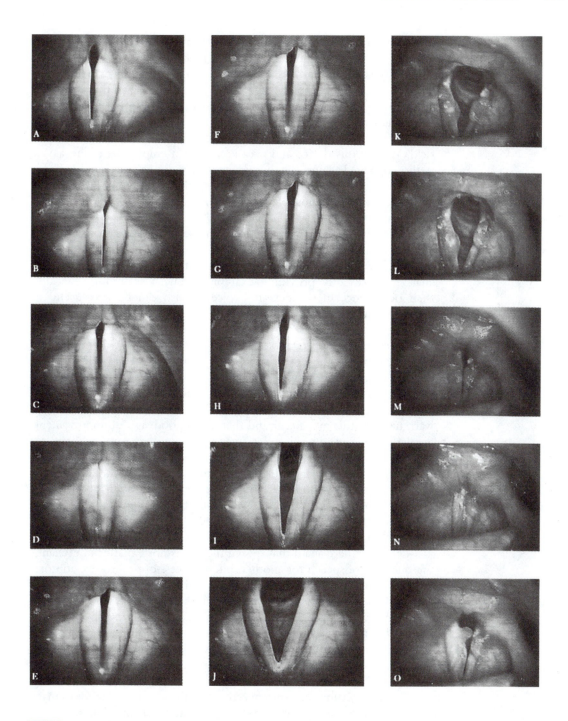

FIGURE 9-6 The vocal fold in action (a-h) phonation, (i-j) respiration, and (k-o) showing laryngeal polyps (used by permission from E. Yanagisawa, J. Casuccio, and M. Suzuki, 1981).

ings, not once but over and over again. It also helps to have a clinician who can imitate almost exactly the voice he hears. We train our own students in this skill so that they can be the echo machine. Since much of the inability to hear one's voice comes from the adaptation to the usual conditions of phonation, almost anything that alters the usual conditions helps one to hear it as it is. Radio announcers long ago found that they could hear their own voices better by cupping one ear to alter the sound field. We use this device and occasionally even employ a hearing aid or stethoscope held against the thyroid cartilage to help the client identify his problem. We have often found that having the person plug his ears with his fingers makes it possible for him to hear his defective voice more clearly and to modify it.

We often find that the person is unable to recognize the deviancy in voice until he is trained in its analysis. One has to know what to listen for. One needs training. The clinician must train the client to do this analyzing, patiently providing examples of what is wrong, checking their occurrence in the person's voice. It also can be very useful to observe visual "feedback" of the voice using instruments such as the VisiPitch.

Unless the person comes to hear what is wrong, she will not correct it. There is one caution we wish to leave with you. Occasionally, a person may feel that she is becoming much worse as the result of this recognition training. All that has happened is that she has become more conscious of what has always been there before; but it is wise, in early treatment, to warn her that this may occur and that it is a good sign of improvement. Similarly, some of our voice cases may become rather emotional and rejecting of themselves as the deviant voice becomes more apparent to them. However, if the clinician is able to share the problem, using the abnormal voice calmly and without anxiety, the person usually soon becomes desensitized to it. We have found it wise from the beginning examination to present the task as a joint endeavor. We explore its causes together, and together we work to modify the voice.

Let us say here again that speech therapy is not a matter of exchanging one type of speech for another, but a process of progressive approximation. Clinicians who have only *good* and *bad* or *yes* and *no* in their professional vocabularies should exchange them for *closer* and *farther* or *hotter* and *colder* as in the old nursery game. In voice therapy, we work with little shifts, and we reinforce with our approval those vocal attempts that come closer to the desired goal. This holds for disorders of pitch, intensity, and quality and for all types of variant human behavior seeking to modify itself.

To aid in getting this concept across (for the client, too, tends to make judgments in terms of black and white), it is well for the clinician to present models of these miniature modifications that change in the direction of the goal. It is the client's task to judge whether they approach or retreat from the goal. By using large changes first, and then smaller ones, the client's perceptions and discriminations are sharpened, and he can then evaluate his own attempts with objectivity.

New voices are weak and unstable. They need careful tending at first. We have found it wise to insist that the client use it at first only in therapy sessions where we can concentrate on its motor and acoustic aspects and make it stronger therein.

Once we feel that the client has the new voice fairly solidly and can use it consistently in therapy when he's listening to himself, we introduce masking noise into his ears so that he can monitor it by proprioception alone, by feeling the vocal postures and muscle tensions. Often at first, this masking tends to create a regression to the old voice, so we introduce the masking noise gradually and intermittently. No one can ever come to use a new voice habitually if he must constantly listen to it. Let's not burden the ears too much. It is also necessary to be sure that the client can use the new voice at his natural tempo or speed of utterance. It must not be labored or too careful. It cannot be confined to a monotone or a chant. All these motor and acoustic variations need some attention.

Next we attempt to stabilize the new voice in display speech, and we like to make recordings of the new voice so that the person can listen to them and feel good. Role playing, orating, readings, all can be used for this purpose. Often at this point we ask the person to give us a verbal autobiography and to use the new voice while doing so. This should run for several sessions. We do this so as to help to identify the new voice with the self. The perpendicular pronoun "I" especially should become colored with the new role. This provides an opportunity for some mild psychotherapy at the same time.

When we feel that definite progress has been made in the foregoing aspects of speech, we stabilize it in communication. We ask the client now to use the new voice outside the therapy sessions—but at first only when he talks to strangers. We do this to avoid the listener's shocked surprise that often greets a voice case when he confronts them with a new voice. The father of a young man who had never known anything but a high falsetto voice stormed into the bathroom one morning to find out what strange man was in the house at seven in the morning. The boy had only said something to the family dog.

Once the new voice has been used easily with strangers, it can be brought out in the circle of acquaintances and friends or family. It is wise to suggest that the person speak of his voice therapy casually or use it as a conversation piece. Most people are very interested. About this time (and perhaps we have protracted the process unduly in describing it, for at times we have changed voices in a single hour), the new voice becomes stabilized and is felt as natural as the old one had been. There will be a few momentary relapses, usually in emotional expression, but the task has been accomplished.

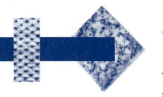

LARYNGECTOMY

When the choice came down to surgery or to die slowly by starvation and strangulation, Francis LeFluer, decided, as he later told us wryly, to "have his throat cut." Here is what he wrote (for he could not speak at all) a few days after the laryngectomy.

> The doctor told me that I had cancer of the throat and that if they removed my voice box immediately—he wanted to schedule surgery for the next morning—the chances were good for complete recovery. My first impulse was to shoot myself and get it over with quickly. Suddenly, my life was in a turmoil—how would I be able to earn a living, or even be able to talk to my family. I was so confused and depressed I just went along with the physician's urgent appeal. And so, after the operation, I found myself lying in a hospital bed with my wife holding my hand. When I tried to tell her I was OK and not to cry, nothing came out of my mouth, just a rush of air out of the hole in my throat under the bandage. I could move my lips but there was no sound. Then I cried—but silently. I was mute. I was not me.

It is indeed a strange, lonely, threatening world for a person who suddenly finds that he cannot utter a sound, cannot speak or laugh or cry aloud, or even kiss normally. Deep depressions often occur and the speech pathologist often finds herself wrestling with many invisible demons of emotion when trying to convince the laryngectomee (the person whose larynx has been removed) that he need not remain mute, that he can learn to speak again.

But how can this be done? How can one possibly speak aloud when the only entrance and exit for the air in the lungs is a hole (stoma) in the neck? To preserve the person's life and because she knows how insidiously cancer can spread, the surgeon usually must remove the entire larynx, and then join the patient's windpipe and (trachea) so that its upper opening is in the stoma through which inhalation and exhalation are now routed. In a few patients in whom the cancer has been caught early and appears to be localized, a partial laryngectomy may be performed so that the usual airway is preserved. But when the disease has spread beyond the vocal folds, the surgeon may perform a radical neck dissection and remove muscles, lymph nodes, and any other impaired structures in the neck region. Although it is difficult to tell precisely, there are approximately 40,000 surviving laryngectomees in the United States at any given point in time; and each year, more than 9,000 individuals undergo surgery for removal of their larynges. More males than females—the ratio is about seven to one—undergo a laryngectomy.

Reasons for Laryngectomy

Because of prompt detection and modern medication, only rarely now is it necessary to remove a person's larynx due to tuberculosis or syphilis, two diseases that sometimes attack the upper respiratory system. **Trauma** resulting from car and industrial accidents or combat injuries may require surgical reconstruction or removal of the larynx. We worked with one adolescent boy whose neck was mutilated by a shotgun blast at close range while hunting.

But most of our laryngectomized clients have been victims of cancer. Typically, they are men in their fifth or sixth decade of life, and all but a very few have been heavy smokers (more than twenty cigarettes a day). The American Cancer Society insists that smoking cigarettes is one of the most deadly and yet preventable causes of disease in our country.

Early Warning Signs of Laryngeal Cancer.   Fortunately, the cure rate for laryngeal cancer is good, second only to that for malignancy of the skin—if the person is alert to the changes in his voice. The most notable symptom is a persistent rough or hoarse vocal quality. But there are other early warning signs, as the wife of one of our clients related in an initial interview.

> Now, I don't see how we could have ignored the early signs of cancer. The hacking cough—smoker's cough he called it. And the throat-clearing habit, when had that started? In fact, his throat clearing was so chronic and so characteristic that his secretary could tell when he was approaching the office; the distinctive sound arrived seconds before he did, like a pervasive perfume or aftershave lotion. Even when he noticed that his voice got tired quickly, Fran blamed it on a chronic postnasal discharge. He simply chewed mildly anesthetic lozenges continually. But when the pitch of his voice began to break upward like an adolescent, that scared him. The next day he made an appointment to see a laryngologist.

The Impact of Laryngectomy

Keep in mind that amputation of the larynx is terribly assaultive surgery; it alters the individual in very basic ways (see Figure 9-7). (1) He now breathes through the opening in his neck, and the air is no longer filtered and warmed by the nasal passages. (2) He cannot blow his nose, and when he coughs, the air is expelled out of the stoma. (3) He will not be able to taste food normally for a while, and usually the sense of smell is lost. (4) He might have difficulty lifting or pushing since he cannot squeeze off the laryngeal valve to fixate his chest. (5) He must be very careful around water, even showers, for unless the stoma is covered, water will pour directly into his lungs. Swimming, of course, is impossible. (6) His body image is changed and he must cope with the aversive reactions of his family, friends, and the public to his altered physical state. But of all the problems the new laryngectomee encounters, the most devastating is the sudden loss of voice.

Trauma.
Shock or injury.

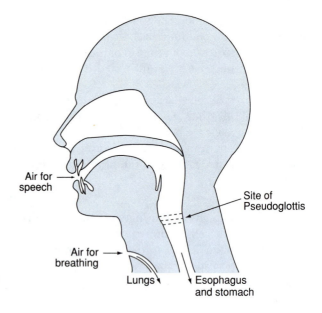

Air for
speech

Site of
Pseudoglottis

Air for
breathing

FIGURE 9-7   After laryngectomy

Lungs

Esophagus
and stomach

New Means of Communication
for the Laryngectomee

The newly laryngectomized person has three options in his quest for a new voice: an artificial larynx, esophageal speech, or a variant of the latter, tracheoesophageal speech.

The Artificial Larynx.   The first method for producing vicarious voice involves the use of an artificial larynx. There are two types: pneumatic and electronic. The first device we ever saw was a cumbersome pneumatic instrument consisting of a bellows held under the arm and a mouth-tube that contained a reed similar to that used in the ordinary harmonica. By inserting the tube into the corner of his mouth and pumping the bellows in his upper arm, the patient who owned it was able to talk intelligibly, though somewhat weakly. But most pneumatic artificial larynges work by lung power (Figure 9-8). The speaker holds the device over his stoma, exhales to activate a reed, and the sound is transported to his mouth by a plastic tube.

We now have much better artificial larynges, most of which can use an electrically activated diaphragm or reed as the sound source.[3] In the instrument illustrated (Figure 9-9), one of the most commonly used, the battery is contained in the case, and the buzzing diaphragm at its end is held against the neck. By articulating carefully, the person can turn the sound thus produced into usable speech.

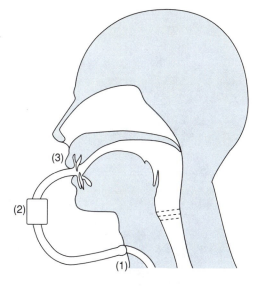

FIGURE 9-8   Pneumatic larynx: Air expelled from the stoma (1) activates a reed (2) and the sound is carried to the person's mouth (3)

Learning to Use the Artificial Larynx.   It is much easier to learn to produce speech by the use of this instrument than it is to master intelligible esophageal phonation. One needs only to press the button on an electrolarynx and hold the diaphragm end of the device flush with the surface of the neck while articulating to be able to achieve some communicative ability. Some users, unfortunately, have had no more training than that provided by the instruction booklet that comes with the instrument. The speech pathologist, however, can make the difference between inferior speech and highly intelligible speech by helping the patient to find the best areas of contact. He can show the patient how to turn on the apparatus intermittently rather than continuously and thereby prevent some of the droning buzz that often interferes with communication. The patient also needs training in mastering the pitch variations that enable him to produce the inflections required by questioning and other prosodic features of normal utterance. Phrasing can also be taught, but perhaps the major contribution a clinician can make is improving the intelligibility of the artificial speech. By helping the patient to articulate the consonants precisely and carefully, the clinician can improve the speech greatly. It is difficult for the user of an electrolarynx to achieve the full potential of the instrument by himself. He needs a clinician.

Esophageal Speech.   It is possible for the laryngectomee to speak again using a different mechanism. As illustrated in Figure 9-7, a *pseudoglottis* (this substitute vibrator for the vocal folds is termed the *pharyngeal-*

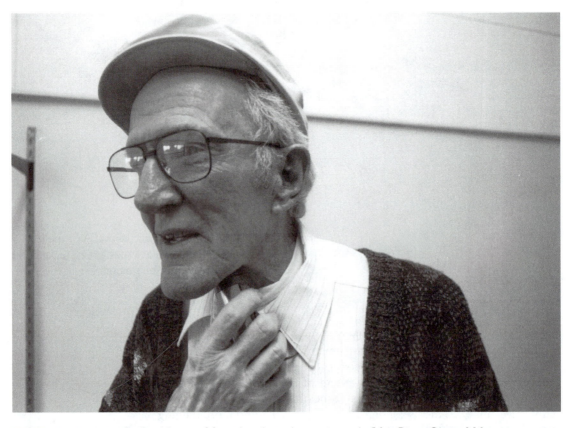

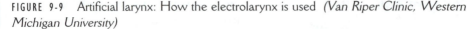
FIGURE 9-9   Artificial larynx: How the electrolarynx is used *(Van Riper Clinic, Western Michigan University)*

esophageal or *PE segment)* can be developed by constricting the muscles along the upper edges of the esophagus, the tube that leads down to the stomach, and setting them into vibration by air that has been taken into the esophagus. It is the speech pathologist's job to teach the laryngectomee how to produce this new and different alaryngeal voice.

We are sure that you have more than once uttered sounds, if not speech, by using this substitute channel, usually after having eaten too well or having drunk too much beer. Certainly as a baby you were burped and those burps were very audible. The difference between those bottle burps and the esophageal (alaryngeal) phonation that we teach the laryngectomized is that the air does not come all the way up from the stomach, but instead it is trapped higher up in the esophagus before it is released. For those who have lost a larynx and are completely aphonic, the esophageal voice may be the way back to a fairly normal life. But it must be learned over the course of many sessions before sufficient control has been mastered to enable the client to communicate effectively.

Learning to Use Esophageal Speech.   The clinician who seeks to help the laryngectomee acquire esophageal speech need not himself be able to produce it, although we have found that our own ability to do so has contributed much to the patient's early progress. What is necessary is the provision of an adequate model such as that by some other skilled esophageal speaker or at the very least some tapes or films of such speakers. Also, the clinician must understand the basic principles for the intake of air into the upper esophagus and have some systematic sequence of subgoals. Clinicians prefer various sequences, but all of them start with the goal of being able to take air into the esophagus segment and to expel it in the production of tone.

In an introductory text such as this one, it would be unwise to go into too much detail; but there are at least three methods for trapping enough air into the esophagus to permit vocalization. In the first, the inhalation method, the sphincters of the esophagus must be relaxed, and then, as the diaphragm descends, air is naturally drawn into the esophagus. Then the sphincters of the cricopharyngeus are tightened and vibrate as the diaphragm returns upward. The second procedure is termed the "injection procedure" or the "glossopharyngeal press." In this method, the lips and soft palate are closed, and the cheeks are contracted simultaneously with an upward and backward bunching of the tongue. This forces or injects the air that was trapped within the mouth cavity down into the esophagus. Good esophageal speakers can use the concomitant constriction of their plosive sounds to pump small amounts of air down into the esophagus, thus continually replenishing the supply, and so speak continuously.

We have found our work with laryngectomees to be challenging and rewarding. It is challenging because there are many problems that must be solved: the need to provide motivation in the face of repeated failure, the need to relieve these patients of their emotional storms, the need for repeated restructuring of tasks and goals. An understanding clinician can make the difference between success and failure and it is very good to know the joy of helping another person to speak again.

Tracheoesophageal Speech.   To speak again, a laryngectomee needs to replace two essential features he has lost: a source of vibration and a power supply. As we have seen, an electrolarynx supplies both vibration and power, but they are *external* to the person. Esophageal speech, on the other hand, replaces the larynx with the pseudoglottis; and power is provided by drawing air in through the oral cavity. Now, since learning to inject air swiftly and easily is perhaps the most difficult aspect of esophageal speech, any method that promotes the use of the clients's own lung power should facilitate the treatment process.

A relatively new form of surgery provides the laryngectomee with a small tunnel between the trachea and esophagus; when he closes the stoma with his finger, the air from his lungs goes upward into the pseudoglottis. Although he must still master a new method of producing sound, his speech is louder and more continuous, and there is no distracting noise from the stoma.

There are some drawbacks in creating a tracheoesophageal shunt: The tube may grow back together, food or drink may leak into the trachea, and there is some surgical risk involved. A small plastic valve called a **voice prosthesis** is inserted in the wall between the trachea and the esophagus. When the patient places his thumb over the stoma, or when using a special respiratory valve over the stoma, air is forced through the prosthesis into the esophagus and up to the pseudoglottis. The valve remains shut during swallowing so there is no problem with aspiration of food and drink.

Perhaps the most sophisticated device—and one that has generated considerable research—is the Blom-Singer Voice Prosthesis (Singer and Blom, 1980). The Blom-Singer valve is a hollow silicon tube that is inserted in the stoma and through the wall of the esophagus (see Figure 9-10). Pulmonary air enters the tube through a hole in the bottom

Voice prosthesis. Actually, any device used to produce voicing (such as an electolarynx), the term now refers most often to a small valve that transports air from the trachea to the esophagus for producing tracheo-esophageal voice.

 FIGURE 9-10 Schematic illustration of the Blom-Singer Tracheostomy Valve and Speech Prosthesis

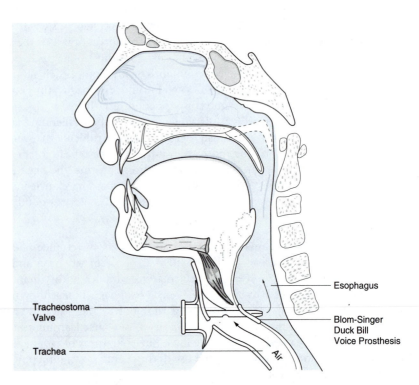

Esophagus

Tracheostoma Valve

Blom-Singer Duck Bill Voice Prosthesis

Trachea

Air

surface of the tracheal portion and then is transferred to the esophagus through a thin slit. The valve is designed to allow air to enter the esophagus, but does not permit food or liquid to return into the trachea. The Blom-Singer system also includes a tracheostoma valve which is activated by breath pressure—it shuts automatically when the person begins to speak so that the stoma does not have to be occluded with the fingers.

Whatever the method of producing pseudovoice may be, a competent speech clinician can do wonders for laryngectomees. By emphasizing precise articulation, by teaching them how to pause and when, and by helping them increase the number of syllables on one air intake, the resulting speech becomes much more intelligible. But beyond these services, the speech clinician is uniquely trained to share the frustrations and anger and helpless feelings that accompany laryngectomy (see Keith, 1984 and Lauder, 1993), and to help the patient cope with them. He will find no more patient listener.

STUDY QUESTIONS

1. Dysphonias may affect what three features of voice?
2. What is the difference between "hysterical aphonia" and "spasmodic dysphonia"?
3. Surgical severing (or sectioning) of the recurrent laryngeal nerve has been used for what purpose in the treatment of voice disorders? How does this differ from the purpose for which botulinum toxin is used?
4. What are some strategies you should suggest to a friend with vocal nodules to help him or her to reduce vocal abuse? And what is meant by "hard attack"?
5. For what reason(s) may some form of counseling or simple psychotherapy be an important element of voice therapy?
6. What factors may account for the occurrence of pitch breaks in the pubescent voice?
7. What are the main disorders of vocal resonance, and what causal factors are associated with each?
8. Why must an individual with persistent hoarseness be referred for medical examination by a laryngologist?
9. In addition to the loss of voice, a laryngectomy has what other immediate effects on the patient's daily activities?
10. What are the advantages and disadvantages associated with each of the three principal types of alaryngeal speech?

ENDNOTES

[1]The incidence of voice disorders in adults is about 1 percent. Surveys show that more school-aged children, as many as 6 percent, have abnormal voices (Senturia and Wilson, 1968; Silverman and Zimmer, 1975; Brindle and Morris, 1979; Miller and Madison, 1984).

[2]Perhaps because people are much more sophisticated about medical ailments than they used to be, the number of hysterically aphonic clients seen in our clinic has declined sharply over the past twenty years.

[3]The electrolarynx was evidently discovered by Gilbert Wright, who noted while shaving that when he pressed his buzzing electric razor against his throat and pantomimed talking while holding his breath, he could produce intelligible speech.

REFERENCES

Aronson, A. (1990). *Clinical voice disorders* (3rd ed.). New York: Thieme Medical Publishers.

Brindle, S., and Morris H. (1979). Prevalence of voice quality deviations in the normal adult population. *Journal of Communication Disorders, 12,* 439–445.

Colton, R., and Casper, J. (1990). *Understanding voice problems: A physiological perspective for diagnosis and treatment.* Baltimore, MD: Williams and Wilkins.

Keith, R. (1984). *Looking forward: A guidebook for the laryngectomee.* New York: Thieme-Stratton.

Lauder, E. (1993). *Self-help for the laryngectomee.* San Antonio, TX: Lauder Publisher.

Luchsinger, R., and Arnold, G. (1965). *Voice-speech-language.* Belmont, CA: Wadsworth.

Miller, S., and Madison, C. (1984). Public school voice clinics I: A working model. *Language,* *Speech and Hearing Services in Schools,* 15, 51–57.

Senturia, B., and Wilson, F. (1968). Otorhinolaryngic findings in children with voice deviations. *Annals of Otology,* 177, 1027–1041.

Silverman, E., and Zimmer, C. (1975). Incidence of chronic hoarseness among school-age children. *Journal of Speech and Hearing Disorders,* 40, 211–215.

Yanagisawa, E., Casuccio, J., and Suzuki, M. (1981). Video laryngoscopy using a rigid telescope and a video home system color camera. *Annals of Otology, Rhinology, and Laryngology,* 90, 316–350.

Zemlin, W. (1981). *Speech and hearing science* (2nd ed.). Englewood Cliffs, NJ: Prentice Hall.

SUPPLEMENTARY READINGS

Aaron, V., and Madison, C. (1991). A vocal hygiene program for high-school cheerleaders. *Language, Speech, and Hearing Services in Schools,* 22, 287–290.

Aronson, A., and DeSanto, L. (1983). Adductor spastic dysphonia: Three years after recurrent laryngeal nerve resection. *Laryngoscope,* 93, 1–8.

Bastian, R. (1987). Laryngeal image biofeedback for voice disorder patients. *Journal of Voice*, 1, 279–282.

Blitzer, A., Brin, M., Fahn, S., and Lovelace, R. (1988). Clinical and laboratory characteristics of focal laryngeal dystonia: Study of 110 cases. *Laryngoscope*, 98, 636–640.

Blitzer, A., and Brin, M. (1991). Laryngeal dystonia: A series with botulin toxin therapy. *Annals of Otolology, Rhinology, and Laryngology*, 100, 85–89.

Blitzer, A., and Brin, M. (1992). The distonic larynx. *Journal of Voice*, 6, 294–297.

Blitzer, A., and Brin, M.F. (1992). Treatment of spasmodic dysphonia (laryngeal dystonia) with local injections of botulinum toxin. *Journal of Voice*, 6, 365–369.

Blom, E., Singer, M., and Hanmaker, R. (1986). A prospective study of tracheoesophageal speech. *Archives of Otolaryngology—Head and Neck Surgery*. 112, 440–447.

Boone, D., and McFarlane, S. (1988). *The voice and voice therapy* (4th ed.). Englewood Cliffs, NJ: Prentice Hall.

Casper, J., and Colton, R. (1993). *Clinical manual for laryngectomy and head/neck cancer rehabilitation*. San Diego, CA: Singular Publishing Group.

Dedo, H., and Shipp, T. (1980). *Spastic dysphonia: A surgical and voice therapy treatment program*. San Diego, CA: College-Hill Press.

Dedo, H., and Izdebski, K. (1983). Intermediate results of 306 recurrent laryngeal nerve sections for spastic dysphonia. *Laryngoscope*, 93, 9–16.

Dedo, H., and Behlau, M. (1991). Recurrent laryngeal nerve section for spastic dysphonia: 5- to 14-year preliminary results in the first 300 patients. *Annals of Otology, Rhinology, and Laryngology*, 100, 274–279.

Ford, C., and Bless, D. (eds.). (1991). *Phonosurgery*. New York: Raven Press.

Gould, W., and Lawrence, V. (1984). *Surgical care of voice disorders*. New York: Springer-Verlag Wien.

Hilgers, F., and Balm, A. (1993). Long-term results of vocal rehabilitation after total laryngectomy with the low-resistance, indwelling Provox voice prosthesis system. *Clinical Otolaryngology*, 18, 517–523.

Hillenbrand, J. (in press). Acoustic correlates of breathy vocal quality: Dysphonic voices and continuous speech. *Journal of the Acoustical Society of America*.

Hirano, M., and Bless, D. (1993). *Videostroboscopic examination of the larynx*. San Diego, CA: Singular Publishing Group.

Hixon, T., Hawley, J., and Wilson, K. (1982). An around-the-house device for the clinical determination of respiratory driving pressure: A note on making simple even simpler. *Journal of Speech and Hearing Disorders*, 47, 413–415.

Kahane, J., and Beckford, N. (1991). The aging larynx and voice. In D. Ripich (ed.), *Handbook of geriatric communication disorders*. Austin, TX: Pro-Ed.

Leith, W., and Johnston, R. (1986). *Handbook of voice therapy for the school clinician*. San Diego, CA: College-Hill Press.

Lindsey, P., Montague, J., and Buffalo, M. (1986). A preliminary survey on the relationship of exogenous factors to laryngeal papilloma. *Language, Speech and Hearing Services in Schools*. 17, 292–299.

Ludlow, C., Naunton, R., Sedory, S., Schulz, G., and Hallett, M. (1988). Effects of botulinum toxin injections on speech in adductor spasmodic dysphonia. *Neurology*. 38, 1220–1225.

Ludlow, C. (1990). Treatment of speech and voice disorders with botulinum toxin. *Journal of the American Medial Association, 264,* 2671–2675.

Ludlow, C., Naunton, R., Terada, S., and Anderson, B. (1991). Successful treatment of selected cases of abductor spasmodic dysphonia using botulinum toxin injection. *Archives of Otolaryngolology—Head and Neck Surgery,* 104, 849–855.

Mason, M. (1993). *Speech pathology for tracheostomized and ventilator dependent patients.* Newport Beach, CA: Voicing.

Passy, V. (1986). Passy-Muir tracheostomy speaking valve. *Archives of Otolaryngology—Head and Neck Surgery,* 95, 247–248.

Reich, A., McHenry, M. and Keaton, A. (1986). A survey of dysphonic episodes in high school cheerleaders. *Language, Speech and Hearing Services in Schools,* 17, 63–71.

Sataloff, R. (1987). The professional voice: Part I. Anatomy, function, and general health. *Journal of Voice,* 1, 92–104.

Singer, M., and Blom, E. (1980). An endoscopic technique for restoration of voice after laryngectomy. *Annals of Otology, Rhinology, and Laryngology,* 89, 529–533.

Stemple, J., Glaze, L. and Gerdeman, B. (1995). *Clinical voice pathology: Theory and management* (2nd ed.). San Diego, CA: Singular Publishing Group.

Weinberg, B., and Moon, J. (1986). Airway resistances of Blom-Singer and Panje low pressure tracheoesophageal puncture prostheses. *Journal of Speech and Hearing Disorders,* 51, 169–172.

Wilson, D. (1987). *Voice problems of children* (3rd ed.). Baltimore, MD: Williams and Wilkins.

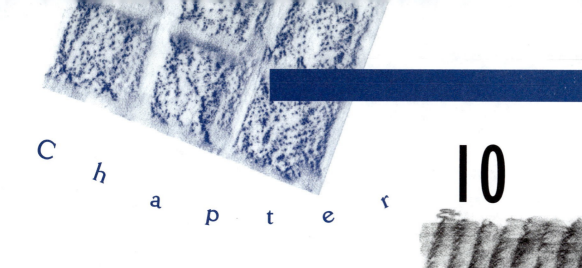

Chapter 10

Cleft Palate

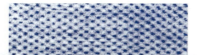

When the obstetrician and delivery room nurses suddenly ceased their chatter, the new mother realized that something was wrong with her baby. Several times she insisted that they tell her if the infant girl had all her fingers and toes. Finally, wrapped in a blanket that framed her badly disfigured face, the child was placed hesitantly in her arms.

> When I saw the gaping black hole and twisted bow-shaped bone beneath my baby's partially developed nose, I cried out, "Dear God, why?" Emotions of fear, guilt, pity, love, and anger flashed over me like lightning slicing the sky, and because of these, another was added . . . shame. Later I learned my reaction was completely normal and exactly what most mothers feel when they first glimpse their cleft-palate infants (De-Longchamp, 1976).

Most babies look pretty good shortly after birth or at least after they have been cleaned up for that first inspection by the happy parents. But there are some, alas, who do not, because they have craniofacial (skull and face) anomalies due to some failure of the bones and tissues of the head to develop normally in the uterus.

It is well known that a cleft of the lip and/or palate may occur as just one of several features of a more involved syndrome. In fact, there may be more than 300 syndromes in which oral clefts of some type can occur (Shprintzen, 1987, cited by Peterson-Falzone, 1989, p. 38). Moreover, according to the American Cleft Palate-Craniofacial Association (1993), approximately one-half of all infants with cleft palate "have associated malformations, either minor or major, occurring in conjunction with the cleft." It is understandable, then, that we may encounter some communication disorders and other problems in this population that go beyond the difficulties that are directly related to oral clefting alone.

Accordingly, those speech-language pathologists who work extensively with cleft palate patients and their families must become familiar with the field of clinical genetics and with the characteristics and effects of many syndromes. In this introductory textbook, however, we will focus just on isolated clefts—that is, clefts that occur in the absence of any additional congenital defects. Even then, of course, possible middle ear infections and hearing fluctuation, along with "the consequences of early hospitalization and surgery, prolonged feeding difficulties, facial disfigurement, and the altered interpersonal interactions they may engender in the extended family and beyond present early management problems predisposing toward speech and language disorders" (Bzoch, 1989, p. 3).

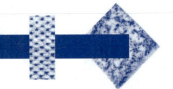

INCIDENCE AND TYPES OF CLEFTS

Although a variety of special classification systems are used to define certain subcategories and to provide other more detailed information, oral clefts are categorized generally with reference to their location and extent.

It can be very important for research and for surgical and other management purposes to specify precise locations, lengths, and widths of clefts; but for our purposes, we will consider just three major categories: *cleft of the lip only, cleft of the palate only,* and *clefts of both lip and palate.* One of these three types of clefting occurs once in about every 700 to 750 live births.

Differential incidence figures vary somewhat from study to study, but it is well established that clefts occur more frequently among American Indians than among Orientals, that they are more frequent in both of those groups than among Whites, and that they occur less frequently in Blacks than in Whites. It also is reported that cleft lip, with or without cleft palate, occurs almost twice as often in males as in females, whereas cleft of the palate without lip clefting occurs about half again more frequently in females than in males. Approximately one-half of all clefts involve both the lip and the palate, while around 25 percent involve the lip only. In the remaining 25 percent only the palate is cleft.

Basically, these clefts each involve a failure or disruption of normal development during the second or third months of gestation. Embryonic processes that will become the face and palate begin to grow together during the fifth to sixth week after conception. The gradual fusing of these structures proceeds from front to back, and by the twelfth week, the development of the soft palate, including the **uvula,** is complete. Perhaps you have noticed in a friend's mouth (or maybe even in your own) what appear to be twin uvulae hanging side by side. If so, you have seen the simplest instance of fusion that was not quite completed. This condition, called **bifid** *uvula,* is believed to occur at a rate of one in 80 Caucasians and, in the absence of other cleft-related factors, causes its owner no particular problems.

When normal development has not occurred, the baby will have a cleft of the upper lip, the upper gum ridge, the hard palate, the soft palate, or combinations of the above (see Figures 10-1 and 10-2). The clefts may be complete or incomplete, meaning that in some cases there was no fusion of the right and left halves of the structures and, in other cases, that the fusion had started but was disrupted before the structure was complete. Gorlin (1993) and McWilliams, Morris, and Shelton (1990), among others, provide detailed discussions of cleft formations as well as further information about associated congenital malformations.

Clefts of the Lip

Clefts almost always involve the upper lip rather than the lower lip, but they may be found in both the lip and the *alveolar ridge* (the upper gum ridge). They may be unilateral and affect only the left or only the right side, or they may be bilateral and affect both sides. If the cleft of the lip is complete, it will extend into the nostril; if the cleft is incomplete, the

Uvula.
The hanging portion of the soft palate.

Bifid.
Divided into two parts, as in a cleft or bifid uvula.

nostril will have been formed by the initial fusion of the structures, but the lip will show a cleft below that area. These possibilities exist because of the way the upper lip is formed. Shortly after conception, one facial process called the frontonasal process joins with two other processes that grow toward the center from each side. These are the maxillary processes of the upper jaw. The frontonasal process eventually forms the middle part of the nose and the middle part of the upper lip, while the maxillary processes form the middle part of the cheeks and the sides of the upper lip. Unless these processes unite and fuse completely, a cleft of the lip will occur.

Clefts of the Palate

Both the hard and soft palates may be cleft, for the palate, like the lip, also requires a fusion of three processes. Somewhat later than the formation of the lip, a small triangular process (structure) that will eventually become the area behind the upper four front teeth joins with the palatine plates to start the formation of the hard palate. As the processes continue to merge, the hard palate, the soft palate, and finally the *uvula* take shape. If the fusion of these processes is interrupted at any time, a cleft of the palate will result. If the processes never started to fuse, the cleft will be complete. Otherwise, an incomplete cleft will be apparent.

Clefts of Both Lip and Palate

Because the structures responsible for the formation of the lip and palate are closely related, some children will have clefts of both the lip and palate. These babies are not pretty to look at because the center of

FIGURE 10-1
Three types of clefts: (A) unilateral cleft of lip and palate, (B) cleft of hard and soft palate, (C) bilateral cleft of lip and palate

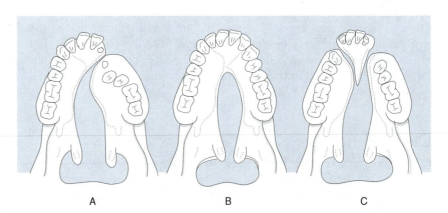

A   B   C

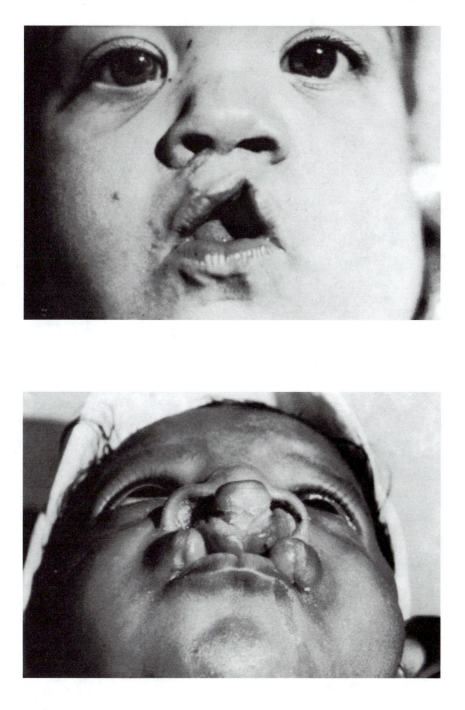

 FIGURE 10-2   Clefts of the lip and palate *(courtesy of Ralph Blocksma, M.D.)*

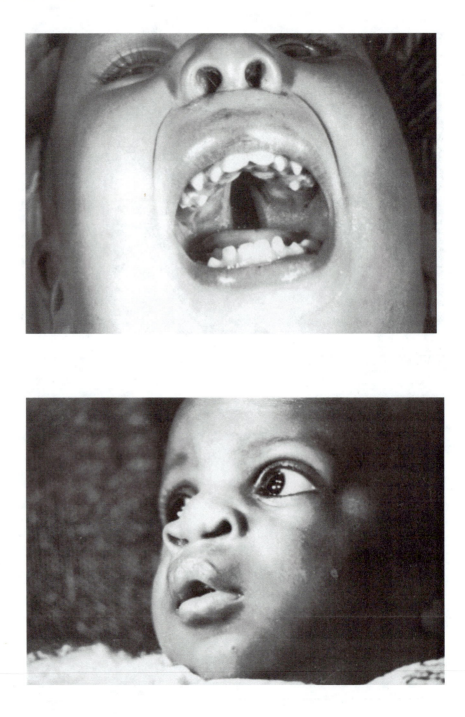

 FIGURE 10-2 CONTINUED

their face is severely distorted. The middle part of their lip and middle part of their palate may even swing freely if no attachment to either side is present.

Submucous Cleft Palate.

Some children (around one in 1,200) do not have any immediately obvious signs of clefts even though a cleft may be present under the mucous lining of the palate. As in the overt clefts we've already described, congenital submucous clefts have been found to be more prevalent among American Indians than among White Caucasians and least prevalent among Blacks. Unlike overt clefts, however, they may be somewhat more common in males than in females.

These hidden clefts seldom are diagnosed at birth and, in fact, might occasionally go without ever being diagnosed. More commonly, however, speech problems such as hypernasal resonance and articulation errors lead to closer examination of the child and revelation of the submucous cleft. In some cases, the speech may be normal unless an adenoidectomy is performed or until adenoidal tissue (which can assist us in closing the velopharyngeal space) begins to atrophy or shrink with maturation.

Signs that a submucous cleft is present include the following: a bifid uvula; a forward notching of the back edge of the hard palate; and a translucent whitish or bluish line in the midline of the soft palate, reflecting the failure of underlying palatal muscles to have fused. The notch may be felt by manual **palpation** even if is not readily visible, but you will have little difficulty seeing the wider and rather deep notches that sometimes are found.

Congenital Palatopharyngeal Incompetence.

Congenital palatopharyngeal incompetence (CPI), once known as congenital palatal insufficiency, refers to a condition in which there is inadequate **velopharyngeal closure** for speech even though there is no overt or submucous clefting of the palate. CPI is not diagnosed at birth and may not even be suspected until a child develops persistent hypernasality after an adenoidectomy, although it certainly can be evident earlier if the problem is severe. It has been shown that many of these children have normally functioning but exceptionally short palates. An unusually deep or enlarged pharynx also may be observed. In some cases the muscles that lift the soft palate may be abnormally positioned. In any event, while adenoids are present, they act like a pad against which the velum may be able to make adequate contact; but when the adenoids are removed, the resulting gap between the palate and the back wall of the throat is too great and leakage occurs.

Palpation.
Examining by tapping or touching.

Velopharyngeal closure.
The more or less complete shutting off of the nasopharynx.

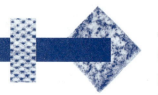

CAUSES OF CLEFTS

It is difficult if not impossible to know why any individual child was born with an oral cleft. As we've seen, the failure of these facial and palatal structures to fuse occurs during the first trimester of pregnancy; so, when a full-term baby is born with a cleft, the cleft has been in existence for over six months. Of interest to parents known to be at risk, it apparently may now be possible to detect the presence of a cleft lip early in the second trimester (Bronshtein, Blumfeld, Kohn, and Blumfeld, 1994).

During medieval times, it was believed that one of the causes of oral clefts was the exposure of expectant mothers to rabbits (who always have **harelips**). There even were local laws prohibiting butchers' shops from displaying rabbits for fear that some unsuspecting pregnant woman might gaze upon the carcass, thereby increasing the likelihood that her child would be born with a cleft lip. Now we know that many oral clefts appear to have a genetic basis. The incidence of clefts in families with no previous occurrence of clefting is very small in live births, but it increases significantly for families in which clefts have occurred. Although hereditary factors are important in both clefts of the lip and the palate, many experts believe that cleft lip is more likely to have a genetic basis.

It generally is believed that genetic factors related to clefting are very complex and that, in fact, *multifactorial inheritance* is involved. In this view, many contributing genes must interact in the presence of negative environmental factors in order to cause a cleft (McWilliams, Morris, and Shelton, 1989). To further complicate the issue, very little is known about specific environmental factors. However, the list of possible *teratogenic agents* is quite extensive. It is suspected, for example, that medications taken during pregnancy, maternal infections and diseases, exposure to radiation, or perhaps even stress, may activate a genetic tendency toward clefting. It also has been suggested that using substances such as alcohol, aspirin, caffeine, cocaine, marijuana, and tobacco during pregnancy can increase not only the risk of clefting but of other **anomalies** as well (Powers, 1986). The clinician who works with the families of cleft palate children should be able to provide general answers to questions about etiology but must refer parents to qualified genetic counselors for specific information and guidance.

The Impact of Clefts

When a baby is born with a cleft, special services are needed immediately. The first problem to be tackled is that of informing the new parents of the less than pleasant news for, unlike many other conditions, the oral cleft is conspicuously apparent from the first. This task requires the skill and compassion of a specialist who knows a lot about the disorder and who un-

Harelip.
A cleft of the upper lip (term is no longer used).

Teratogen.
Any agent or substance that acts prenatally to cause a congenital abnormality.

Anomaly.
An anatomic deviation from normal structure or form.

derstands the devastating impact of the event. It is not an easy task and some physicians and nurses shirk their responsibility or perform poorly. For example, we have had mothers of cleft-palate children tell us that they were kept under anesthesia for hours after the birth of their child until someone was able to muster enough courage to talk with them. Fortunately, the situation is improving. Most obstetricians now call in a specialist, probably a plastic surgeon, who will both inform and reassure the parents immediately that the child can be helped. Some hospitals also have files of other parents who can be called in to assist the new parents to overcome their initial shock. But most parents, once the initial anguish is over, have myriad practical questions: How will they be able to feed the child? When will the lip be closed? The palate? Will he have dental problems? How can they prepare him for stares and negative comments? Will he be able to talk normally? Responding appropriately to these concerns obviously requires the concerted effort of several different professionals.

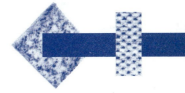

THE ORAL CLEFT TEAM

The mere participation of appropriate specialists in counseling, evaluation, and treatment, however, does not ensure that a child with an oral cleft will receive the best possible professional care. As an old adage reminds us, "too many cooks can spoil the broth," and this cautionary advice is particularly applicable when several different specialists seek independently to pursue their own treatment plans. No matter how qualified and well-intentioned each specialist may be, their joint efforts must be closely coordinated in order to obtain the best final outcome.

In years past, we were saddened far too often by seeing adolescents and adults whose early treatments had been fragmented and uncoordinated. As a result, they came to us with badly distorted facial features, very poor dentition, nearly unintelligible speech, and frequently with heavy burdens of negative emotion. Happily, we now see fewer of such treatment failures, due largely to the growing availability of interdisciplinary oral cleft teams.

The team approach to cleft palate management actually started over fifty years ago when some professionals began to realize that truly successful results were more likely to be obtained through open communication, cooperative planning, and integrated treatment. Gradually, this concept gained widened acceptance, and today there are well over 200 oral cleft teams functioning in the United States.

Not all teams are structured identically, nor do they work in exactly the same way. Basically, though, a team includes a core of professional members who meet regularly to examine patients and to develop together a comprehensive plan of treatment for the individual patient. When specialists are free to discuss their respective points of view, and if the team process is not dominated by any one specialist, the complex of problems associated with oral clefts is likely to be addressed more sensitively and systematically. Moreover, the team approach saves time and money for the parents and spares them the anguish of going from one specialist to another and sometimes getting conflicting advice.

While the compositions of cleft teams vary, most authorities agree that the minimum "core" should consist of a plastic surgeon, a speech pathologist, and an **orthodontist.** For an "ideal" team, however, McWilliams (1992) would add the following: anesthesiologist, audiologist, coordinator, educator, endodontist, geneticist, genetic counselor, nurse practitioner, oral surgeon, otolaryngologist, parents, pediatrician, periodontist, **prosthodontist,** psychiatrist, psychologist, radiologist, and social worker. Most actual teams no doubt fall somewhere between the minimum and the ideal, with many smaller teams depending upon consultation, as needed, by professionals not actually represented in regular team meetings.

Speech pathologists who become members of these teams must understand the responsibilities and capabilities of the other members. Here we are interested only in providing a brief overview of a few of the other specialties commonly encountered, but detailed information about professional roles and responsibilities may be found in references such as Brodsky, Holt, and Ritter-Schmidt (1992).

The *plastic surgeon* specializes in the modification of soft tissue, including closure of the lip and repair of the palate. Typically the first specialist the parents meet, the plastic surgeon often coordinates the team approach to the entire treatment. The *otolaryngologist*—or *ear, nose, and throat (ENT)* specialist—will evaluate and treat, if necessary, the tonsils and adenoids and will perform ear surgery, if indicated. The ENT physician often is involved in **nasendoscopic** studies of velopharyngeal closure. The *orthodontist* is responsible for the positioning of the teeth. He or she may use devices to straighten teeth and to ensure as normal an occlusion as possible. The *prosthodontist,* or *prosthetic dentist,* designs and builds prostheses—appliances to replace missing dental and oral structures. These may include dentures, speech bulbs, palatal lifts, and **obturators**. A *radiologist* is the physician who makes and interprets x-ray studies of the oral and nasopharyngeal structures, including still x-rays (lateral head plates) and videotaped motion x-rays (videofluoroscopy).

The *pediatrician* oversees the general medical condition and physical development of the child; and, since both the child and the parents face many emotional problems associated with the cleft, a *psychologist* may be called upon to provide appropriate testing and treatment. Children with oral clefts have such a high incidence of middle ear problems and hearing loss that regular monitoring is absolutely essential, and so a variety of types of hearing evaluations are administered and interpreted by the team's

Orthodontist.
A dentist who specializes in repositioning of the teeth.

Prosthodontist.
A dental specialist who makes prostheses.

Nasendoscopy.
A technique for viewing velopharyngeal and/or laryngeal structures from above with a flexible fiberoptic instrument.

Obturator.
An appliance used to close a cleft or a gap.

audiologist. Finally, the *speech pathologist* not only works directly with clients and parents to improve the child's speech, but may be involved in evaluating and coordinating the efforts of other specialists, since the facilitation of normal speech development should be one of the most important early management considerations of the oral cleft team.

General Management Principles

Although treatment approaches have improved greatly in recent decades, unfortunately there still are children with oral clefts who receive substandard care. Consequently, a nationwide process was initiated in 1991 to develop and promote uniform guidelines for practitioners who treat clefts and other craniofacial anomalies. That "consensus" process has provided detailed recommendations for case management, all of which are based upon ten basic principles that were identified as being essential to optimal patient care.

1. Management of patients with craniofacial anomalies is best provided by an interdisciplinary team of specialists.
2. Optimal care . . . is provided by teams that see sufficient numbers of patients each year to maintain clinical expertise in diagnosis and treatment.
3. The optimal time for the first evaluation is within the first few weeks of life and, whenever possible, within the first few days. However, referral for team evaluation and management is appropriate for patients at any age.
4. From the time of first contact with the child and family, every effort must be made to assist the family in adjusting to the birth of a child with a craniofacial anomaly and to the consequent demands and stress placed upon the family.
5. Parents/caregivers must be given information about recommended treatment procedures, options, risk factors, benefits, and costs to assist them in (a) making informed decisions on the child's behalf, and (b) preparing the child and themselves for all recommended procedures. The team should actively solicit family participation and collaboration in treatment planning. When the child is mature enough to do so, he or she should participate in treatment decisions.
6. Treatment plans should be developed and implemented on the basis of team recommendations.
7. Care should be coordinated by the team but should be provided at the local level whenever possible; however, complex diagnostic and surgical procedures should be restricted to major centers with the appropriate facilities and experienced care providers.
8. It is the responsibility of each team to be sensitive to linguistic, cultural, ethnic, psychosocial, economic, and physical factors that affect

the dynamic relationship between the team and the patient and family.

9. It is the responsibility of each team member to monitor both short-term and long-term outcomes. Thus longitudinal follow-up of patients, including appropriate documentation and record keeping, is essential.

10. Evaluation of treatment outcomes must take into account the satisfaction and psychosocial well-being of the patient as well as effects on growth, function, and appearance (American Cleft Palate-Craniofacial Association, 1993).

It is to be hoped that adherence to these principles and to the practice standards accompanying them will soon help to ensure that all individuals with oral clefts receive the best possible professional care.

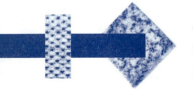

SURGERY FOR CLEFTS

Surgical treatment for the oral cleft patient may be classified either as primary or secondary. Primary surgery for the cleft of the lip, for example, attempts to close the cleft. Lip surgery can almost always improve the facial appearance of the infant greatly, and it usually is done very early in life—often between one and two months of age. Some surgeons believe it is important to begin the repair of bilateral lip clefts even before the baby is one month old, while the premaxilla still can easily be moved back into a more normal position (Shons, 1993). The primary repair of nasal deformities sometimes is undertaken at the same time as the primary lip surgery is done, although the more extensive nasal surgery (*rhinoplasty*) tends to be delayed until greater facial growth has occurred.

Primary surgery on the palate is designed to close the cleft while interfering as little as possible with later growth and development of the middle portion of the face. For years, many surgeons closed the palate in two stages. They performed early repair of the infant's soft palate but postponed hard palate surgery until later childhood, hoping thereby to avoid middle face abnormalities. However, it now has been demonstrated that normal speech is much more likely to develop when total surgical closure is completed at a very young age (12 to 18 months). Furthermore, facial growth appears to be only minimally disturbed by the modern surgical procedures used in these early closures. Complete closure even earlier (at 6 to 12 months of age) has been recommended by Nguyen and Sullivan (1993). They acknowledge the importance of minimizing growth disturbance but observe that facial distortions usually can be satisfactorily managed with further surgery, while speech impairments can often be irreversible.

Understandably, most parents are anxious to have the palate repaired as soon as possible so that their infant can suck and eat properly and not develop abnormal speech habits. The likelihood of speech impairment increases dramatically when closure is delayed even until the age of two years, and good speech results reportedly have been obtained when closure was done as early as sixteen weeks. There is some evidence, too, that complete surgical closure before the age of one year may facilitate relatively normal development of the **maxillary** region of the face (Ross, 1987). So, except in the case of extremely wide clefts of the hard palate, it is becoming increasingly common for complete closure of the hard and soft palates to be completed prior to 18 months of age.

Secondary surgery on the palate is performed only when primary surgery has not enabled the youngster to achieve effective closure of the passageway from the throat to the nasal cavity. This inadequate velopharyngeal closure is evident when the voice sounds excessively nasal or when air escapes through the nose during the production of consonants requiring high amounts of oral air pressure.

Adequate velopharyngeal closure requires sufficient length and movement of the soft palate. It also requires that the lateral pharyngeal walls move toward one another, and that the posterior pharyngeal wall move forward, at the level of the elevated velum. Deficiencies may remain yet following primary surgery, and so secondary palatal surgery is performed to try to remediate remaining problems. This should take place as soon as possible after it has been determined that the child is unable to achieve the closure required for speech, hopefully before too many undesirable articulatory compensations become habituated.

The most common secondary procedure involves the surgical construction of one or another type of **pharyngeal flap** (see Figure 10-3). This involves the creation of a narrow flap of pharyngeal tissue that remains attached to the back wall of the throat. The other end of the flap is then pulled forward and sutured into the back edge of the soft palate, thus forming a bridge of tissue that partially blocks the rear entrance to the nasal cavity. If the lateral walls of the pharynx can move toward this midline flap, good closure may be obtained for speech. Morris, Spriestersbach, and Darley (1995) at the University of Iowa studied 65 recipients of pharyngeal flap surgery and reported that 54 (83 percent) had normal velopharyngeal function, with 43 (66 percent) showing normal or "near normal" speech production. Care must be taken that the tissue flap is not too wide, however, for if it occupies too much of the horizontal velopharyngeal space the patient will find it difficult to breathe normally through the nose and may well produce *de*nasal speech. Extremely loud snoring may be another outcome!

When lateral wall movement is absent or too limited, some version of *sphincter pharyngoplasty* may be performed. In this procedure, segments of the palatopharyngeus muscle are surgically separated from each side of

Maxilla.
Upper jaw.

Pharyngeal flap.
A tissue bridge between the soft palate and the back wall of the throat.

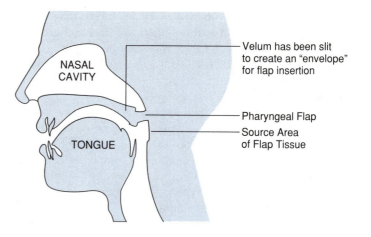

Velum has been slit to create an "envelope" for flap insertion

Pharyngeal Flap
Source Area of Flap Tissue

NASAL CAVITY

TONGUE

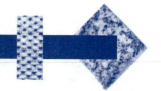

FIGURE 10-3   One type of superiorly based pharyngeal flap (from Westlake and Rutherford, 1966)

the pharynx and then are sutured together in the middle of the back wall of the throat. The result is a sphincter that, if constructed properly and at the level where the velum most closely approximates the back wall of the throat, can be closed and opened as required for normal speech.

Teflon, silicone, and other substances, including cartilage from the patient's own body (see, for example, Denny, Marks, and Oliff-Carneol, 1993), also have been injected or positioned surgically in the posterior pharyngeal wall to bring the wall of the throat forward and make it easier for the velum to effect a closure.

Finally, we should mention that surgical correction of submucous clefts is not done unless the condition is causing hypernasal resonance of the voice or nasal escape of air during consonant production.

Major advances in surgery continue to occur, and great strides have been made in reconstructing the structures needed to shut off the nasal airway. We are not seeing nearly as many persons with cleft-palate speech as we did twenty or thirty years ago, and those we do see do not show the facial deformations and grossly deviant speech that were common at that time. Nevertheless, not even the best surgeon using the most modern techniques may always achieve total success with all these persons.

PROSTHESES

Certain clefts are so wide and extensive, or the tissue remaining so scant or poorly developed, that the surgical prognosis for improved speech, easy swallowing, and good facial appearance is not very promising. Occasionally, too, some surgical closure already may have been unsuccessfully attempted. There also are individuals for whom the medical risks associated with any type of surgery are unacceptably high; and sometimes the religious or other beliefs of a family may prohibit surgery. Particularly in these types of circumstances, the prosthodontist may be called upon to fit a prosthetic device to assist in separating the nasal from the oral cavity.

Essentially, prostheses are artificial substitutes for missing or deficient parts. In the case of oral prostheses, we have a substitute for one of the structures of the mouth, such as the teeth or the palate. We may have a device that is used to obturate, or occlude, an opening in the hard palate, or we may have a device that is designed to assist existing structures in doing their jobs, such as in the case of a speech bulb or a palatal lift.

Prostheses have been made of many materials. There are accounts in ancient Greek literature of individuals filling their clefts of the hard palate with fruit rinds, cloth, leather, tar, and wax so that they could eat and drink. In the late 1800s artificial hard palates anchored to the teeth were provided with hinged gates, rubber bulbs, rubber tubes, silver balls, and other devices to plug or narrow the nasopharyngeal airway. All of these were very unsanitary, often prevented nasal breathing or interfered with it, and at times produced marked denasality on some sounds while failing to eliminate the nasality on others.

The modern appliance uses acrylic resin that can be molded and worked and reshaped by the designer so that it will fit and function appropriately. It is more sanitary, easily cleaned, and relatively light in weight. When necessary, the appliance can even be modified without the need for new impressions to be taken or new casts made.

The dental portion of a prosthesis may be designed to improve the cosmetic appearance as well as to improve speech. In addition to the obvious improvement that comes from having the teeth look better, a dental prosthesis may be so designed as to provide needed bulk to the upper lip portion of the face. The portion of the appliance that is designed to plug or block the opening in an unrepaired palatal cleft is referred to as an obturator. Obturators usually attach to existing teeth or may be attached to a dental prosthesis. If the patient has very few teeth or badly misaligned teeth, it can be difficult to keep these and other prosthetic devices in place, but advances in the use of dental implants may help to solve such problems.

When a device is needed to assist in velopharyngeal closure, the prosthodontist may design what sometimes has been called a "speech bulb." This prosthesis extends from the palatal portion into the nasopharynx to help fill the deficient velopharyngeal space. One such prosthesis is shown in Figure 10-4. As mentioned earlier, a speech bulb may be recommended when surgery is contraindicated or for health purposes or when previous surgery has failed. Its purpose, of course, is to decrease hypernasality and to eliminate the nasal escape of air during oral consonant production. In some cases it appears that the prosthesis helps to stimulate increased muscular contraction of the pharyngeal walls, and it

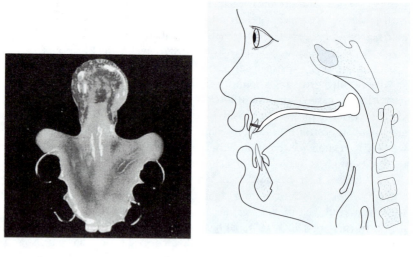

 **FIGURE 10-4** A velopharyngeal prosthesis and how it is placed at level of normal closure (from Westlake and Rutherford, 1966)

becomes possible gradually to reduce the size of the bulb while still maintaining good oral speech.

Attention has been given also to the use of palatal lifts designed to elevate the middle section of the velum in cases where there is little evidence of enough muscular potential for velopharyngeal closure, even though the palate seems long enough. It has been suggested that the presence of a lift also may stimulate increased muscle activity (in this case, of muscles that elevate the velum) of a type that enhances velopharyngeal closure.

Regardless of the type of appliance that may be used, a speech pathologist and prosthodontist should work closely together in evaluating its effects on speech—both positive and potentially negative. The desired reduction of nasality may be achieved, for example, but because of the altered shape and sensations of the oral cavity the child could begin to experience some new articulatory difficulty. For a more detailed discussion of prostheses and their implications for speech, you will find Leeper, Sills, and Charles (1993) a readable and informative reference.

COMMUNICATION PROBLEMS ASSOCIATED WITH CLEFT PALATE

Clefts of the lip and palate affect speech in two major ways: The voice quality becomes deviant, and the articulation is impaired. With regard to the voice quality, the most prominent impression is that of excessive nasality. The person seems to be speaking through the nose. In addition to a hypernasal vocal quality, there is audible turbulence created by air escaping from the nostrils. Moreover, when closely analyzed, the voice quality differences shown by cleft-palate speakers are not confined to excessive nasality. Some of our clients also have had hoarse voices, which we believe stemmed from their strained attempts to control the airstream in their throats or at the larynx. A curious, flat, muffled vocal quality—termed *cul de sac resonance*—is sometimes present if a speaker's anterior nasal passages are blocked.

There are also rather unique types of *articulation errors* present in cleft-palate speakers. They have more trouble with the plosives, fricatives, and affricates since these require the storing up of air pressure behind the closure or the narrowed opening. Voiced sounds seem to be easier than the unvoiced ones, but the consonant blends present considerable difficulty. In contrast to the errors made by other young children, young cleft-palate children (and often adults) tend to substitute glottal stops and pharyngeal fricatives for the standard sounds. Their speech seems to be punctuated by the little "catches of the breath" they use instead of such sounds as /p/, /b/, /t/, /d/, /k/, and /g/, or clearing-of-the-throat noises that replace the fricatives. The distortion errors are almost unique to the cleft-palate speaker. They are primarily due to nasal emission, the person snorting the sounds out of his nose. In severe cases, the intelligibility is very poor, and often one of the major tasks of the speech pathologist is to help the cleft-palate speaker to be understood. Fortunately, even without therapy, many persons with cleft palate manage to discard some of their gross errors and improve their intelligibility somewhat as they grow older. Keep in mind that children with clefts can also have articulation and phonology difficulties because of delayed maturation, hearing loss, or dental abnormalities.

Some cleft-palate children may also be slow to develop certain language skills. Language deficiencies, when they do exist, are generally pretty mild (Long and Dalston, 1982; Heinenman-DeBoer, 1985) and, in our experience, usually stem from lack of early stimulation, hearing loss, low parental expectations, or a disinclination to talk because of negative listener reactions.

We mentioned earlier the common occurrence of hearing loss among cleft palate children. Unfortunately, precise data regarding prevalence or degree of hearing loss are not available, nor is it known just how often a loss is present in only one ear as opposed to both. We do know, however, that nearly all hearing losses associated with cleft palate are related to the presence of a middle ear disease, **otitis media.** In Chapter 13 we provide information about otitis media and conductive hearing loss and their implications for speech and language development.

Even if it might not literally be true that "everyone who has a palatal cleft starts life with otitis media," as asserted by McWilliams, Morris, and

Otitis media. Inflammation of the middle ear; when accompanied by accumulation of fluid, called *serous otitis media.*

Shelton (1990, p. 109), it is very clear why neonatal hearing assessments are urged by workers in this field. Children with clefts often have intermittent episodes of hearing loss, with the loss ranging anywhere from mild to severe. In some cases, especially if the problem is not identified early and medically treated, a hearing loss can become permanent. It is crucial that the hearing of a cleft palate child be tested regularly by an audiologist, and that this testing routinely include *tympanometry* (again, see Chapter 13), even when the results are negative, from infancy through adolescence. When indicated, of course, the audiologist will make appropriate recommendations regarding possible use of a hearing aid and, in some instances, seek to ensure that the child's school provides suitable educational accommodation.

It commonly is held that otitis media occurs so often in these children because of the impaired function of their **eustachian tubes.** In order to provide proper pressurization, ventilation, and drainage of the middle ear, the pharyngeal end of the eustachian tube must periodically be open. The quick opening gesture, which normally occurs automatically when we swallow or yawn, is brought about by action of our palatal tensor musculature—musculature that typically is disrupted by an oral cleft. It is to provide ventilation following surgical drainage of the middle ear, of course, that small plastic tubes sometimes are inserted through the eardrum as part of the treatment for otitis media.

Without doubt, an inherent dysfunction of the eustachian tube plays a most critical role in these otitis media cases. In addition, however, Paradise, Elster, and Tan (1994) have reported that cleft palate infants who were fed only cow's milk or soy formula were much more likely to show middle ear effusion than were those who fed, exclusively or in part, on their mothers' harvested breast milk. They concluded that impaired eustachian tube function is not the only causal factor in the infants' initial development of a middle ear problem. So, as more is learned about other factors, perhaps it no longer will be inevitable that every child with a cleft palate starts life with otitis media.

Assessment by the Speech Pathologist

The speech pathologist wants to begin to see a child with a cleft palate as soon as possible. During this early contact, the parents can be informed about the need for normal speech and language stimulation, what to expect from their child regarding speech production, and, to some extent, the anatomical requirements for speech. Some clinicians use established language-stimulation programs as a preventive measure with these children.

Presumably, even when she is not a member of an oral cleft team, the speech pathologist will have access to the comprehensive assessment information accumulated by such a team. If the client has not been seen previously by an interdisciplinary team, the speech pathologist should make

Eustachian tube. The passageway connecting the throat cavity with the middle ear.

arrangements as soon as possible for referral to a team, whatever the client's age.

But let us assume, for purposes of further discussion, that our speech pathologist is a team member. Like other teams, it regularly conducts a variety of examinations and evaluations that are needed in order to develop, implement, and evaluate a comprehensive treatment plan. How then will she proceed? Most likely her approach will not differ greatly from the practice guidelines of the American Cleft Palate-Craniofacial Association (1993), which we have condensed.

The child's speech and language will be evaluated at least annually until the age of four years. Thereafter, if no speech-language problems are observed, the clinician will do at least brief screening examinations, annually until the child's adenoids have atrophied, and then every three years until dental and skeletal maturity are reached. For those who do have speech-language problems, she will conduct pre- and posttreatment evaluations related to any behavioral, surgical, or prosthetic management procedures that are implemented. In addition, she will conduct, or at least participate in, any necessary evaluations of the client's ability to achieve adequate velopharyngeal closure. More specifically, the following types of assessments are among those expected of the team's speech pathologist.

General Communicative Effectiveness.

The first task involves simply listening to the child's speech for the degree of nasality. After noting the degree of nasality, the clinician then listens to the general articulatory pattern without recording actual errors. Is there an obvious preponderance of a particular type of error (glottal stops, pharyngeal fricatives)? Does the articulation appear to alter with different communication situations, rates, or stress patterns? Next, she listens to the language of the child and checks for word choice, sentence complexity, and structure. The rate and rhythm of the youngster's speech should be noted. Finally, are there any particular mannerisms that attract attention? Is there a facial grimace, a constriction of the nares, or any other behavior that detracts from the child's total communicative effectiveness?

The Oral Examination.

The clinician will need to get a gross picture of palatal shape and length and movement of the soft palate in relation to the pharyngeal walls. It is not possible to actually view the site of velopharyngeal closure because it is above the lower portion of the soft palate; however, it is possible to make a general judgment regarding the mobility of the soft palate during various vowel productions. The examiner also looks for any other oral cavity deviations, especially dental disruptions or malocclusion, which may interfere with speech.

Psychological and Social Adjustment.

As you might expect, cleft palate, like any chronic disorder, tends to make psychological and social adjustment a bit more difficult for an individual. There is, however, no such thing as a "cleft-palate personality," nor do persons with this disorder exhibit behavior that may be characterized as deviant (Rollin, 1987). Still, in our clinical experience, some children and adults with cleft palate were more introverted, had more difficulty with peer relationships, were less satisfied with their occupational achievements, and, in general, tended to function slightly less adequately than did their contemporaries without oral clefts. Consequently, we usually include some evaluation of a client's adjusting characteristics, even though this may be explored in greater depth by the psychologist or social worker. We find it equally profitable to investigate the parental and family adjustments, since environmental reaction is often directly linked to the child's self-concept.

Language Assessment.   Many children with cleft palates develop language at a normal rate and in a normal sequence. However, since some cleft-palate children have difficulty acquiring language, the speech pathologist will at least administer a screening test during an evaluation. She pays particular attention to the child's expressive skills and phonology.

Articulation Testing.   We can get some impression of the adequacy of the velopharyngeal closure mechanism by analyzing the speech itself. First, we should check for articulation errors. If we find key words in which all or most of the defective sounds are used correctly, we can be pretty sure that enough closure is present. Again, if at times these errors are not accompanied by nose twitching or nasal emission of air, we can conclude that the valve probably is all right. If the person can speak very well with her nostrils closed but has much nasal distortion when they are open, we would suspect inadequate closure. Finally, if the consonants that require extra mouth pressure /p-b; t-d; s-z; tʃ-dʒ/ are those that are nasally distorted, while the *r* and the *l* or the *f* and the *v* are quite adequate, we would conclude that the closure was poor. Among the articulation inventories that we might use with a cleft palate client are the Iowa Pressure Articulation Test (Morris, Spriestersbach, and Darley, 1961) and the preschool articulation test described by Van Demark and Swickard (1980).

Velopharyngeal Competency

Surgery and prosthetic appliances do not always guarantee that normal speech can be obtained even with the best of speech therapy. The person may come to us with a closure mechanism that will not close sufficiently to permit normal speech no matter how long and hard we work. We may be able to improve the person's articulation and intelligibility, but he will still sound hypernasal, and abnormal. We have known clinicians and clients who struggled for years to do the impossible, years that might better have been spent in designing a better prosthesis or in new surgery. How can we be sure that this client of ours can really close the rear passageway to the nose? How can we know that he has a competent velopharyngeal valve?

In the past, speech pathologists have used such simple tests as the ability to suck liquids through a straw or to blow out candles to determine the client's capacity for velar closure. Or they have visually observed the uvular movement or the constriction of the pharyngeal walls. Unfortunately, tests of this nature have proved inadequate. Participation on an oral cleft team requires that a speech pathologist have some familiarity with a growing number of much more sophisticated techniques for evaluating velopharyngeal function.

Many of the newer techniques involve attempts to directly visualize the structures of the throat and palate. The radiologist may contribute any one of a number of x-ray techniques, including cinefluoroscopy or video fluoroscopy. These are especially useful since they show the structures in motion during speech production. Also, traditional lateral views have been augmented by basal and frontal cineradiography that can add to our ability to see the structures involved in velopharyngeal activity.

Other nonradiological attempts to see what is happening have approached the structures from above. Nasendoscopy involves the insertion of a viewing scope into the nasal cavity (see Figure 10-5). Without inter-

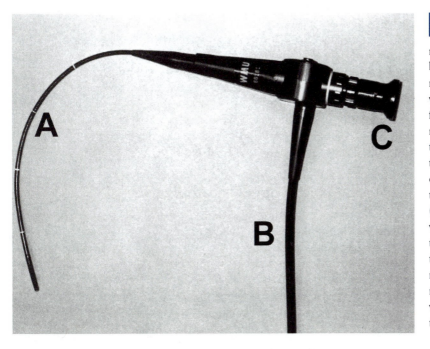

FIGURE 10-5   A flexible fiberoptic nasendoscope that can be inserted through the nares to observe velopharyngeal valving from above: (A) the narrow endoscopic tube that actually is placed into the nasal cavity; (B) the cable that provides light to illuminate the view; (C) the eyepiece for live viewing can be attached to a videotape recorder to produce a permanent record of observed movements of the velum and the walls of the pharynx.

fering with the speech structures, one is thereby able to see clearly the movements of the velum and throat during spontaneous speech.

The nasendoscope can be attached to videotape equipment, thereby allowing the imaging of velopharyngeal valving during speech to be displayed and replayed for careful analysis on a TV monitor. This not only permits the examiner to do very detailed studies of closure inadequacies but makes it simpler to share this important information with other members of the oral cleft team.

Nasometry is another procedure that is gaining increasing popularity among clinicians who work with cleft palate clients. It does not involve direct observation of the velopharyngeal mechanism but, rather, provides a relatively objective basis for measuring the "nasalance" present in a speech sample. In brief, the nasometer uses one microphone to detect acoustic energy radiated from the nose and another microphone to detect simultaneously the acoustic energy radiated from the mouth. These two signals are computer-analyzed and the results are reported as a nasalance score: the percentage of the total (*oral PLUS nasal*) sound energy that was radiated just from the nose. This measure tells us only how well the client was using velopharyngeal valving during the particular speaking task, so we must be careful not to infer *capability* or physiologic adequacy just from a nasalance score. Nevertheless, nasometry data provide a useful supplement to other observations. Moreover, the nasometer can assist us in evaluating the results of therapy, surgery, and prosthodontia. And, since it provides graphic displays of nasalance in real time, the nasometer can be a very useful instrument for biofeedback during speech therapy.

A wide array of other instrument systems employing such techniques as *ultrasound, electromyography, photodetection, spectrographic signal analysis,* and *differential analyses of air pressures and air flow rates* have been used to evaluate velopharyngeal closure. Few are routinely used clinically by many oral cleft teams, however, and some are practical only for research purposes. Nevertheless, you may wish to learn more about these technologies; if so, you will find further details discussed in Bzoch (1989) and in McWilliams, Morris, and Shelton (1990).

Treatment by the Speech Pathologist

Electromyography (EMG).
Recording of electrical activity associated with muscle contraction.

It is impossible to outline a program of speech therapy techniques that would be applicable to all cleft-palate clients, or even a majority, since the problems presented by the clients are so different. We deal with speech that reflects the personality of the client, with her concept of self. The basic attitude of a client who feels that, because she has an organic disability, there is nothing that can be done to alter her speech has a profound effect upon therapy. Most of these clients know little about the nature of their problem or the possibilities for improving speech. They come as passively and as unenthusiastically as they go to the surgeon, the prosthodontist, or the orthodontist, because they have been told that they should. Few of them feel any powerful urge to accept some of the responsibility for their speech improvement.

It is also necessary, quite apart from the individual's attitudes toward his speech and its therapy, to take into account the actual organic disability which may be present. Some cleft-palate persons with very defective speech may have complete closures and the potential for completely normal speech. Some of these are already using their closures in activities other than speech or on other speech sounds except those that are defective. Others of the same group may have the potential to use their soft palate or pharyngeal musculatures but have not learned to do so. But we must also recognize that there are some cleft-palate clients whose structures or prostheses are not adequate for normal speech, and for whom we may be able to do very little. In cases of "borderline" adequacy it often requires a period of trial therapy to differentiate these groups.

Again, let us state our melioristic philosophy of speech therapy: We make the person's speech better and we make him a happier person; we do not have to make his speech perfect or make him a completely happy human. Within the limits of our time and energy and knowledge, and with an awareness of the limitations that the client also possesses, let us do our utmost and be content with that. Our clients must learn to speak as well as they can, with as little interference to communication as possible and as little abnormality as possible.

The Goals of Therapy.   Our basic points of attack are the following. We must decrease the nasal emission, the hypernasality, and the defective articulation. We must improve the oral air pressure and oral airflow. We must eliminate abnormal foci of tension and abnormal nostril contractions. We must activate the tongue tip, lip, and jaws. We must improve speaking respiratory rate and control. We must improve velar and pharyngeal contraction.

We once examined a person with an unrepaired unilateral cleft of both the hard and soft palates who had fairly normal speech. How he managed this we were unable to tell, but he did use wide jaw movements, slow speech, short phrases, and dentalized most of his frontal sounds. All plosives were made with very loose contacts. He spoke softly and did become nasal when he spoke loudly. At any rate, he demonstrated how much we might be able to do in speech therapy. This case also illustrates an important principle. We should work for altering the direction of airflow so that it flows toward the mouth rather than upward through the nose. And we should teach the cleft-palate person to articulate with a minimum of oral air pressure.

Air-Pressure Controls.   Air pressure within the mouth varies with the various speech sounds. The plosives and the sibilants require the most air pressure. Voiced sounds require less than do the unvoiced sounds due to the increased audibility of the former. The /t/ and /d/ require less than do the /k/ and /g/. People vary widely one from another in the degree of closure used in producing the plosives and the fricatives. Certain individuals use very tight closures and sudden releases; others do not. Cleft palate clients often use very tight closures and sudden releases. This is very unwise since much more air pressure is required for such plosives than for the loose-contact, slow-release type.

The fricatives, which employ a narrow opening or channel for the airflow, are also produced differently by different people. Some use a very narrow channel; others a broader one. Cleft-palate individuals tend to use the narrower ones that require a greater air pressure, and so nasal emission tends to occur. We therefore should teach them differently.

Much of the stimulus value of a sound can be increased by prolonging its duration. If cleft-palate persons are to soften their contacts in order to make use of the lessened air pressure in the mouth due to the palatal air leak, they must prolong these sounds somewhat. Weaker s sounds should be held longer. A slightly prolonged /f/ in the word *fish,* even if weaker in airflow, will be understood as readily as a quicker, stronger one.

Concentration in therapy upon these factors also emphasizes the direction of airflow through the mouth rather than the nose. People with clefts are nose-conscious, as the contraction of their nostrils demonstrates. By concentrating on the longer, slower, looser contacts and the shallower channels of articulation, the airflow tends to go mouthward. This emphasis upon the mouth, rather than the nose as the major channel for speech and airflow, is among the major objectives of any speech therapy. We have known cleft-palate children to speak much better as soon as they held a megaphone to their lips. Most speech clinicians do lip and tongue training. We have given lip exercises with profit to cleft-palate persons who already had perfect lip control, primarily so that they would become mouth-conscious. One of our children spoke much better when he put on a clown's mask that had a monstrous mouth that he watched in a mirror. He just became more mouth-conscious, and the air came out of that opening, We have improved the speech of cleft-palate clients by teaching them to read lips. One of our majors got better speech from a cleft-palate girl by putting lipstick on her mouth and having her watch it in the mirror. Cleft-palate clients must think of speech as coming out of the mouth.

Many speech pathologists teach their cleft-palate clients to open the mouth widely in speech, as far as they can without appearing abnormal. This is often difficult to teach, and resistance is almost sure to be found; but when it can be used it does seem to improve speech. Air must take a tortuous course when it must go upstairs through the filters of the nasal caverns and then down and out through the narrow slits of our nostrils. It would much rather come out of the mouth, especially if that pathway is open. Moreover, larger mouth openings for the vowels tend to produce looser contacts of lips and tongue, and they certainly increase the consciousness of the mouth rather than the nose.

Muscle Training.   It is also possible of course, in many cases, to improve the state of air pressure within the mouth by shutting off the air leak, by improving velopharyngeal closure. Many of the muscles are weak and can be strengthened through appropriate exercises *if surgery or a prosthesis has been successful in creating the conditions for a possible closure* (Karnell and Van Demark, 1986). If the cleft-palate client can blow up a balloon or whistle, or if inspection with a dental mirror shows good occlusion of the nasopharynx, we should be able to help him use some closure in speech. Even when this is not possible but when, in phonation, yawning, or other activities, we can see the velum lift or the side walls of the pharynx contract or the rear wall come forward slightly, we must presume that we can improve this functioning until we find otherwise. (This may not be true if the velum is too short or taut or the pharynx so enlarged that no closure seems possible.)

Such muscle training requires two major items besides devoted practice: location of the musculatures by the patient and perception of their movement. In physical therapy where comparable tasks are present, the physical therapist, through massage, positioning, and passive movement, is often able to get movement of muscles as inert as those of the cleft-palate patient's repaired velum. Unfortunately, a limb is easier to manipulate than is a palate. Nevertheless, speech pathologists have employed some of the same principles of physical therapy in activating the velar and pharyngeal muscles. Light massage with a finger cot (covering of rubber) first along one side of the uvula, then on the other, and then with two fingers straddling the midline, has helped to localize the area. The stroking must be done very lightly and both away from the midline in a horizontal direction, and anteroposteriorly. These exercises must also be done with caution lest tissues be injured; but when they are done lightly and the patient attempts to feel and predict the location and direction of movement, they can be very effective.

We may also use the visual sense. Many cleft-palate clients have no visual imagery of their palates with which to correlate movement. They should study and describe the action of the clinician's palate in action. They should watch both their own and their clinician's palates in mirrors. They can be shown large pictures of the palate on charts and be taught to point to the area that the clinician touches. When there is residual movement, it should be viewed visually, and then imagined. A very clear picture should be possessed by every cleft-palate patient of the nature of his problem. Even little children can be given this in imaginative terms: "the little red gate or door."

Since most repaired cleft-palate clients have some movement of the levator and tensor muscles as well as of the constrictor muscles in certain activities, they must be taught to isolate and to identify the experience. Certain key words should be conditioned to palatal activity: "up . . . down . . . squeeze . . . let go . . . open . . . shut." These must be used by the clinician only when the activity actually occurs. They should first be used by the client when observing the clinician's palatal movements, then when observing his own, then with intermittent eye closing with attention to kinesthesia.

Weak palatal movement, when present, can be made more effective in closure by having the patient lie on a cot with his head held far backward so that the force of gravity aids rather than resists the palatal movement. When there is asymmetrical pull on the palate, turning the head or the jaw to one side seems to be of some assistance.

Dry swallowing, when repeated, often helps the patient to activate and localize the velopharyngeal contractions. Often a state of localized strain or fatigue may help the client to become aware that he has such muscles. Very slow chewing may also produce certain muscular contractions of the pharynx and velum. Sudden sucking of air through various sizes of tubes will also initiate velar activity.

Blowing Exercises.   Perhaps blowing exercises have been used more frequently than any other single device for strengthening the palate. Blowing takes air pressure, and if the air is to come out of the mouth, a velopharyngeal opening will reduce that pressure enough to reduce the airflow through the mouth to a considerable degree. We must be certain, however, that we are having an increasingly greater ratio of mouth airflow to nasal airflow if we can hope that the palate is being strengthened. Various devices have been employed to demonstrate this ratio: double shelves to be placed under nose and mouth openings with feathers or fringes to indicate airflow, tubes from the nose to the ear, candle flame affected by tubes from the nose and mouth, clouded mirrors, and many others.

We should emphasize that blowing exercises performed with great tension and the constriction of the nostrils are most unwise. They merely inform the client that palatal contraction is too laborious to be used in speech. We also doubt the efficacy of blowing air out of the mouth while holding the nose shut, since we may make the client too nose-conscious and in any event, closure of the nostrils does not help the velopharyngeal valve to shut. Indeed, there seems to be a sort of inverse reciprocal reaction in the action of the **nares** and the velar musculatures. Even in normal speakers, voluntary contraction of the nares often produces an increase in nasality. As the front door shuts, the back door opens. Often there is very little transfer of training from blowing to speech. This is especially true if the blowing is too strained, if air pres-

Nares.
Nostrils.

sures far exceeding those used in normal speech are used, and if set mouth openings and passive tongue postures are employed. We could hardly expect much transfer with so many variables in the training. Nevertheless, the palatal and pharyngeal activity in blowing (especially in soft blowing) is more like that used in speech than is shown in such activities as yawning, swallowing, and so on. We must not throw the baby out with the bath. Blowing exercises can help the client to become mouth-conscious; they can help her discriminate the two airflow channels; they can help her to increase the amount of oral air pressure needed for good articulation; and they can improve the contraction of the velar and pharyngeal muscles. But they must be used wisely rather than indiscriminately.

For example, we have found the treatment plan devised by Shprintzen, McCall, and Skolnick (1975) a good way in which to use blowing and whistling to achieve velar closure for speech. The client is first taught to whistle (or blow) and phonate at the same time. Gradually, using successive approximations, the whistle is faded out until she is able to produce a nonnasal vowel (/i/ is used initially because it is similar to the posture for whistling). The vowel is then surrounded by two nonnasal consonants (such as in the word "leak"). Finally, sentences and conversation are utilized. At each step in the program, the client is asked to hear and feel the difference between nasal and nonnasal utterances.

Articulation Problems.   The backward playing of samples of speech of various degrees of nasality has demonstrated that the listener judges a given sample as being more nasal if it has poorer articulation. The voice quality itself seems more nasal when it is played forward than when it is played backward. Thus, the improvement of articulation can also produce a decrease in perceived nasality. We have also seen that the majority of cleft-palate speakers have speech sounds that are defective.

The basic problems in articulation are three: incorrect tongue placement, the substitution of glottal stops and fricatives, and the nasalization or nasal emission of many consonants. Most articulation errors shown by speakers with cleft palates are due to abnormalities of the oral mechanism and to the efforts these speakers make to compensate for the structural defects. However, hearing loss and environmental factors must not be overlooked during evaluation and treatment. And, of course, the cleft palate child is not immune to linguistically based phonology problems (Hodson, Chin, Redmond, and Simpson, 1983).

By and large, many of the processes and procedures outlined in our chapter on articulation and phonology will be applicable in our work with this population, although some of the difficulties encountered by the cleft palate child require more focused attention. Tongue placement may be particularly problematic.

Correcting Tongue Placement.   Many of our cleft-palate clients have had sluggish or inactive tongue tips; they seemed to carry their tongues high in their mouths and tried to produce sounds with the broad blade or back of their tongues. The treatment for this involves training the client to increase the mobility of the tongue tip; to raise the points of anterior contact for the /ʧ/, /d/, /l/, and /ʤ/ sounds; and to differentiate tongue lifting from simultaneous jaw movement.

Exercises for increasing the mobility of the tongue include sensitization of the tongue tip—curling, grooving, lifting, lowering, thrusting, arching, tapping, sustaining postures, pressing, scraping, fluttering, and many others. These should not be practiced while holding the breath but while blowing gently both voiced and unvoiced air if the training is to generalize to speech. Undue tension is to be avoided. Speed gains should be made in terms of rhythmic patterns. Different sizes of mouth opening and lip postures should also be practiced with the tongue training. Many of these clients have never explored the many possibilities of tongue movement or action. It is wise to use these exercises as warm-up periods for consonant practice. Often the production of certain consonants is sandwiched between two tongue-training exercises.

The differentiation of tongue movement from the accompanying jaw movements can be done by immobilizing the jaw with various heights of tooth props until enough independence is achieved to permit the activity without this aid. Frequent checking is necessary. Visual feedback from a mirror is also useful. Lateral movements of the mandible during tongue tapping and consonant production will also be useful. The use of the first two fingers forked to monitor the location of both lips will help. Also, if the client will place one finger on his nose and his thumb under his chin, any accompanying movement of the jaw will be noticed immediately.

Eliminating Glottal Stop Errors.   The use of the glottal stop or fricative substitutions requires a state of localized tension of the larynx, and therefore we try to create some relaxation in this area. The use of slight coughs to teach a /k/ sound is very unwise. Instead, the back of the tongue must be raised, and this can be accomplished more easily on the /k/ and /g/ sounds by pressing hard with the tongue tip against the lower teeth and closing the jaws partially. Ear training is essential. We have also been able to eliminate this difficult error by having the client produce the consonants on inhalation.

Decreasing Nasality and Nasal Emission.   While much of the success of articulating the consonant sounds without nasality or nasal emission will depend upon the success of establishing oral airflow and better velopharyngeal closure, we find that by teaching the plosives with very loose contacts, great improvement can be made. Using a nasometer for biofeedback, as mentioned earlier, can be very effective in decreasing nasality.

For the fricatives, the use of wider mouth openings on the following or preceding vowels tends to decrease the nasality. We also suggest the prolongation of these sounds with decreasing air pressure, thus using the duration rather than the clear quality of the fricative as the message-carrying feature.

It is important, of course, to use the usual ear training to identify the defectiveness of a given sound and to contrast it with the correct sound. Then we must teach the proper production of the isolated sound, strengthening and stabilizing it. We have mentioned before that cleft-palate clients often speak very rapidly so as to conserve the breath pressure. Slowing down the speed of utterance with proper phrasing and breathing often produces immediate improvement in all of the articulation even when little attention is paid to the isolated sounds.

Other Concerns.   Perhaps the most pronounced of all the ticlike mannerisms that characterize cleft-palate speech is the nostril contraction or flaring. This often serves as an equivalent for velar contraction, and often prevents the latter from taking place. It is cosmetically unattractive, often interferes with the utterance of the labial plosives, and helps to produce the snorting-snuffling that is so unpleasant in these persons. It has no effect upon nasality or nasal emission except to make them worse. We therefore always do as much as we can to eliminate this habit. We first attempt to bring this nostril tic up to consciousness, to help the client become aware of its unpleasant stimulus value, and then through negative practice, canceling, pull-outs, and preparatory sets to eliminate it. Usually it is responsive to this treatment, especially when mirror work is used. In the more severe cases a nucleus of nonnostril-contraction speech can be achieved by contracting the lips in a wide tight smile, stretching them so far that the upper teeth are bared. The clinician must be sure that he does not penalize contraction and thus suppress it before it is weakened (Warren, 1986).

Many cleft-palate clients have as poor eye contact as do stutterers, a behavior that makes the speech and condition more noticeable. They also may have unusual head postures and lip bitings, or they may cover their mouths in speaking. All these should be reduced.

Speech therapy with cleft-palate clients is usually long-term therapy. Few of these persons show any dramatic improvement in a short time. There are many problems to be solved and many avenues to be explored. The work is time consuming and often difficult. Nevertheless, we can do much to help the persons with cleft-palates speak better (Albery and Enderby, 1984).

STUDY QUESTIONS

1. Describe the basic sequence of processes involved in normal development of the lip and palate. Approximately when during pregnancy are these processes completed?
2. What are the three basic categories of oral clefting? Which of these is least likely to cause speech problems, and why?
3. How frequently are infants born with some type of oral cleft? What differences in incidence are reported between sexes and among different races?
4. What is meant by a "submucous" cleft, and what are the signs suggesting that such a cleft is present?
5. What is meant by "multifactorial inheritance" and what are five suspected teratogenic agents that may play a role in the creation of oral clefts?
6. Describe the professional specialties that comprise a "core" interdisciplinary oral cleft team. What additional professions would be represented on an "ideal" team?
7. For what reason(s) is it now recommended that total surgical repair of the cleft palate be completed before the infant is eighteen months old?
8. Under what conditions might prosthetic management of an oral cleft be preferred over the surgical approach?
9. Why are children with cleft palates particularly likely to experience at least intermittent hearing loss?
10. What major speech characteristics are associated with inadequate velopharyngeal closure?

REFERENCES

Albery, L., and Enderby, P. (1984). Intensive speech therapy for cleft palate children. *British Journal of Disorders of Communication*, 19, 115–124.

American Cleft Palate-Craniofacial Association. (1993). Parameters for the evaluation and treatment of patients with cleft lip/palate or other craniofacial anomalies. *Cleft Palate-Craniofacial Journal*, 30 (Suppl 1).

Brodsky, L., Holt, L., and Ritter-Schmidt, D. (1992). *Craniofacial anomalies: An interdisciplinary approach*. St. Louis, MO: Mosby-Year Book.

Bronshtein, M., Blumenfeld, I., Kohn, J., and Blumenfeld, Z. (1994). Detection of cleft lip by early second-trimester transvaginal sonography. *Obstetrics and Gynecology*, 84, 73–76.

Bzoch, K. (ed.). (1989). *Communicative disorders related to cleft lip and palate* (3rd ed.). Boston: College-Hill Press.

DeLongchamp, S. (1976). Our Cathy was special. American Cleft Palate Education Foundation Essay Contest, First Prize, 1.

Denny, A., Marks, S., and Oliff-Carneol, S. (1993). Correction of velopharyngeal insufficiency by pharyngeal augmentation using autologous cartilage: A preliminary report. *Cleft Palate-Craniofacial Journal*, 30, 46–54.

Gorlin, R. (1993). Development and genetic aspects of cleft lip and palate. In K. Moller and C. Starr (eds.), *Cleft palate: Interdisciplinary issues and treatment*. Austin, TX: Pro-ed.

Heinenman-DeBoer, J. (1985). *Cleft palate children and intelligence: Intellectual abilities of cleft palate children in a cross-sectional and longitudinal study*. Lisse, Switzerland: Swets and Zeitlinger.

Hodson, B., Chin, C., Redmond, B., and Simpson, R. (1983). Phonological evaluation and remediation of speech deviations of a child with a repaired cleft palate: A case study. *Journal of Speech and Hearing Disorders*, 48, 93–98.

Karnell, M., and Van Demark, D. (1986). Longitudinal speech performance in patients with cleft palate: Comparisons based on secondary management. *Cleft Palate Journal*, 23, 278–288.

Leeper, H., Sills, P., and Charles, D. (1993). Prosthodontic management of maxillofacial and palatal defects. In K. Moller and C. Starr (eds.), *Cleft palate: Interdisciplinary issues and treatment*. Austin, TX: Pro-ed.

Long, N. and Dalston, R. (1982). Paired gestural and vocal behavior in one-year-old cleft lip and palate children. *Journal of Speech and Hearing Disorders*, 47, 403–406.

McWilliams, B. (1992). Rationale for an interdisciplinary team approach. In L. Brodsky, L. Holt, and D. Ritter-Schmidt, *Craniofacial anomalies: An interdisciplinary approach*. St. Louis, MO: Mosby-Year Book.

McWilliams, B., Morris, H., and Shelton, R. (1990). *Cleft palate speech* (2nd ed.). Philadelphia: B.C. Decker.

Morris, H., Spriestersbach, D., and Darley, F. (1961). An articulation test for assessing velopharyngeal closure. *Journal of Speech and Hearing Research*, 4, 48–55.

Nguyen, P., and Sullivan, P. (1993). Issues and controversies in the management of cleft palate. *Clinics in Plastic Surgery*, 20, 671–682.

Paradise, J., Elster, B., and Tan, L. (1994). Evidence in infants with cleft palate that breast milk protects against otitis media. *Pediatrics*, 94, 853–860.

Peterson-Falzone, S. (1989) Basic concepts in congenital craniofacial defects. In K. Bzoch (ed.), *Communicative disorders related to cleft lip and palate* (3rd ed.). Boston: College-Hill Press.

Powers, G. (1986). *Cleft palate*. Austin, TX: Pro-ed.

Rollin, W. (1987). *The psychology of communication disorders in individuals and their families*. Englewood Cliffs, NJ: Prentice Hall.

Ross, R. (1987). Treatment variables affecting facial growth in complete unilateral cleft lip and palate. *Cleft Palate Journal*, 24, 5–77.

Shons, A. (1993). Surgical issues and procedures. In K. Moller and C. Starr (eds.), *Cleft palate: Interdisciplinary issues and treatment*. Austin, TX: Pro-ed.

Shprintzen, R. (1987). Syndromic cleft lip and palate. Presented in the Symposium on the Etiological Heterogeneity of Cleft Lip and Palate. American Cleft Palate Association, San Antonio, TX.

Shprintzen, R., McCall, G., and Skolnick, M. (1975). A new therapeutic technique for treatment of velopharyngeal incompetence. *Journal of Speech and Hearing Disorders*, 40, 69–83.

Van Demark, D., and Swickard, S. (1980). A preschool articulation test to assess velopharyngeal competency. *Cleft Palate Journal*, 17, 175–179.

Warren, D. (1986). Compensatory speech behaviors in individuals with cleft palate: A regulation/control phenomenon. *Cleft Palate Journal*, 23, 251–260.

Westlake, H., and Rutherford, D. (1966). *Cleft palate*. Englewood Cliffs, NJ: Prentice Hall, 1966.

SUPPLEMENTARY READINGS

Moller, K., and Starr, C. (eds.). (1993). *Cleft palate: Interdisciplinary issues and treatment*. Austin, TX: Pro-ed.

Morris, H., Bardach, J., Ardinger, H., Jones, D., Kelly, K., Olin, W., and Wheeler, J. (1993). Multidisciplinary treatment results for patients with isolated cleft palate. *Plastic and Reconstructive Surgery*, 92, 845–851.

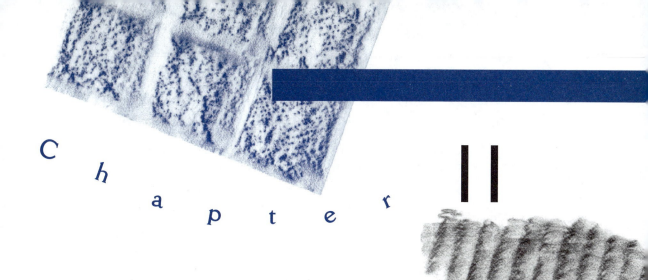

Aphasia and
Related Disorders

When an adult suddenly loses the easy use of words, it must be a devastating experience. Indeed, perhaps only the person abruptly deprived of language—and thus of the communicative bond to others—can really understand aphasia. Here is how one of our clients, a Presbyterian minister, described the devastating impact of his stroke.

> I woke up in a hospital bed with a paralyzed right side, no control over my bowels or bladder, and, worst of all, I couldn't communicate—except to curse and sob. When I left the hospital three weeks later, I had regained about 3 percent of my former vocabulary. I could not read, write, or even tell you the name of the city I lived in. The story of Zacharias (St. Luke 1:5–22) being struck dumb by the angel Gabriel kept cycling and recycling in my thoughts. Later I learned that I had aphasia.

Another client described his difficulty understanding speech in this way: "It's like trying to read by the flickering light of a single firefly."

Speech pathologists who work in hospital speech and hearing clinics, in community speech and hearing centers, or in private practice find that many of their clients come to them with aphasia. Generally, these individuals are adults of fifty years or older who have suffered a left hemisphere **stroke,** or **cerebrovascular accident (CVA).** Some are younger persons who have been in automobile or other accidents that caused brain damage. It has been estimated that approximately 2 million Americans are handicapped to some degree as the result of strokes. While many people survive this common hazard of aging (about 200,000 die from strokes each year), they often are, as we shall see, disastrously handicapped, and one of the major features of that handicap is an impairment in the ability to use language.

THE DISORDER

"The term 'aphasia' refers to a family of clinically diverse disorders that affect the ability to communicate by oral or written language, or both, following brain damage . . . . Aphasia is an umbrella concept combining a multiplicity of deficits involving one or more aspects of language use." (Goodglass, 1993, pp. 1–2). The aphasic client has difficulty in (1) formulating, (2) comprehending, or (3) expressing meanings. Often there is some impairment in all of these functions; it may range from a very mild disruption in the reception of complex messages to almost total loss of encoding and decoding ability. Along with these difficulties there may be associated problems of defective articulation, inability to produce voice, and broken fluency; but the basic problem in aphasia lies in handling *symbolic* behavior. Aphasic clients not only have difficulty in speaking, they also find it difficult to read silently, to write, to comprehend the speech of others, to calculate mathematically, or even to gesture. Let us illustrate some of this behavior in a severe case of aphasia.

Stroke.
Stoppage of bloodflow to the brain, usually due to a blood clot or hemorrhaging (see *cerebrovascular accident*).

Cerebrovascular accident (CVA).
Injury to blood vessels of the brain (see *stroke*).

A week after her forty-ninth birthday, Mrs. Bowerman suffered a stroke. A blood vessel in her brain ruptured, leaving her with a paralyzed right arm and leg, defective vision, and many symptoms of aphasia. For example, she is able to speak a little but gropes continually for words. Here is how she tried to ask her husband about some money she had hidden in the refrigerator: "Ah, you know, in food . . . ah, oh, I mean, eggs . . . and, oh . . . shit! . . . save for mekum . . . no, no, meat . . . ice, ah. . . ." Sometimes Mrs. Bowerman lapses into a rapid gibberish.

She is unable to tell time, make change, or even to follow a simple recipe. She reads only the headlines in the newspapers but enjoys watching television, particularly the game shows. Sometimes she will try to sound out words in an article but becomes frustrated very easily. She can write her name, the phrase "I love you," and a few common words.

The client seems able to understand what is said to her if the speaker talks slowly and simply. Her husband noted that it may take Mrs. Bowerman as long as 20 seconds to recognize some words spoken to her. Before her stroke, the client was an active, outgoing, and well-liked member of the small community in which she resides. She was a leader in the League of Women Voters and a volunteer reader for the blind. Now she is withdrawn and depressed. She cries frequently and does not seem to be able to stop crying once she has begun.

There are some terms that are commonly used to describe some of this behavior. Mrs. Bowerman's inability to write is termed *agraphia;* her inability to read, *alexia;* her inability to handle mathematics, **acalculia;** her jumbled sentences, **paraphasia.** When she lapses into verbal gibberish, it is designated as *jargon.* The inability to stop crying, the repetition of words in speaking or letters in writing is called *perseveration.* People with aphasia perseverate more when their frustrations become chronic or when they are pushed to do a difficult task—this is called *noise buildup.* The client's inability to remember or find a necessary word is called **anomia.** The long delay she showed in recognizing certain words is termed slow *rise time.* Recovered clients tell us that often they can see the letters but that they appear to have no meaning, or they see the picture of an object but cannot tell what it is. This is termed a *visual **agnosia.*** Or they can hear someone talking to them but cannot comprehend. The speech sounds "jumbled." This is called an *auditory agnosia.* There is one other major term we must provide you: *apraxia.* This refers to an inability to command a part of the body to make a willed movement. An individual who may understand perfectly what you mean when you ask him to protrude his tongue or to pick up a pencil may not be able to command his tongue or hand to do so. Perhaps he lacks the inner speech that determines voluntary movement. At any rate, this inability to make a voluntary movement is termed apraxia. There are many other technical words, but these are the most common.

Different aphasics show different patterns of impairment. Mrs. Bowerman was severely affected not only in the *expressive* and receptive aspects of handling meaningful symbols but also in their *formulation.* Most vic-

Acalculia.
Inability to do simple arithmetic problems due to brain injury.

Paraphasia.
Aphasic behavior characterized by jumbled, inarticulate words.

Anomia.
Inability to remember familar words due to brain injury.

Agnosia.
Inability to interpret the meanings of sensory stimulation due to brain injury; may be visual, auditory, or tactual.

tims of aphasia show some general loss in language ability, and it becomes more marked under fatigue or stress. However, some may show their difficulty *primarily* in only one area.

It also has been observed that deaf individuals who rely upon signing and who suffer left hemisphere brain injury are susceptible to communication impairments. The production and understanding of manual gestures break down. Clearly, we may not think of aphasia as a language problem expressed only in disturbed speech, hearing, writing or reading. Rather, it is a more central disability.

Goodglass provides the following brief sketches that may help you further to appreciate the types and degrees of communication difficulties found in aphasia.

Case 1. The patient, whose right arm and leg remain paralyzed from a recent stroke, communicates with a small vocabulary of nouns and verbs that he rarely combines into two-word phrases. A typical response to a question, for example, How did you get here today? is "Drivin . . . wife . . . yeah . . . drivin." These words are produced somewhat effortfully, but are clearly pronounced. He can recite the numbers up to 21 and the days of the week with perfect facility. He understands conversation and commands when they relate to his current situation, but is often left behind by a change in topic. He can read and understand many words and easy sentences, but cannot write more than his name.

Case 2. A patient who suffered an embolic stroke during open-heart surgery produces speech with effortless articulation and grammar, but rarely succeeds in completing a thought because he cannot retrieve the key nouns and verbs of his intended message. He recognizes these words when they are supplied by the examiner, but he cannot repeat them himself. He understands speech almost perfectly, but makes errors in both reading and writing. A sample of his account of his hospital experience goes like this: "I had one of those . . . they did it on my . . . my . . . ort . . . my art . . . I can't say it . . . there are two of them." (Examiner: The aortic valve?) "That right. Then I was in the . . . where they put three or four people. . . ."

Case 3. This patient proved to have suffered a stroke when he was found confused and unable to make sense in talking. On examination, he is socially appropriate in response to greeting, but answers routine questions with a largely irrelevant and voluble flow of speech. His speech output has no coherent content and is sprinkled with neologisms and incorrectly used words, and although he is attentive and takes turns in conversation, he appears to grasp only fragments of questions and his answers have only tangential allusions to the subject matter. For example, when asked, Who lives at home with you? his response is "My wife, she goes her work to work on it but her heffle is all about it." On testing for comprehension of single words, he can point to only one of six objects that are named for him. He can name none correctly on request. His attempts to write result in a jargon similar to his speech. (Goodglass, 1993, pp. 1–2)

Years ago in a veterans hospital we had occasion to encounter a fifty-eight-year-old gentleman whose stroke had not resulted in significant or lasting physical impairment but whose communication abilities were severely affected. He seemed to understand most of what was said to him, but his reading had not been tested since he never had learned to read or write. Eight months after his CVA he was able to say only one word: *boom-boom*. He said it distinctly, and he said it often, both to initiate a conversation and to answer any and every question. Nearly always he said it happily and enthusiastically; always he said it emphatically. And he seemed to have no doubt that we understood perfectly whatever it was that he was trying to communicate—in spite of the fact that we obviously were unable to respond in any meaningful way.

Hopefully, you are beginning to see that it would be impossible to characterize a "typical" client with aphasia. However, in spite of the wide variations encountered, there appear to be clients who share symptom patterns that are different than the symptom clusters of other clients. So for many years some *aphasiologists*—clinicians, researchers, and other scholars who study the topic—have devised (and then discarded) systems for classifying subtypes of aphasia. Other aphasiologists have argued, in effect, that "aphasia is aphasia" and that classification serves no useful purpose. In any event, no single system yet has enjoyed universal acceptance.

Many clinicians, nevertheless, do use the classification system described by Goodglass and Kaplan (1983), which seeks to categorize aphasic patients in terms of seven "syndromic" groupings: *Broca's aphasia*, primarily an **expressive** disorder; *global aphasia*, all modes of language severely affected; *transcortical motor aphasia*, similar to Broca's but able to repeat after you with little difficulty; *Wernicke's aphasia*, primarily sensory impairment; *conduction aphasia*, inability to repeat after you, but spontaneous speech is more intact; *anomic aphasia*, primary difficulty with word retrieval; and *transcortical sensory aphasia*, where echolalia is common (Davis, 1993). This foregoing brief synopsis clearly cannot do justice to the system, but even those who are very familiar with it do not always find it easy to categorize a client.

For our introductory purposes, we will limit our "classification" just to the following two primary patterns of aphasia (see Figure 11-1). (1) *Broca's*, or "motor" (nonfluent), *aphasia* is due to damage to the anterior portion of the brain. Patients have halting, groping speech. For example, one individual with nonfluent aphasia, when asked to define "money," responded, "Mon-mon-monag. . . . No! Ah . . . ah . . . spendy . . . go to . . . ah . . . ah . . . sore (store). . . ." (2) *Wernicke's*, or "sensory" (fluent), *aphasia* is due to a lesion in the posterior part of the brain. These patients have difficulty understanding speech. When asked to define the word "money," a fluent aphasic responded, "How did you say that again? Money? You mean like, you put it in a pocket? What was that again?"

Expressive aphasia. The difficulty in sending meaningful messages, as in the speaking, writing, or gesturing difficulties of the aphasic.

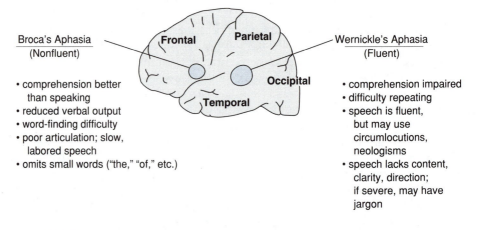

Broca's Aphasia
(Nonfluent)

- comprehension better
  than speaking
- reduced verbal output
- word-finding difficulty
- poor articulation; slow,
  labored speech
- omits small words ("the," "of," etc.)

Wernickle's Aphasia
(Fluent)

- comprehension impaired
- difficulty repeating
- speech is fluent,
  but may use
  circumlocutions,
  neologisms
- speech lacks content,
  clarity, direction;
  if severe, may have
  jargon

 FIGURE II-I   Left cerebral hemisphere showing general sites of two major types of aphasia (from Emerick and Haynes, 1986)

Most neurologists agree, however, that there is a great deal of inconsistency of brain organization from person to person, and it is therefore very difficult to fit clinical cases into specific categories. Difficulty in comprehension is one of the major features of all aphasia; and some impairment is usually present in one or another of the sense modalities, although in some patients it appears only under stress. A clear picture of this receptive disability is provided by Boone.

> One man who recovered fully from aphasia described his inability to understand spoken language in this way: He knew that his wife was talking to him as he could hear her voice, but all the words she said were meaningless. When she asked him if he wanted a cup of coffee, he said it sounded like "ba boo la cakka somma ba boo?" It was without sense. When she finally poured him a cup of coffee and pointed to it, he knew immediately what she meant. The same thing was true when he tried to read the morning paper. He remembered the name "Johnson," which was the only word he could recognize. He could see the various letters and even the grouping of the letters into words, but the words didn't mean anything to him. It was like trying to read a foreign language. As he improved, he was able to understand a spoken command if it were simply stated. Then, if his wife said, "Have a cup of coffee?" he could understand it. But had she said something more complex like "The coffee pot's on the stove; why don't you let me pour you a cup?" he would not have been able to understand all that she had said. (1965, p. 18)

Keep in mind that the impoverishment of language observed in aphasia is *not* due to loss of mental capacity, impairment of sensory organs, or paralysis of the speech apparatus. Aphasia also is not, however, merely a loss of words. It can be shown clinically—by the use of open-end sentences, oral opposites, or other forms of cueing—that even severe aphasics are capable of uttering words. They can often tell when sentences are grammatically correct. Often the problem seems to be *retrieving* words. The more common a word, the more probable that it will be retained. For example, an aphasic may understand or use the words "kiss" or "rain" but not "osculation" or "precipitation," even though all four might have been in his premorbid vocabulary (Wallace and Canter, 1985; Williams, 1983).

CAUSES OF APHASIA

As we have said, one of the most common causes of aphasia is a cerebrovascular accident (CVA), or stroke, that results in damage (lesion) to the left side of the brain (see Figure 11-2). Such damage, however, may be due not only to an impairment in the blood supply to the brain, but also to tumors, traumatic injuries, or infectious diseases such as **encephalitis.** When language is impaired, the lesion is almost always located in the left or dominant hemisphere. In left-handed people, right hemisphere damage may cause aphasia.

When brain damage occurs as the result of a CVA, the restricted or blocked blood flow may be due to (1) a **thrombosis,** in which a blood clot forms in one blood vessel within the brain; or (2) an **embolism** in which a blood clot arising in some other area of the body (such as an injured limb) travels upward and lodges in one of the brain's blood vessels; or (3) an **aneurysm,** a blood-filled pouch formed by dilation of a diseased artery wall; or (4) a **hemorrhage** in which an essential blood vessel breaks.

Most of the aphasias produced by direct head injuries result from automobile or motorcycle accidents, gunshot wounds, or brain surgery.

DIFFERENTIAL DIAGNOSIS

Workers in the health professions are called upon to make **differential diagnoses** to distinguish aphasia and a number of other conditions involving abnormality in language in adults. We include now a brief overview of three disorders (resulting from injury to, or degeneration of, the brain) that might be confused with aphasia.

Right-Hemisphere Damage

As we pointed out in Chapter 2, the left cerebral hemisphere is the dominant hemisphere for processing and planning language events. Very few people have language capability—at least productive language capability—

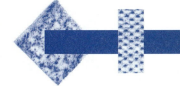

Encephalitis.
A disease characterized by inflammation or lesions of the brain.

Thrombosis.
Blood clot formed in place that does not move.

Embolism.
A clogging of a blood vessel as by a clot that moves.

Aneurysm.
A swelling or dilation of an artery due to weakening of the wall of the blood vessel.

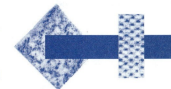

Hemorrhage.
Bleeding.

Differential diagnosis.
The process of distinguishing one disorder from another.

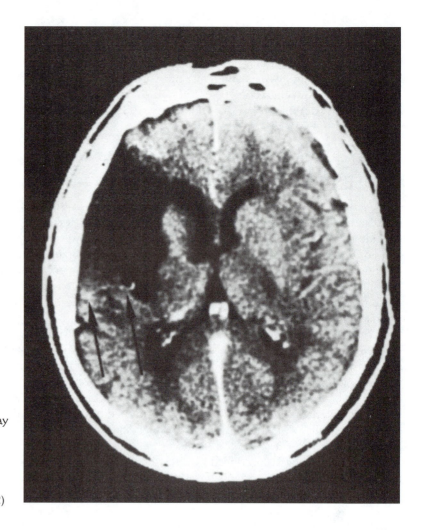

FIGURE II-2
Computerized tomographic (CT) scan (x-ray pictures taken from many angles and computerized) showing lesion in left hemisphere (from Seines, Rubens, Risse, and Levy, 1982)

located in the right side of the brain. The two cerebral hemispheres differ in cognitive "style"; whereas the left hemisphere tends to be analytical, rational, and logical, the right hemisphere functions in a holistic, intuitive, and emotional manner. A person with speech centers in the left hemisphere, however, does suffer rather distinctive deficits if the damage is isolated in the right side of his brain. Here are some of the most salient characteristics seen in right-hemisphere damage (Lowe and Webb, 1986).

Language-Speech Deficits.
1. Receptive skills:
   - impaired capability to understand humor, metaphors, or nuances of meaning
   - impaired pitch discrimination

- impaired ability to perceive emotions of other persons; may know what they are saying but not be able to recognize the emotional tone
- impaired ability to appreciate music

2. Expressive skills:
   - impaired articulation
   - errors in naming
   - verbosity, i.e., may use excessive number of words to express an idea

For an excellent personal account of right hemisphere stroke, see Johnson (1990).

Visual Perception Deficits.
1. Left visual field cut (**hemianopsia**)
2. Impairment of left-right directionality
3. May neglect left side of page in reading or writing
4. Impairment of part-whole relationships and detection of visual incongruities
5. May have difficulty recognizing familiar faces and places

Denial of/or Unconcern about the Disability.
The person may act as if he or she is not paralyzed on the left side.

Conceptual/Cognitive Deficits.
1. The person may be disoriented as to time/date/place.
2. He or she has difficulty grasping an event as a whole.
3. He or she finds it hard to complete a task that requires a series of discrete steps.

Language Confusion

Persons suffering from diffuse brain damage manifest a number of cognitive dysfunctions that, on cursory appraisal, might be mistaken for aphasia. Because the injury to the brain is widespread (and often due to trauma), many higher intellectual capabilities are disturbed (Sarno and Levita, 1979; Holland, 1982; Davis, 1993, Chapter 6), as the following case example illustrates.

> Tom Snively, a twenty-year-old college junior, suffered a closed head injury in a skiing accident. He was in a coma for two weeks. Now, two months post onset, he is an inpatient in the Rehabilitation Center. When evaluated with a standard test of aphasia, Tom showed no disturbance of vocabulary or syntax, though he did have some limited word-finding difficulty. The examiner noted, however, that the young man had trouble attending and staying in touch with the test situation. The patient tended to give responses that, although syntactically correct, often were irrelevant. Additionally, Tom was disoriented and, particularly in response to

Hemianopsia.
Blindness of one-half of the visual field.

open-ended questions, gave rambling, fabricated answers. Here is a portion of an interview conducted by a medical social worker that reveals the patient's disorientation and tendency to confabulate.

Worker: Where are you?

Tom: Ah, in training camp. Colorado Springs. And tomorrow we do time trials for the giant slalom.

Worker: But, what is this place?

Tom: A training center. I had a hamstring pull and need whirlpool treatments.

As the label suggests, patients with language confusion do not think clearly, have memory loss, and tend to be disoriented (Mentis and Pruting, 1987). Many of them show changes in personality as well; apathy, impulsiveness, and lability are common. The confusion may range from mild and temporary, as in concussion or hypothermia, to profound, as in traumatic head injury or drug overdose. Traumatic head injuries are increasing—as many as half a million children and adults suffer such injuries annually—and there is currently a great deal of interest in cognitive rehabilitation. Closed head injury is the leading cause of disability and death among people under age 35 in this country (Salazar, 1990). The reader will want to consult the rapidly developing literature on the topic. Ylvisaker (1985) and Davis (1993) would be good places to begin.

Dementia

Dementia refers to a group of disorders all of which feature generalized intellectual decline. The deterioration of emotional control, cognitive skills, and language use stems from diffuse bilateral subcortical and cortical brain injury or atrophy (Bayles and Kaszniak, 1987). Dementia is caused by, among other factors, infectious diseases, tumor, multiple strokes, and Parkinson's and Alzheimer's diseases. In its later stages, human immunodeficiency virus (HIV) also may produce language and speech deterioration. Unlike language confusion, dementia often has a gradual, insidious onset (Cummings and Benson, 1983; Davis, 1993, chap. 6).

Before a clinical diagnosis of dementia can be confirmed, several key features must be present (Berg et al., 1982).

1. There must be a sustained deterioration of *memory*, plus a disturbance in at least three of the following areas: (a) orientation in time and place; (b) judgment and problem solving (dealing with everyday situations); (c) community affairs (shopping, handling finances); (d) home and avocations; and (e) personal care.

2. There must be gradual onset and progression.

3. Duration must be at least six months.

Dementia.
General mental deterioration.

In order to illustrate the salient behavioral and communicative symptoms observed in dementia, we include a portion of a diagnostic report on a patient in the second phase of Alzheimer's disease (Powell and Courtice, 1983).

> This 64-year-old patient manifested the following behaviors: lowered drive and energy level; memory loss; slow reaction time; and difficulty making decisions. Her personality has changed in the past year so that now she typically is dull, bland, and unresponsive socially.
>
> Mrs. Davis' language abilities are only mildly impaired at this time. She can match objects, point to and name pictures, and repeat words, phrases, and short sentences.
>
> Phonologically and syntactically her speech is within normal limits. She does have limited output, however, and restricted usage. The patient's speech performance is slow and often, after trying to respond to a task, she will say, "I don't know."
>
> The patient's language disturbance was more evident on tasks requiring greater intellectual effort and abstraction. For example, Mrs. Davis was unable to find and correct semantic errors in sentences ("My sister is an only child") or discern the ambiguity in sentences ("Visiting relatives can be a nuisance," "The shooting of the police was awful").

Although we must curtail our discussion, the prevalence of Dementia of the Alzheimer's Type (DAT) is great enough, affecting some 2.5 to 3 million Americans (Subcommittee on Brain and Behavioral Science, 1991), that speech-language pathologists increasingly are involved with such patients. If you plan to join the profession—or if, perhaps, DAT has become an unwelcome visitor in your own home—we urge you to examine such references as Bayles and Boone (1982), Nicholas et al. (1985), and LeBrun, Devreux, F., and Rousseau (1987). In addition, the books for families and nonprofessionals by Mace and Rabins (1991) and Rau (1993) are especially informative and well written.

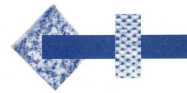

APHASIA TESTS

The first task of the speech clinician who seeks to help the person with aphasia is to determine the nature and extent of his disability. Shortened versions of published language inventories may he used as screening tests (Eisenson, 1954; Powell, Bailey, and Clark, 1980; Whurr, 1983) to get some general impressions of the aphasic's problem behavior. However, most clinicians agree that more comprehensive tests are necessary if an effective treatment plan is to be designed. Three of the more frequently used diagnostic tests are the Porch Index of Communicative Ability (PICA) (Porch, 1981), the Minnesota Test for Differential Diagnosis of Aphasia (Schuell, 1972), and the Boston Diagnostic Aphasia Examination (Goodglass and Kaplan, 1983).

The Porch or PICA test is a test that stresses a systematic presentation of ten stimuli. There are eighteen subtests designed to evaluate verbal, gestural, and graphic skills, but the major innovation is a multidimensional scoring system that replaces the more traditional right-wrong method of scoring. Thus Porch's system is based on a clinical evaluation of *accuracy* (the degree of correctness or rightness of a response); *responsiveness* (the ease with which the response is elicited, especially in terms of how much information the patient requires in order to complete the task); *completeness* (the degree to which the patient carries out the task in its entirety); *promptness* (the presence or absence of significant delay in making a response); and *efficiency* (the degree of facility the patient demonstrates in performing the motoric aspects of the response). The clinician scores the client's reactions to the test materials on a scale that extends from 1 (no response) to 16 (complete, complex response). Composite percentile scores derived from the PICA make it possible to quantify the severity of the client's language disorder and to predict the prospects for improvement.

The Schuell test evaluates the aphasic's performance in five major areas: auditory disturbances, visual and reading difficulties, speech and language difficulties, visuomotor and writing disturbances, and deficits in handling mathematical concepts. A brief and incomplete outline of the subtests in each area may be illustrative.

> *Auditory Disturbances.* The examiner evaluates the patient's abilities in recognizing common words, understanding sentences, following directions, repeating digits and sentences.
>
> *Visual and Reading Difficulties.* This part examines the patient's ability to match forms, letters, pictures, and words with visual symbols, and checks for comprehension of silent and oral reading passages.
>
> *Speech and Language Difficulties.* This section of the test explores the aphasic's difficulties in expressing himself in oral language. Speech movements and articulation patterns are checked, and the presence or absence of dysarthria and dyspraxia are confirmed.
>
> *Visual and Writing Difficulties.* This section requires writing numbers, spelling, copying, and other such activities.
>
> *Mathematical Deficits.* The testing here examines the patient's ability to handle the simple mathematical skills, knowledge of coin values, ability to tell time, and other similar skills.

The Boston Diagnostic Aphasia Examination includes a five-factor analysis of the patient's performance on the examination. Factor I relates to reading and writing; factor II concerns performance on spatial-quantitative-body parts tests; factor III appears to be highly related to speech fluency; factor IV is related to auditory comprehension; and factor V to the presence of paraphasia. The authors, Goodglass and Kaplan, suggest that these factors are useful in identifying major types of aphasia, including

Broca's aphasia, Wernicke's aphasia, anomic aphasia, conduction aphasia, and transcortical aphasia. To some extent, this test is based on research in psycholinguistics.

There are other tests besides these three for diagnosing and appraising the extent of the aphasic involvement, but these are representative. Perhaps in the future we will have better, more naturalistic, ways of assessing the language abilities of aphasics. After all, how much real communication is involved in pointing to pictures, naming objects, or writing words to dictation? Relatives tell us that the aphasic person communicates much better at home than the examinations reveal. By analyzing samples of the client's spontaneous speech for the amount and efficiency of message transmission, we may get a much clearer picture of his communicative abilities. To that end, we have found that the assessment device prepared by Holland (1980) is an excellent way of determining how an aphasic actually communicates in everyday situations. The tasks on this instrument include simulated (role-played) everyday situations—responding to social greetings, using an elevator, shopping, and keeping a doctor's appointment. Two other useful tools for identifying how the aphasic communicates in everyday settings are the checklists prepared by Sarno (1969) and Skinner et al. (1984).

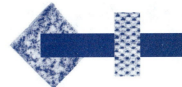

PHYSICAL AND PSYCHOSOCIAL ELEMENTS

Most aphasic clients show a one-sided paralysis (hemiplegia) or weakness of one arm and leg on the side opposite the brain injury, usually the right side. This may persist in some patients, but often the patient regains the use of the leg enough to permit walking. Some patients suffer a loss of sensation on the afflicted side. They sometimes also show hemianopsia, a visual disturbance that makes it impossible for them to see more than half of the field of vision. Some of them have convulsions. We must keep in mind that brain injury is a serious health problem and that those who work in aphasia rehabilitation inevitably must work in close coordination—preferably in a team fashion—with physicians and practitioners from other health and human service professions.

The language tests we described do not show the frustrations, anxiety, and helplessness experienced by people who have suffered a loss in the ability to handle symbols. They are lost souls. Consider a disorder which drastically alters those very attributes most critical to normal human functioning—communication with others, control of body functions and physical ability, the orderly processing of reality and of one's own life. A longtime friend and colleague, a professor of literature, underscored her feeling of disunity with a verse in her well-worn copy of Emily Dickinson's poems.

I felt a Cleaving in my Mind—
As if my Brain had split—
I tried to match it—Seam by Seam,
But could not make them fit.

Now, imagine the terrible impact on a person when all these profound changes happen precipitously, when the victim has had no warning, no chance to prepare for the ordeal. Some patients show personality changes—an outgoing, happy person may become despondent and moody, while another may become aggressive and controlling—but usually the basic personality traits persist despite tremendous frustration and change in self-concepts. Some victims laugh or cry without reason. All fatigue very easily, find it difficult to concentrate, and tend to perseverate. Speech pathologists must also explore these areas if they hope to help the person with aphasia. We find that the adjustment inventories devised by Müller, Code, and Mugford (1983) and Robinson et al. (1985) help identify problems in the client's psychosocial functioning. The personal experiences reported by Buck (1968) can provide much of the needed understanding.

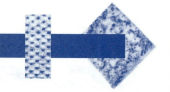

PROGNOSIS

Immediately after the injury, the patient often shows a picture of extreme helplessness, but much of the impairment may subside within three or four months when what is known as *spontaneous recovery* occurs, although it is seldom complete and residual signs of aphasic disturbance can usually be found even in those who apparently have become well. Some authorities feel that spontaneous recovery seldom can be expected after six months, and any improvement thereafter must be viewed as due to the relearning efforts of the patient himself or the teaching efforts of his clinicians. Individuals suffering traumatic brain injury may have a much longer period of spontaneous recovery and their improvement in communication tends to follow a "staircase" pattern of dramatic gain–plateau–dramatic gain.

The extent and location of the brain damage is, of course, a critical factor in a patient's prospects of recovery. Individuals who show persistent problems in auditory recognition and comprehension or severe motor speech impairment are less likely to make significant improvement. The younger and the more intelligent and the more motivated the person is, the better are her chances for regaining her place in a communicative world. Wise handling of these patients immediately after the injury is absolutely essential if the terrific frustration that produces depression and defeatism is to be avoided. Often the attitudes of the members of the family, doctors, and nurses can create unfavorable prognoses. Families can be helped to understand and to be supportive by reading books such as that of Hess and Bahr (1981). With professional speech therapy and the co-operation of all those who tend the patient, many individuals suffering from milder forms of aphasia can regain much of their ability to communicate. Even those who are severely impaired (global) aphasics can make enough recovery to improve their quality of life during the years remaining to them (Marshall and Phillips, 1983; Davis 1993, chap. 11).

TREATMENT

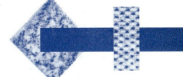

In the section of this chapter devoted to diagnostic testing, the various deficits and impairments in reception, formulation, and expression were explored. In therapy we begin with those functions that have remained comparatively unaffected—we begin with what the patient can do. If he can gesture but not talk, we would start by strengthening that gesture language, then seek to attach simple verbalizations to the gestures. If he cannot write but has less difficulty in reading simple material, we would begin with reading and then later have him start copying. If there is a pronounced difficulty in word finding, we may instead have him identify pictures or words by pointing. Or we may start with the automatic speech that remains—"How are you?" "Good morning," "bread and butter," or counting or naming the days of the week. Most aphasics retain some subsymbolic or automatic speech such as social ritual utterances ("Hello," "How are you?"), items that occur in a series (poems, prayers), and of course, emotional expressions. If he has difficulties in comprehension, as most aphasics do, we make sure that we speak simply and slowly, though naturally. Aphasics are very susceptible to time pressure.

We make sure that we make silence comfortable so that he has time to search. Often he may get only one or two words of a sentence we say to him, and he must have time to guess how they are related. When we repeat what we say, we wait, and then repeat it exactly so that he will not have to decode a new message when he's just beginning to comprehend the old one. We avoid abstractions as much as we can. We talk about the things related to his major interests. Discovering one day that one of our patients had been a racing buff—a fact that had not appeared in our case history or family interviews, we procured some racing forms and had him help us select the horses to win, place, and show. At first he could only point, but from this nucleus we were eventually able to help him recapture some of the speech and mathematical skills he had lost.

Aphasia therapy consists of building bridges from the things the patient can do to those he cannot. We show the person how to reach out for language as a natural extension of ideas and concepts from his past; we do not so much teach words as stimulate and re-energize old associations to work again (Jennings and Lubinski, 1981). One of the surprising features of aphasic therapy is that when the patient begins to progress in one area of his language handling, that progress often spreads to other areas. We do not have to teach these people new skills of symbolic processing; we have to help them *find* the ones that they have lost. We have to teach them to search without becoming frantic and frustrated. Our role is that of an immensely patient guide and companion to one lost in a wilderness not of his own making.

Although it is often difficult to get the person with aphasia, so overwhelmed is she by the catastrophe of the sudden change, to accept some responsibility for her own recovery of language, it is of paramount importance that this be done. As soon as we can, therefore, we try to encourage her to do her homework, setting up the tasks that she can perform by herself or with the help of her family: copying, writing, memorizing, naming pictures in a catalogue, describing, echoing—whatever is within her capacity and can be reinforced. Prerecorded drill material is a useful tool for this purpose, but the daily newspaper and television have been used by some of our aphasics in their determined effort to regain some of their speech and comprehension. In achieving this self-therapy, the speech pathologist must work closely with the family of the patient. As McKenzie Buck says, "Aphasia is a family illness as well as a family catastrophe." By helping the members of the family understand the nature of the problem, by helping them make the necessary adjustments, they can aid the aphasic greatly in his self-therapy.[1]

It is very difficult to describe the treatment for aphasia in general terms because the patterns of disability vary so much from case to case. As we have said, most of our early work with these patients consists of strengthening and improving the least impaired symbolic skills so that they can feel that they are not helpless and hopeless but beginning to improve (Figure 11-3). But we also work hard on the whole general language disability, building foundations for improvements in all areas; it is this that we wish to consider next.

Stimulation

The world of an aphasic client must be a most confusing place. Depending upon the particular functions affected, she may hear sounds or people talking to her but be unable to comprehend them; she may pick up the morning paper and see only meaningless squiggles running across the page. She may try to write her name in her checkbook and be unable to do so. She tries to ask for a cigarette and either she cannot remember its name or she speaks gibberish. She looks at the clock and cannot tell the time. She puts her hand in her pocket and feels something but does not know that what she feels is a coin. It is a blooming, buzzing confusion without rhyme, reason, or meaning. Here and there are moments of clarity, but they flit by too swiftly or are lost in frustration and depression.

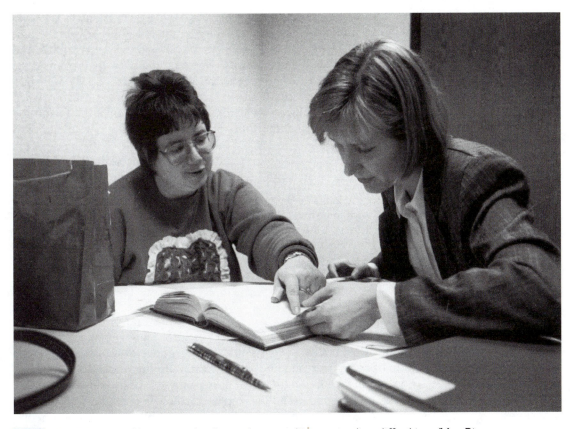

One of the major tasks of the speech pathologist is to provide islands of consistency in this sea of uncertainty. Patiently she explores her patient to determine the things he can do. Perhaps he can copy letters from the alphabet; or if he cannot, perhaps he can trace over those she provides. Very well, she begins with this activity and continues with it until he knows that this function at least is within his powers. Then she stimulates him with other things. She may have him echo her words, animal noises, or gestures. They may put their spoons in their coffee cups in unison and stir the sugar and cream. She may ask him to point predictively to which one of the objects—knife, fork, or spoon—she will use in a moment to spread his bread. She may ask him to read her lips as she stimulates him with the number "three" for the three peanuts in her hand, then help him count them aloud. She may guide his hand in writing a few sentences to his wife. She will take his hand and touch it to his nose, his ears, his mouth, his feet, saying these names as she does so. Every attempt is made to combine as many cues as possible—auditory, visual, tactile—in this stimulation. Always she uses self-talk and parallel talk in very simple words, phrases, or sentences, providing the spoken symbols for every experience, for every activity. Day after day, she reviews this patient stimulation, tolerant of failure and happy when success comes. For success will come as the confusion subsides and the aphasic begins to find the functions he has lost (Aten, Caligiuri, and Holland, 1982).

Let us give an example of stimulation therapy with a homebound client who felt isolated and neglected.

> Since Mr. Fontaine had been a policeman for twenty-nine years, he knew the town intimately. The clinician drove slowly down side streets while the client gave directions, first by hand gesture and gradually using street names. They read signs, both traffic and commercial, did some shopping, and dropped by the police station for coffee and chats with the client's former fellow workers.

Inhibition

Brain injury makes it hard to inhibit oneself. The lower centers of the brain miss their old brakes, as we see in the frequent overflow of emotion in the form of crying and laughing spells or **catastrophic responses.** Perseveration continues too long. One of our aphasics, once he had begun a sentence with "I think" could not stop saying these two words, over and over, over and over, over and over. Another was unable to speak what she desired to utter because all speech attempts began with "Yes, yes, yes," and the broken record went round and round on that single word. Accordingly we train our clients to inhibit themselves, to stop doing what they are doing, first upon our command, and then upon their own. We train them to inhibit any attempt to speak until we give the signal, or until they tap their foot five times. We teach them to wait, to pause, to say "No more that." We give them time to reorganize. We have them wait until we smile before they try again. We ask them to rehearse silently or in a mirror or in pantomime what they are about to do or say. We have them duplicate on purpose their crying or laughing jags and to stop them when the second hand of the watch points down. For the aphasic who can read, we provide "inhibition cards" that might, for example, read as follows: "Stop laughing!" "Wait!" "Whisper first!" We have them confess and cancel the perseveration which does occur.

Catastrophic response. A sudden extreme change in behavior by the aphasic characterized by irritability, flushing or fainting, withdrawal from random movements.

Translation

The person with aphasia often gets blocked in formulating, receiving, or sending messages because he keeps going up the same blind alley over and over again. We must teach him to shift when he meets these dead ends, to try another tack.

The speech pathologist is always alert for strategies by which the aphasic tries to retrieve words or correct his errors. Davis (1985) describes two useful ways to implement the translation process: deblocking and PACE. *Deblocking* involves using the most intact language function to trigger use in impaired modalities. For example, one client could not recognize words if they were presented auditorily, but did recognize them instantly when they were written. First, we showed him the written word "chickadee" (he was an inveterate bird watcher); then, immediately, the same word was given auditorily and he was able to respond correctly.

PACE stands for *Promoting Aphasic Communicative Effectiveness.* The essence of this approach is simply to get the client *communicating* any way he can—pointing, gesturing, drawing, writing, even pantomiming. Again, we give an example with our client whose hobby was watching birds. A pile of cards depicting a number of bird species was placed face down on a table. Both clinician and client then took turns trying to transmit clues—giving the bird song, showing its flight pattern with hand gestures, drawing its unique feather color—that would identify a particular bird.

The basic point of translation is to train the person to shift from one type of symbolization to another. We may ask him to spell aloud, then print the name of the animal he hears meowing on the tape recorder. We have him count to three by the taps, again by drawing vertical lines, again by clapping hands, again by tracing the numeral, and finally by saying it. We say "Sit down!" and he must try to point to the appropriate picture, then to pantomime it with his lips silently, then to act it out, then to find the phrase on a card (Figure 11-4). We don't overwhelm him with too many translations at first; we let him lead us; but we always work to give him experiences in shifting from one set of symbolic meanings to another.

Memorization

One of the best ways of creating islands of consistency in the hurly-burly world of aphasia is to teach clients to memorize. Often we begin by having them memorize sequences of movements as in a calisthenic exercise or a sequence of lines to be drawn or the selection of a set of objects in a definite order. We demonstrate such sequences as opening the window, then closing the door, then saying "Too hot!" and then ask them to duplicate our performance. We have them find us three desired objects in a catalogue in the order in which we write them on the board. We arrange wood block letters in a row on the table so that they spell the client's name. We have him memorize the cards of different sizes and shapes that have written upon them such phrases as "Good morning," "Nice day," "How are you?" "Goodbye," so that he can show them to us appropriately long before he can say these things. We have him write from memory, draw from

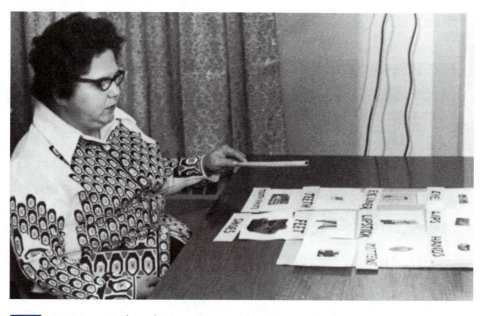

FIGURE 11-4   An aphasic patient matches written words to pictures

memory, using flashcards to stimulate him and varying the exposure and delay time so he succeeds more than he fails. Finally, we ask him to learn by rote such passages as this:

> I have been sick. I had a stroke. I must learn to read and write and speak again. Getting better. Takes time. Must work hard. No use feeling sorry. Get to work now.

Later on, we have the client memorize poems and prose passages of increasing complexity. These not only help to provide associations between words, but also help in relearning the basic syntax of language.

Parallel Talking

We emphasize stimulation with simple materials, not complex ones. We speak simply and clearly, supplementing with gesture or written or pictured materials when needed. We do a great amount of parallel talking in this stimulation, telling him, simply and in short phrases or sentences, what he is doing, feeling, or perceiving. We use not only this sort of commentary but also prediction and recall. Often, as we do this parallel talk, we find the patient will almost unconsciously join in and say a word for us on which we fumble or postpone the utterance. We have come to make this technique the basic part of our therapy. It is a bit difficult to learn to do this well, for the clinician must make sure that he does the appropriate verbalization and hesitates at exactly the moment when the patient is experiencing the thought expressed. It is also necessary to keep from making too much of the client's spontaneous utterance when it does occur under these conditions. We merely say yes, and then restimulate him with what he has spoken in the context of the entire utterance. This is especially effective with the *expressive* aphasic, but we have also used a whispered or pantomimed form of parallel talking to help those who have trouble understanding spoken speech to read our lips. Often these individuals, if they learn to pantomime the speech they *see,* can then comprehend it, and some of the auditory agnosia subsides. The wife and other associates of the patient can be taught to do much of this parallel talking. We have found it most useful.

Scanning and Concentrating

The aphasic patient is like a man who suddenly finds himself in a strange country. He is overwhelmed by strange sights and sounds. He may hear people talking and be unable to understand what they are saying. He cannot write their language. He does not know what purposes some of the objects about him serve. Even a spoon is something strange. What he must do, in such a situation, is learn to observe and scan for meanings and consistencies. He must come to concentrate on things that look alike or on meaningless words that always seem to appear in the same context. Only in this way can such a person, suddenly transported to a strange land, come to find a place in it. But it is difficult for him to concentrate and difficult for him to observe closely. He needs help in scanning and concentration.

Accordingly, the clinician assists him to create order out of his chaos by training him in sorting out things that look alike, feel alike, sound alike. She may give him a magazine and ask him to find all the pictures in which shoes are portrayed, to tear them out, and to put them under one of his own shoes. She may say some words for him and ask him to signal every time he hears one that begins with an /s/ sound. She may have him feel a series of objects with his eyes closed and select those that are smooth to the touch. She may work with opposites: big things and little things; hot foods and cold foods. She asks him to choose, to match, to classify. He needs categories. She helps him reacquire them.

Organization

The client needs order in his disordered cosmos. He needs definite routines of daily living, consistent schedules of events. When we come to our daily sessions with an aphasic, we use the same greeting each time and begin our therapy with the same sort of activity before we try something new. The other people about him must help in this same ordering of his life so that a portion of it will become familiar and organized rather than confused.

But he must also learn to organize his own life, his own thoughts, and outward behaviors. He needs help in patterning his consciousness. Accordingly we train him to make patterns of all types. We may begin by merely asking him or showing him how to set the table, or to turn the pages of a magazine left to right, or to arrange a few scrambled numbers in the proper order. We may have him raise his arm in a series of gradual steps. We may ask him to count the number of windows in the room, to draw a house, to roll a clay model of the cigarette he cannot ask for. We give him form boards to assemble. We give him some cards, each with a word on it, and ask him to place them serially so they make a sentence that commands us to do something. We get him to sing some old tunes. We ask him to read aloud a sentence through the window of a shield that exposes only one word at a time. We ask him to correct our mispronunciations, our use of wrong words, his own mistakes. All these activities require scanning and concentration. The clinician helps, always using her self talk and parallel talk to provide a running commentary for his thinking.

Formulation

The person with aphasia often has trouble not only in sending her messages or in receiving them; she also cannot formulate them with precision. Sometimes she cannot find the exact word she needs; and instead of searching for another almost as good, or revising the whole utterance, she stops right there, helplessly, fixed on the thorn of her frustration. Basically, what she needs is the freedom to make new wholes, to try it again in a different way, so that this different way also makes sense.

Although, as we have indicated, we use self talk and parallel talking constantly throughout all of these various approaches to therapy with the aphasic, we use these techniques with greatest effectiveness in helping her to formulate. Here is a brief excerpt from such a therapy session.

Clinician:	All right, Mary. Let's begin. Talk to yourself. Say what you do. Like this. (*Clinician opens her purse, takes out pencil, writes her name. As she does so, she speaks in unison with her activity.*) Open purse . . . here pencil . . . write name. (*She hands Mary the purse and signals her to repeat her behavior.*)
Mary (opens purse):	Open puss . . . no . . . poos . . . no . . . oh dear, oh my . . .(*gives up*)

Clinician:	OK. You got mixed up on "purse". . . . Purrrrrse. . . . Never mind. Say the whole thing. (*She repeats action.*)
Mary:	Open puss . . .
Clinician:	And here pencil . . .
Mary:	Pencil . . . and now I write mame . . . no . . . mama . . . no . . .
Clinician:	Write name . . . name . . . like this. (*Demonstrates.*)
Mary:	Write name like . . .(*writes Mary*). . . Mary . . . Mary. . . . Write no good . . .
Clinician:	Fine! You did it. Now let's do it again. Talk to yourself. Say what you're doing.

A thousand experiences of this sort, based on the experiences of daily living, can aid the patient to improve in formulation. Her husband and children can easily learn to do these things. They should use simple self-talk so she knows what they are doing, perceiving, or feeling. Through parallel talking, they can put the words in her ears at the moment she needs them, thus reauditorizing her thinking and giving her the verbal symbols that have become lost or scrambled. Sooner or later, the client will begin to talk to herself as she does things, sees things, or feels things. This should be highly rewarded by all about her.

We may also help a client to formulate in other ways. We ask him to complete unfinished figures, to assemble toys, to repair a broken electric cord, to weave a rug, to complete the writing of unfinished sentences, to prewrite what he is about to say, or to rehearse it in pantomime. We have him do simple description and exposition on paper or aloud. We teach him to fill in the hands of a series of blank clock faces to indicate the hours. We teach him to make change; to do mental arithmetic, or if he cannot do so, to do the operations on paper. We give him simple problems to solve. We teach him to paraphrase, to tell us what he has read in the paper or heard on the radio. We encourage a free flow of ideas and words by having him perform divergent semantic tasks, such as naming things that roll, kinds of transportation, types of fruit. The fascinating thing about all of this is to discover how each new achievement seems to unlock the doors to other new achievements.

Body Image Integration

It is not only the outside world that is strange to the patient. He also is a stranger to himself. He has changed. He is not the person he used to be. The various members of his family often show this by their reactions. They may treat him like a child or as a nuisance or as though he were an imbecile. Good counseling can prevent much of this, but it is difficult for a family to become adjusted to a handicapped stranger in the house.

We have said that the aphasic person is also a stranger to himself. Often there is paralysis of the arm or leg. A part of him will not obey his bidding; he has suddenly sprouted a dead limb. Any one of us who has lain too long on an arm in bed and awakes to find it "gone to sleep," a strange and inert thing there in bed with him, will vaguely understand how important this experience must be. But there are a thousand other changes in the person too. He has trouble reading, writing, talking, telling time, comprehending, counting. Who is this person who suddenly has come to inhabit his skin? It is the clinician's job to help him become acquainted, to reintroduce him to his new self and to get him to like this new person. It isn't easy but it can be done.

We begin by reintroducing him to his body. We touch his feet and name them as we do so. We lift his arm and tell him what we are doing. We have him stroke his face and find his eyes and ears and mouth. We get him to move his lips and his tongue as we do. We do much of our work with the body image in front of the mirror. We command the helpless hand to squeeze on the exercise ball, and we squeeze it. We take his picture in all sorts of therapeutic activities and show them to him. We look together in old albums at the snapshots of his childhood and youth. Perhaps all the king's horses couldn't do it, but a good clinician often can put Humpty Dumpty together again.

Psychotherapy

It should be obvious by now that these patients need psychotherapy. They meet many penalties, experience frustrations so intense they would break up almost any physically normal person. They find their cups overflowing with anxiety, guilt, and hostility. They worry about the hospital bills, about the paycheck that is no more, about their possible future in a nursing home. They become furious with anger, often over trifles. And yet, fortunately, the same brain injury that creates these storms of emotion also makes them transient. They do not last, do not reverberate. Furious one moment, the next moment a patient is laughing.

We do not have the space in this introductory text to describe psychotherapy options for adult aphasics. The book by Rollin (1987) provides an excellent overview of counseling for patients and their families. We have found Stroke Clubs, which are support groups for brain-injured persons and their relatives, to be of inestimable value in dealing with the emotional aspects of the disorder. You may find out more about Stroke Clubs by contacting the American Heart Association in your area.

Such an outline of therapeutic activities is far from being comprehensive, but it may provide a starting platform. It does not indicate how the clinician works especially on the functions of one area in which progress seems most likely to occur. And it does not show, except by implication, the need for ingenuity and, above all, the patient perseverance needed to rehabilitate these persons. Personally, we have found our work with aphasics to be more fascinating and rewarding than that with many other communicative disabilities. This is true not only with children with aphasia but also with the many adults who have been brought to us for help. To see a person who has been stricken down at the entrance to the valley of death rejoin the human race, and to feel that perhaps you have had a humble part in the rejoining, is reward enough for all the failure and frustrations aphasia therapy brings.

STUDY QUESTIONS

1. Define the term "aphasia" as you would in explaining the disorder to a next door neighbor who asks what you're studying.
2. What is meant by "CVA" and what are the principal causes of CVAs?
3. Why is it that a left hemisphere stroke is more likely than a right hemisphere stroke to produce aphasia?
4. What fundamental characteristics differentiate "Broca's aphasia" from "Wernicke's aphasia"?
5. What types of symptoms might you expect to observe in a person who has suffered right hemisphere damage?
6. To what does "DAT" refer, and about how many Americans are estimated to suffer this problem?
7. How should you respond to a person who says "My spouse had a stroke last week and, it seems to me, must have become mentally retarded because there's no speech at all except some gibberish"?
8. For what reason(s) may brain injury suffered in, for example, an automobile accident result create problems that resemble, but are not actually, aphasia?
9. Define the term "apraxia" and explain how this problem is different than "agnosia."
10. Why do you suppose it has been said that "aphasia is a family illness as well as a family catastrophe"?

ENDNOTES

[1]For a comprehensive review of family therapy in aphasia, see the chapter by Rollin (1984) and the article by Watson (1986).

REFERENCES

Aten, J., Caligiuri, M., and Holland, A. (1982). The efficacy of functional communication therapy for chronic aphasic patients. *Journal of Speech and Hearing Disorders, 47*, 93–96.

Bayles, K., and Boone, D. (1982). The potential of language tasks for identifying senile dementia. *Journal of Speech and Hearing Disorders, 47,* 210–217.

Bayles, K., and Kaszniak, A. (1987). *Communication and cognition in normal aging and dementia.* San Diego, CA: College-Hill Press.

Berg, L., et al. (1982). Mild senile dementia of Alzheimer type: Research diagnostic criteria, recruitment, and description of a study population. *Journal of Neurology, Neurosurgery and Psychiatry, 11,* 962–968.

Boone, D. R. (1965). *An adult has aphasia.* Danville, IL: Interstate Printers and Publishers.

Buck, M. (1968). *Dysphasia.* Englewood Cliffs, NJ: Prentice Hall.

Cummings, J., and Benson, D. (1983). *Dementia: A clinical approach.* Stoneham, MA: Butterworths.

Davis, G. (1993). *A survey of adult aphasia and related language disorders* (2nd ed.). Englewood Cliffs, NJ: Prentice Hall.

Davis, G. (1985). *Adult aphasia rehabilitation: Applied pragmatics.* San Diego, CA: College-Hill Press.

Eisenson, J. (1954). *Examining for aphasia.* New York: Psychological Corp.

Emerick, L., and Haynes, W. (1986). *Diagnosis and evaluation in speech pathology* (3rd ed.). Englewood Cliffs, NJ: Prentice Hall.

Goodglass, H. (1993) *Understanding aphasia.* San Diego, CA: Academic Press.

Goodglass, H., and Kaplan, E. (1983). *The assessment of aphasia and related disorders* (2nd ed). Philadelphia: Lea and Febiger.

Hess, L., and Bahr, R. (1981). *What every family should know about strokes.* New York: Appleton-Century-Crofts.

Holland, A. (1982). When is aphasia aphasia? The problem of closed head injury. In R. Brookshire

(ed.), *Clinical aphasiology conference proceedings.* Minneapolis, MN: BRK.

Jennings, E., and Lubinski, K. (1981). Strategies for improving thinking in the language impaired adult. *Journal of Communication Disorders, 14,* 255–271.

Johnson, F. (1990) *Right hemisphere stroke.* Detroit, MI: Wayne State University Press.

Lebrun, Y., Devreux, F., and Rousseau, J. (1987). Disorders of commmunicative behavior in degenerative dementia. *Folia Phoniatrica, 39,* 1–8.

Lowe, R., and Webb, W. (1986). *Neurology for the speech-language pathologist.* Stoneham, MA: Butterworths.

Mace, N., and Rabins, P. (1991). *The 36-hour day: A family guide to caring for persons with Alzheimer's disease, related dementing illnesses, and memory loss in later life* (rev. ed.). Baltimore, MD: Johns Hopkins University Press.

Marshall, R., and Phillips, D. (1983). Prognosis for improved verbal communication in aphasic stroke patients. *Archives for Physical Medicine and Rehabilitation, 64,* 597–600.

Mentis, M., and Prutting, C. (1987). Cohesion in the discourse of normal and head-injured adults. *Journal of Speech and Hearing Research, 30,* 88–98.

Müller, D., Code, C., and Mugford, J. (1983). Predicting psychosocial adjustment to aphasia, *British Journal of Disorders of Communication, 18,* 23–29.

Nicholas, M., et al. (1985). Empty speech in Alzheimer's disease and fluent aphasia. *Journal of Speech and Hearing Research, 28,* 405–410.

Porch, B. (1981). *Porch Index of Communicative Ability, Vol. II: Administration, scoring and interpretation* (3rd ed.). Palo Alto, CA: Consulting Psychologists Press.

Porch, B. et al. (1980). Statistical prediction of change in aphasia. *Journal of Speech and Hearing Research, 23,* 312–321.

Powell, L., Bailey, S., and Clark, E. (1980). A very short form of the Minnesota Aphasia Test.

British Journal of Social and Clinical Psychology, 19, 189–194.

Powell, L., and Courtice, K. (1983). *Alzheimer's disease.* Reading, MA: Addison-Wesley.

Rau, M. (1993). *Coping with communication challenges in Alzheimer's disease.* San Diego, CA: Singular Publishing Group.

Robinson, R., et al. (1985). Social functioning assessment in stroke patients. *Archives of Physical Medicine and Rehabilitation,* 66, 496–500.

Rollin, W. (1984). Family therapy and the adult aphasic. In J. Eisenson (ed.), *Adult aphasia.* Englewood Cliffs, NJ: Prentice Hall.

Rollin, W. (1987). *The psychology of communication disorders in individuals and their families.* Englewood Cliffs, NJ: Prentice Hall.

Sarno, M.T. (1969). *The functional communication profile.* New York: New York University Medical Center Monograph 42.

Sarno, M.T., and Levita, E. (1979). Recovery in the aphasic in the first year post-stroke. *Stroke,* 10, 663–670.

Schuell, H. (1972). *Minnesota Test for Differential Diagnosis of Aphasia* (rev. ed.). Minneapolis: University of Minnesota Press.

Seins, O., Rubens, A., Risse, G., and Levy, R. (1982). Transient aphasia with persistent apraxia. *Archives of Neurology,* 39, 122–126.

Skinner, C., et al. (1984). *Edinburgh functional communication profile: An observation procedure of the evaluation of disordered communication in elderly patients.* London: Winslow Press.

Subcommittee on Brain and Behavioral Sciences. (1991). *Maximizing human potential: Decade of the brain 1990–2000* (NTIS Publication No. PB91–133769). Bethesda, MD: National Institutes of Health.

Wallace, G., and Canter, C. (1985). Effects of personally relevant language materials on the performance of severely aphasic individuals. *Journal of Speech and Hearing Disorders,* 50, 385–390.

Watson, P. (1986). Stroke in the family: Theoretical consideration. *Rehabilitation Nursing,* 11, 15–17.

Whurr, R. (1983). Whurr Aphasia Screening Test. London: M. Phil.

Williams, S. (1983). Factors influencing naming performance in aphasia: A review of the literature. *Journal of Communication Disorders,* 16, 357–372.

Ylvisaker, M. (ed.). (1985). *Head injury rehabilitation: Children and adolescents.* San Diego, CA: College-Hill Press.

C h a p t e r **12**

Cerebral Palsy and Other Neuropathologies

Most infants learn to sit, stand, walk, and talk with very little real trouble. To be sure, for a time they totter about unsteadily and fall down frequently, but eventually they acquire smooth, virtually automatic control of their muscles, and they begin uneventfully to master even the rapid and fine coordinations required for speech. But for children with cerebral palsy, even turning the head, or swallowing food, or lifting an arm can be a struggle; truly intelligible speech may forever be unattainable. The weaknesses, the paralysis, and the incoordinations shown by the cerebral palsied child stem from injury to the motor control centers of the brain—injury that occurs before, during, or shortly after birth.

All professionals who work with physically handicapped children or adults will encounter cerebral palsy. Certainly the speech-language pathologist will, for half or more of the persons with this condition have some difficulty in speaking. All the dimensions of speech—articulation, language, voice, and fluency—may present abnormalities of greater or lesser degrees. Breathing for speech also can be quite disturbed. In brief, the speech of the child with cerebral palsy can be severely dysarthric; apraxia may be present; and normal language acquisition may be deterred.

A few of the less severely involved individuals may be able to speak fairly well and to function with relative or complete independence. Some very few may even have very good speech, but the many whose ability to communicate is markedly impaired are in urgent need of the services speech pathology can offer. Seldom do we work alone, however, with such clients. In association with cerebral palsy it is not uncommon to find feeding-swallowing, perceptual, sensory, mobility, intellectual, learning, attention deficit, social-emotional, and other "comorbid" difficulties (Blondis, Roizen, Snow, Accardo, 1993) requiring an interdisciplinary team approach. As one member of the rehabilitation team a speech pathologist often works closely with special and regular education teachers, physical and occupational therapists, pediatricians, orthopedists, social workers, psychologists, and other specialists.

As must these other professionals, the speech clinician needs to understand the nature of the group of disorders that traditionally have been classified under the general label of cerebral palsy. Here, for example, is one fairly typical current definition of cerebral palsy:

> A term used to describe a number of permanent neuromotor impairments acquired before the age of 3 years; subcategories of cerebral palsy that describe the type of neuromotor involvement resulting from damage to specific areas of the brain are spasticity, ataxia, athetosis, rigidity, and mixed; . . . Because normal patterns of neuromotor maturation occur over time, it may take up to two years to confirm a diagnosis of cerebral palsy. (Billeaud, 1993, p. 163)

If that definition seems a bit imprecise to you, you already have begun to understand why some clinicians and researchers question the utility of the label. It seems to reflect a lumping together of problems that can be quite different from one another. As a diagnostic label, it does little more than distinguish between early developmental and later acquired neuro-motor disorders (admittedly an important distinction, but one which can be made in other ways). As at least one observer has noted, injuries that cause dysarthria in children tend to be pooled under the term cerebral palsy, while injuries that cause dysarthria in adults tend to lead to a search for specific causes (Wertz, 1985, p. 72). And we would agree that a fuller understanding of specific causes is fundamental both to improved treatment and to more effective prevention. In the future we may see growing dissatisfaction with the use of "cerebral palsy" as a common designation for this group of disorders. Perhaps even now we should speak of cerebral pals*ies,* just as we speak of dysarthr*ias,* in any general discussion of the topic.

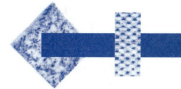

VARIETIES OF CEREBRAL PALSY

Just as the general diagnostic label continues to be widely used, so do various terms that seek to identify subcategories of the disorder. There is some movement away from the classification system cited in the above definition, but the subcategories **spasticity, athetosis,** and *ataxia* still are frequently cited as the three major varieties of cerebral palsy, with recognition that more than one of these symptom complexes is often found in the same individual and that such symptoms as *rigidity, tremor,* and **flaccidity** also occur in some cases. According to Hardy (1994), though, "the term *dyskinesia* (a disorder of excessive and involuntary movement) is becoming preferred . . . (over) the older term *athetosis,*" and *ataxia* is rarely used any more.

Spasticity

Spasticity itself has been defined as the paralysis due to simultaneous contraction of antagonistic or reciprocal muscle groups accompanied by a definite degree of hypertension or hypertonicity. It is due to a lesion or injury in the pyramidal nerve tracts and is by far the most common form of cerebral palsy. The muscles overcontract; they pull too hard and too suddenly. Slight stimuli will set off major contractions. The person with spasticity who tries to move his little finger may jerk not only the hand, but the arm or trunk as well. He may have a characteristic manner of walking—the typical "scissors gait." The hands may be clenched and curled up along the wrists in their extreme contraction, or the whole arm may be drawn upward and backward along the neck. He may tend to contract his chest muscles and thus enlarge the thoracic cavity during the act of speaking,

Spasticity.
One of the varieties of cerebral palsy; characterized by highly tensed contractions of muscle groups.

Athetosis.
One of the forms of cerebral palsy characterized by writhing, shaking, involuntary movements of the head, limbs, or the body.

Flaccidity.
State of passive relaxation; uncontracted, limp in appearance.

which compels him in turn to compress the abdomen excessively in order to force out some air. He thus may be said to inhale with the thorax at the same time that he exhales with the abdomen. Great tension is thereby produced and this reflects itself in muscular abnormality all over the body. It also shows up in speech in the form of unnatural pauses and gasping and weak or aphonic voice. Many of the "breaks" in his speech are due to this form of faulty breathing.

Since it is difficult to make gradual and smooth movements, spastic speech is often explosive and blurting. Often the extreme tension that characterizes spasticity will produce **hard** articulatory **contacts** that resemble or engender stuttering symptoms. The sounds involving complex coordinations are, of course, usually defective; and the tongue tip sounds that make contact with the upper-gum ridge are very difficult. Where there is some facial paralysis, the labial sounds are much more difficult than might be expected. In cases where there are both symptoms of spasticity and athetosis, the articulation is prone to be more distorted than if spasticity alone is present. Finally, the **diadochokinetic rate** of tongue lifting is a pretty good indication of the number of articulation errors to be found in any one case.

Athetosis (Dyskinesia)

By *athetosis* or *dyskinesia* we refer to motor abnormalities caused by damage to relay stations (extrapyramidal structures) located deep within the brain. Athetosis may be described as involuntary writhing contractions that affect one muscle after another. These contractions may be fast or slow, large or small. The head may swing from side to side. The arm may shake rhythmically. The jaw and facial muscles may show a rhythmic contortion or repetitive grimaces, but in some individuals, these movements disappear in sleep or under the influence of alcohol. There seem to be two major types of athetosis, the nontension type and tension athetosis, which is often mistaken for spasticity. The latter may be distinguished from true spasticity by moving the arm against the person's resistance. The tension athetoid arm tends to yield gradually; the spastic arm releases with a jerk.

Speech in athetosis often becomes weak in volume. The final sounds of words and final words of phrases are often whispered. A marked tremulo may be heard. Monotones are very common, and in athetosis tension, the habitual pitch can be near the upper limit of the range. Falsetto voice is not unusual. Another common voice quality is that of hoarseness, especially in the males. Persons with athetoid cerebral palsy make many articulation errors; and the finer the coordination involved in producing the sound, the more it is likely to be distorted. Tongue-tip sounds are especially difficult. Breathing disturbances are common, as are hearing and vision problems.

Hard contacts.
Hypertensed fixed articulatory postures, such as those assumed by stutterers in attempting feared words.

Diadochokinesis.
Rate of repetition of a spoken syllable.

Ataxia

Ataxia manifests itself mainly in a lack of ability to balance oneself or to coordinate the movements of muscle groups. Muscle tone is also very low. The person with ataxic cerebral palsy finds it very difficult to perform any complex activity—walking, writing, speaking—in a smooth, integrated series of motions. Her movements characteristically lack the appropriate rate, sufficient force, and proper direction. Ataxic speech is slurred and arrhythmic. This condition seems to be due to a lesion in the cerebellum and is very rarely the primary symptom in cerebral palsy.

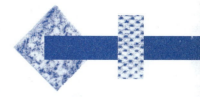

CLASSIFICATION BY BODY PARTS

Cerebral palsy is also classified in terms of how much of the body is affected. If one limb is spastic or athetoid, the term *monoplegia* is used; if half the body (right or left) is affected, the word *hemiplegia* designates the condition. *Diplegia* refers to involvement of both upper *or* both lower limbs; *quadriplegia* to spasticity or athetosis in all four limbs. The greatest number of articulatory errors are shown in quadriplegia involving combined athetosis and spasticity.

CAUSES OF CEREBRAL PALSY

Cerebral palsy is due to a brain injury occurring before birth (**prenatal**), at the time of birth (**perinatal**) or shortly after birth (postnatal). Although an exact cause often cannot be identified for the individual occurrence of cerebral palsy in at least one in 1,000 live births, the most common causes relate to brain hemorrhage and to lack of oxygen. In turn, many possible precipitants and risk factors are relatively well known. It is important to note here that modern medical knowledge and technology assure the survival of infants who, because of the severity of their congenital disorders, would not have survived at all just a few years ago. Thus it is reasonable to expect that the incidence of cerebral palsy and other developmental disabilities may be considerably greater than suggested by current data.[1]

In any event, prenatal brain insult may be due to the mother's suffering from an infectious disease (particularly rubella, or measles), or from diabetes. Exposure to lead or mercury can result in fetal malformations such as cerebral palsy, and other agents suspected as possible causes include nicotine, alcohol, drugs, and exposure to radiation. The importance of good prenatal health care is evident; but as observed by Billeaud (1993), "increasing numbers of pre-term, very-low-birth-weight, sick infants are

Ataxia.
Loss of ability to perform gross motor coordinations.

Prenatal.
Before birth.

Perinatal.
During the birth process.

being born to women who have had inadequate (or no) prenatal care." Unwed teenage mothers, also on the increase, no doubt account for many of these babies who will require special services for years to come.

Perinatal causes may include premature, difficult, or prolonged labor, and instrument injuries. As pointed out by Sparks (1984):

> Although the risk of injury due to obstetrical trauma is greatly reduced from former times, these injuries do occur. The infant at greatest risk for injury to any part of the central nervous system is the infant in breech presentation. . . . High incidence of asphyxia (or **anoxia**) and cerebral hemmorrhage associated with the delivery of the head occurs in this group. . . . Perinatal brain damage may also be the result of injury to blood vessels in the brain and consequent bleeding . . . (and) infants in a breech presentation are 10 times more likely to have subdural **hematomas** (blood clots due to bleeding from ruptured blood vessels) than those born in head-first presentation. . . . Large infants of mothers having their first baby and infants who are delivered rapidly of mothers who have had multiple deliveries are at risk for developing a subdural hemorrhage.
>
> Anesthetic agents given to the laboring mother may affect the fetus. Any agent that produces maternal hypotension may decrease the gas exchange between mother and fetus, resulting in reduction of oxygen to the fetus, which, in turn, may damage the brain. (pp. 127–128)

Postnatally, certain diseases in the very young child that are marked by a high fever (pneumonia, for example, or meningitis) also can result in cerebral palsy.

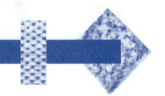

IMPACT OF CEREBRAL PALSY

Although some cerebral-palsied individuals are also retarded—perhaps as many as 50 percent (though it is very difficult to assess severely impaired persons with standard tests)—many possess normal intelligence. However, because they may stagger, drool, and make strange noises and bizarre grimaces when attempting to talk, some people get the wrong impression. Geri Jewell, a comedienne who is cerebral palsied, describes it this way in her autobiography:

> The disability makes you *appear* as if you haven't got a brain in your head, so many people mistake cerebral palsy for some kind of mental retardation. But our minds *are* alive and learning and questioning and doing what everybody else's mind is doing. It's because our lights aren't on, nobody thinks we're home. (From *Geri* by Geri Jewell, published by William Morrow and Co., 1984. Quoted by permission of the publisher.)

Intelligent cerebral-palsied individuals meet so many frustrations during their daily lives that they tend to build emotional handicaps as great

Anoxia.
Oxygen deficiency.

Hematoma.
Localized swelling filled with blood.

as their physical disabilities (Marinelli and Orto, 1984). They develop fears about walking, talking, eating, going downstairs, carrying a tray, holding a pencil, and a hundred other daily activities. These often become so intense that they create more tensions and hence more spasticity or athetosis. Thus one girl so feared to lift a coffee cup to her lips that she could not do so without spilling and breaking it; yet she was able to etch delicate tracings on a copper dish.

Many of these children are so pampered and protected by their parents that they never have an opportunity to learn the skills required of them for social living. Their parents are constantly afraid that they will hurt themselves, but as one adult with tension athetosis said to us, "My parents never let me try to ride a bicycle and now at last I've done it. Better to break your neck than your spirit." Many cerebral palsied people come to a fatalistic attitude of passive acceptance of whatever blows, kindnesses, or pity society may give them. Others put up a gallant battle and succeed in creating useful and satisfying lives for themselves.

A former client, now a doctoral student, described how academic success helped to enhance his feeling of self-worth.[2]

> I used to feel that my mind was imprisoned in this twisted body . . . but no longer, not since I discovered statistics. Now, despite the contractures from prolonged tension on my limbs, my slow, labored speech, I am treated as an equal in the arena of mathematics. I can even laugh now at the impossible situations my jerky movements create—like the night last weekend when I was arrested by a rookie campus security officer. I was coming home very late from the computer lab and lurching along the sidewalk in my usual fashion. Thinking I was an inebriated collegian, the officer stopped his patrol car and confronted me. When he heard me talk, he simply hustled me into the car and back to the station. It turned out that he thought my jerky spastic movements were signs of resisting arrest! Well, when it all got sorted out, we had a good chuckle and I think the officer and the university security department learned a good lesson: to become more aware of the handicapped.

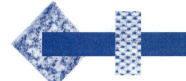

SPEECH THERAPY

At times the cerebral-palsied child is first presented as a case of delayed speech. These children often do not begin to talk until five or six, but many of them could learn earlier with proper parental teaching. In general, the same procedures used on other delayed-speech cases and in teaching the baby to talk are employed. Imitation must be taught. Sounds must come to have meaning and identity. Words must be taught in terms of their sound sequences and associations. Babbling games using puppets are especially effective in getting a young spastic child to talk. It is especially necessary that the child be praised for all vocalization, since he is likely to fall into a whispered or mere lip-moving type of speech. When possible, the first speech teaching should be done when the child is lying on his back in bed. Recordings with singing and speech games are very useful in stimulating these children.

In most cases of cerebral palsy the physical therapist and occupational therapist will have done a great deal of work with the child before the speech pathologist is called in. In some treatment settings, the entire therapy team carries out prespeech oromotor training through a carefully planned feeding program. The premise guiding this particular approach is that speech depends in part on the vegetative use of the tongue, lips, and jaws and that eating abnormalities may affect later attempts at sound production. In some cases, brain-injured children and adults may have *dysphagia,* a swallowing disorder "characterized by difficulty in oral preparation for the swallow or in moving the material from mouth to stomach" (Logemann, 1987, p. 57). Since the speech pathologist is familiar with the function of the oral area, she will be called upon to assess and perform therapy on individuals who have swallowing disorders.[3]

Many of the activities used in physical therapy can be made more interesting to the child if vocalization is used in conjunction with them. Thus one child whose very spastic left leg was being passively rotated in a whirlpool bath was taught to say "round and round; round and round" as the leg moved. He was unable to say these words at first under any other condition; but soon he had attained the ability to say them anywhere, and the distraction seemed to ease some of the spasticity. In some programs, general relaxation of the whole body forms a large part of the treatment of spasticity and tension athetosis, and even these exercises may be combined with sighing or yawning on the various vowels. Relaxation of the articulatory or the throat muscles seems to be very difficult for these cases, and we often indirectly attain decreases in the tension of these structures by teaching the child to speak while chewing.

Among several interesting approaches to the treatment of clients with cerebral palsy is that advocated by the Bobaths. Instead of using the traditional methods to induce general relaxation, the Bobath method, essentially a physical therapy approach, seeks first to inhibit the pathological reflex activity by holding the child firmly in a posture that prevents the usual abnormal motor activity. Then the primitive but normal reflexes are stimulated and facilitated, and finally, voluntary motor control is evoked. Some very surprising changes occur when this sequence is successfully carried out. We have seen young children with cerebral palsy who were thrashing around and unable to produce anything but strangled bursts of tortured vocalization become quiet and relaxed and able to babble normally when treated by a skillful Bobath practitioner.[4]

Some speech pathologists work closely with physical therapists using the Rood technique. This involves a systematic sequence of stimulation and relaxation of the muscular groups required for more effective coordination. By using such tools as ice, brushes, and other surface stimulators to stimulate or relax certain muscles, patterns of more normal motor behaviors can be developed. We have witnessed some remarkable improvement when these are introduced and reinforced. Articulation and voice changes resulting from the joint efforts of the speech pathologist and physical therapist working together in the application of these techniques are often very impressive.[5]

Rhythms of all kinds seem to provide especially favorable media for speech practice, if the rhythms are given at a speed that suits the particular case. In following these rhythms it is not wise to combine speech with muscular movements because of the nature of the disability. Visual stimuli such as the rhythmic swinging of a flashlight beam on a wall are very effective in producing more fluent speech. Tonal stimuli of all kinds are also used. Many children with cerebral palsy can utter polysyllabic words in unison with a recurrent melody whether they sing them or not.

In general, the child with cerebral palsy has inadequate control of her tongue. Most of the sounds that require lifting of the tongue tip are defective. When the /t/, /d/, and /n/sounds are adequate, it will be observed that they are dentalized. The tongue does not make contact with the upper-gum ridge but with the back surface of the teeth or it may be protruded. Several of our cases were able to acquire good /l/and /r/sounds without any direct teaching. Instead, we taught them to make the /t/, /d/, and /n/sounds against the upper-gum ridge, and the tongue-tip lifting carried over into the /l/and /r/sounds.

In most of these cases, the essential task is to free the tongue from its tendency to move only in conjunction with the lower jaw. The old traditional tongue exercises have little value, but those that involve the emergence of a finer movement from a gross one are very useful. Just as we have been able to teach a client to pick up a pin by beginning with trunk, arm, and wrist movements, so we can finally teach him to move his tongue tip without closing his mouth.

It should be obvious that no speech pathologist can hope to solve the many problems of giving the child with cerebral palsy usable speech unless the parents and other professional members help in the process. Much of the work of the speech clinician will involve demonstration and consultation. We cannot simply tell others how to facilitate speech. We must show them. In turn, in our work we also must reinforce the treatment being provided by other members of the team (Thompson, Rubin, and Bilenker, 1983; Tarnowski and Drabman, 1986).

At times one of the major obstacles in achieving useful speech in the person with cerebral palsy is the inability to produce voice without great struggle. When he tries to talk, he may exert great physical effort; and this may induce closures of both the true and false vocal folds. So we rarely work directly on voice production for this reason. Instead, we try to combine sounds and movements, and we stimulate him with pleasant sounds. We do a lot of singing and humming in our early speech therapy with these children, making speech pleasant, making sound production desirable. Often the breathing of the child with cerebral palsy shows great abnormality, especially when he tries to produce speech. He may inhale far too deeply, then exhale most of this air prior to speech attempt or in the utterance of just one syllable, and then strain from that time onward. He may even try to speak while inhaling, an activity that will evoke strain even in a normal speaker. These persons must be trained to eliminate these faulty procedures.

The breaks in fluency that are so characteristic of spasticity are often eliminated by this training, but it is usually wise to teach these children a type of phrasing that will not place too much demand upon them for sustained utterance. The pauses must be much more frequent than those of the normal individual, and they should be slightly longer. If he trains himself to speak short phrases on one breath, his fluency will improve. Moreover, since no untimely gasps for breath will occur, his voice will be less likely to rise in pitch, or to be strained, and the final sounds of the words will be better articulated.

Fluency may be improved also by giving the child training in making smooth transitions between vowels or consecutive consonants. Thus, he is asked to practice shifting gradually rather than suddenly from a prolonged /u/ to a prolonged /i/ sound to produce the word *we*. At first, breaks are likely to occur, but they can be greatly improved through practice; and the child's general speech reflects the improvement. Again the plosives often cause breaks in rhythm because the contacts are made too hard and consequently set up tremors. We have had success in treating these errors with the same methods we use for the stutterer's hard contacts. In one case, who always "stuck" on his /p/, /t/, and /k/ sounds and showed breaks in his speech, we were able to solve the problem by simply asking him "to keep his mouth in motion" whenever he said a word beginning with these sounds.

It may, of course, be necessary to supplement this speech therapy with informal psychotherapy, especially in adult clients. They must be taught an objective attitude toward their disorder. They must whittle down the emotional fraction of their total handicap; they must increase their assets in every way. As fear and shame diminish, the tensions will decrease. In many cases, greater improvement in speech and muscular coordination will come from psychotherapy than from the speech therapy itself (Rollin, 1987).

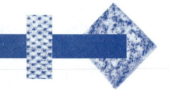

MOTOR SPEECH DISORDERS

All the diverse structures and systems that combine together to produce speech are regulated by the nervous system. Any damage or disease involving this regulatory system will disrupt the normally swift movements of the speech mechanism. This disruption is reflected in distortion of the speech signal, primarily in the utterance of speech sounds.

Basically, there are two types of motor speech disorders: dysarthria and apraxia. These two disorders may coexist or they may occur separately. When paralysis, weakness, or incoordination resulting from neuropathology disturbs the motor control centers, all facets of speech production—respiration, laryngeal control, resonance, articulation, and prosody—may malfunction. The resultant disorder is called *dysarthria,* or more properly, dysarthrias, since the term includes a group of motor speech impairments that stem from disturbance of the muscular control of the speech apparatus.

The Mayo Clinic research shows that six types of dysarthria can be differentiated from each other by listening carefully to how the afflicted person talks. Each neurological disorder attacks the nervous system at a particular site, causes specific motor impairments, and most important for differential diagnosis, produces characteristic patterns or clusters of speech symptoms. The specific features of the abnormal speech assist the neurologist in locating the lesion in the client's **peripheral** or **central nervous system.** We include Table 12.1, which delineates the six types of dysarthria according to neurological condition, site of lesion, neuromuscular symptoms, and major speech characteristics. To these types, a seventh, *Unilateral upper motor neuron* (UUMN), recently has been added. It involves weakness and incoordination, and it virtually always is associated with imprecise articulation of consonants. Phonation is disturbed in more than 50 percent of such patients; rate and prosody, in about one-quarter; and resonance, in only about 14 percent (Duffy, 1995).

As we pointed out in the last chapter, *apraxia* is the disruption of the capacity to program voluntarily the production and sequencing of speech sounds; although the individual does not show muscular paralysis, her articulation is garbled and she seems to have forgotten how to execute speech-related movements. In fact, the more volition involved in the execution of a particular act, the worse the client's performance seems to be.

Differential diagnosis is not an easy task because of the possible overlap between the two disorders. To assist you in distinguishing between dysarthria and apraxia, we include Table 12.2.

For further current information regarding motor speech disorders, consult the comprehensive works of Beukelman and Mirenda (1992), Duffy (1995), and Johns (1985).

Peripheral nervous system.
The nerves outside the brain and spinal cord; carries messages to and from the central nervous system.

Central nervous system (CNS).
The brain and spinal cord.

THE SEVERELY IMPAIRED

There are some clients with such severe cerebral palsy or other motor disabilities that the acquisition of intelligible speech is virtually impossible. Despite years of competent professional help, they lack the motor control needed for effective oral communication. In such cases it is both appropriate and necessary for the speech clinician to help the speechless client communicate through nonvocal means, using either high- or low-technology strategies.

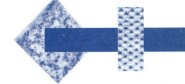

TABLE 12.1 Six Types of Dysarthria

Type	Site of Lesion	Neurological Disorder	Neuromuscular Condition	Speech Characteristics
Flaccid	Lower motor neuron (cranial nerves V, VII, IX, X, XII)	Bulbar palsy	Flaccid paralysis, hypotonia, atrophy	Imprecise consonants, hypernasality, breathy voice
Spastic	Upper motor neuron	Pseudobulbar palsy	Spastic paralysis, limited range of motion, slow movements	Strained-strangled harsh voice, slow rate, hypernasality, imprecise consonants
Ataxic	Cerebellum	Cerebellar ataxia	Inaccurate movements, hypotonia, slow movements	Excess and equal stress, irregular articulatory breakdown, prolongation of sounds
Hypokinetic	Basal ganglia	Parkinsonism	Slow movements, limited range of movements, rigidity, tremor	Monopitch, monoloudness, reduced stress, imprecise consonants, short rushes of speech
Hyperkinetic	Basal ganglia	Chorea	Quick involuntary movements	Imprecise consonants, variable rate, distorted vowels, monopitch
		Dystonias	Slow, twisting movements	Irregular articulation breakdown, monopitch, monoloudness
Mixed	Upper and lower motor neuron	Amyotrophic lateral sclerosis Multiple sclerosis	Gradual, progressive loss of motor control	Slow rate, reduced loudness, breathy voice, tremor in vowels

Based upon Darley, Aronson, and Brown (1975); see also, Duffy (1995)

TABLE 12.2 Differential Diagnosis of Dysarthria and Apraxia

	Dysarthria	Apraxia
Definition	Distinct patterns of speech due to weakness, slowness and incoordination of speech muscles. Oral movements are disrupted and reflect different types of neuropathology	Articulation errors, in the absence of muscle slowness, weakness, incoordination, due to disruption of cortical programming for the *voluntary* production of speech sounds
Oral peripheral examination	Obvious defectiveness: slow, weak, and incoordinated. *Vegetative* functions (sucking, chewing), disturbed as well as speech movements	No obvious dysfunction except when requested to execute *voluntary* movements. Vegetative functions performed adequately.
Articulation	Simplifications a. distortions b. substitutions Errors consistent More complex units (clusters of consonants) are more difficult More errors in final position Errors consistent with neurological record Severity related to extent of neuromuscular involvement	Complication a. transpositions, reversals b. perseverative and anticipatory errors c. few distortions, more substitutions, intrusive additions Errors increase proportionate to word weight (grammatical class, difficulty of initial consonant, position in sentence and word length) Fewer errors in spontaneous performance Inconsistency is key sign
Repeated utterance	Same performance	Makes repeated attempt and may achieve correct performance. Appears to grope or struggle.
Rate	Deterioration of performance with increased rate Slow rate of speech	Performance improves at faster rate Disturbances of prosody: stuttering-like struggle reactions; slow, labored speech during voluntary attempts
Response to stimulation	May alter performance slightly to match auditory-visual model. Best response to demonstration of specific articulatory gestures	Best performance if sees and hears model. Does better if provided one stimulation and given several chances to match the model

From Emerick and Haynes (1986); also see Haynes, Pindzola, and Emerick (1992)

Humans have used nonvocal modes of communication for a long time—smoke signals, Morse code, semaphore flags, and the hand signals used in professional sports are just a few examples. What is relatively new, however, is the application of nonvocal systems to help the handicapped share what they think and feel. The helping professions, with speech pathology leading the way, are now providing two basic types of nonoral systems: (1) modes of communication that *replace* the vocal tract, typically for those individuals who have little or no prospect of ever talking, and (2) modes of communication that *augment* or supplement the limited speaking abilities of the individual; hence, the terminology Augmentative and Alternative Communication (AAC) is often encountered. The augmentative approach is often used with young children because it fosters social exchange, which in turn enhances a youngster's desire to communicate both orally and by nonvocal means.

A number of factors are included in making the decision as to whether an individual is a suitable candidate for an AAC system and to determine the *type* of system to employ. The client's visual, auditory, and motor skills, his level of cognitive development and intelligence, and his motivation and need for communication are some of the variables that a treatment team will use in determining if a child can utilize an alternative gesture or symbol system. We include now a portion of a clinical report in which a speech pathologist establishes the rationale for developing a nonoral communication system for an eight-year-old with quadriplegic spasticity.

> Sally has received conventional speech therapy for five years with no appreciable improvement. She is able to produce only a weak, tense, and erratic phonation. Attempts at consonant sounds elicit an exaggerated mandibular extensor thrust.
>
> According to the child's case history, all prespeech oral activity—sucking, chewing, swallowing—were delayed. At the present time she still has abnormal oral reflexes.
>
> Sally's receptive language skills are in the low-normal range. A test of verbal intelligence placed her at the seventy-eighth percentile for receptive vocabulary.
>
> The child seems very eager to communicate; at the present time she taps with an unsharpened pencil to indicate "yes" and "no" in response to questions directed to her. Her parents are willing to cooperate in any program which will enhance their ability to communicate with Sally.

Augmentative and Alternative Communication Systems

In the past few years, many ingenious devices and techniques have been adapted or invented to help the speechless communicate. We describe only a few of the most commonly used nonvocal communication systems.

Gestures.   Messages transmitted visually by means of movements of body parts are the most direct form of nonvocal communication. Gestures may be as simple as coded eye blinks or foot taps (1 blink = no; 2 = yes; 3 = need to use bathroom) or as complex as a system of hand signals such as the American Manual Alphabet or the American Indian Sign Language (Amerind). The manual alphabet consists of finger movements that depict letters, while Amerind comprises pictographs that portray whole concepts or ideas (Figure 12-1).

Communication Boards.   Communication boards of various types have been designed to aid in the communication process. Sometimes the person can point to the appropriate spot with his hand or perhaps his foot. At other times, for this pointing he may be able to use a headstick as illustrated in Figure 12-2. For those who cannot even point, the desired picture symbol or word may be located by scanning first the horizontal and then the vertical columns, the client indicating by his yes or no signal which one contains the item needed. Very simple boards are used at first and more complicated ones later.

Communication boards that utilize symbols rather than a limited set of pictures offer greater communicative potential because the client can combine the items into phrases and sentences. There are many nonalphabetical symbol systems available and Figure 12-3 illustrates three of the more frequently used types. The Rebus symbols are somewhat easier to learn because they look like the action or object they represent. However, the **Blissymbolics** can be combined in various ways to present almost any message; not all of the symbols are **iconic,** as Figure 12-4 illustrates.

Although the Blissymbols at first appear rather abstract, they seem to be easily learned. Moreover, since the word represented by the symbols is presented underneath it, many severely handicapped children learn to read this way, and other people who do not know the system can use the printed words to communicate with them.

Electronic and Computer Enhancement.   Biomedical engineers have created ingenious devices and techniques to allow the speechless

Blissymbolics.
A set of pictographs for the nonverbal person.

Iconic.
Words, signs, that resemble what they represent.

FIGURE 12-1   Examples of the American Manual Alphabet and Amerind

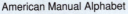

American Manual Alphabet   Amerind Pictograph for "Cry"

C   A   T   T

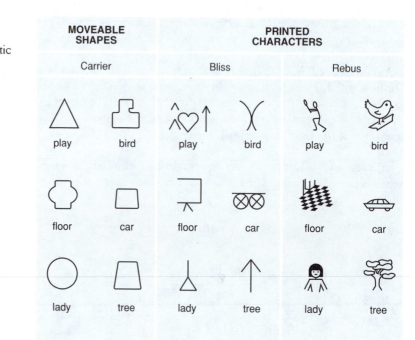

 FIGURE 12-2   A communication aid for the severely handicapped

 FIGURE 12-3
Examples of
symbols from nonalphabetic
systems   (Clark, 1981)

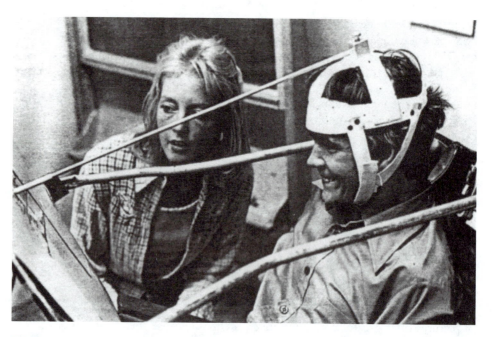

Ear	(To) Hear	Book	Before, In Front Of	After, Behind

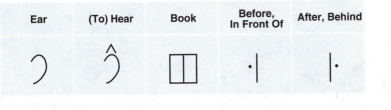

 FIGURE 12-4 Some representative Blissymbols (Blissymbolics used herein, Blissymbolics Communication Institute 1981, Toronto, Canada)

individual to communicate.[6] The signaling can be done through the use of electronic switches coupled to the breathing or head, eye, arm, or trunk movements, even the slight tensing of a muscle that does not move (Fishman, 1987). There are several models of electronic synthesizers that emit audible signals when the person presses appropriate buttons on a keyboard. Miniaturized electronic "typewriters" have been used to produce messages on a continuous paper display or on a television monitor.

AAC options also include a variety of dedicated computer-based devices and a wide array of software programs that allow any personal computer to be used as an assistive device for communication (Figure 12-5). The interested student will find comprehensive discussions of many AAC methods, strategies, and technologies in Blackstone (1986) and Beukelman and Mirenda (1992).

All members of the healing professions will encounter speechless clients sooner or later, for they include not only the cerebral palsied but also persons who are tracheotomized, who have suffered spinal cord injuries, who have severe motor speech disorders, and who present other debilitating and often progressive neurologic problems. In some instances, as we noted in Chapter 6, even autistic children may utilize AAC systems (Mirenda and Mathy, 1989). The speech-language pathologist in particular must remember that effective communication is his goal, not simply better speech.

STUDY QUESTIONS

1. The vast majority of cerebral-palsied individuals fall into what two major varieties of the disorder?
2. What are the two principal causes of cerebral palsy?
3. What prenatal factors are believed to cause an infant to be at risk for developmental disability?
3. For what reasons might we expect to see increasing numbers of cerebral palsied and other developmentally disabled youngsters in coming years?

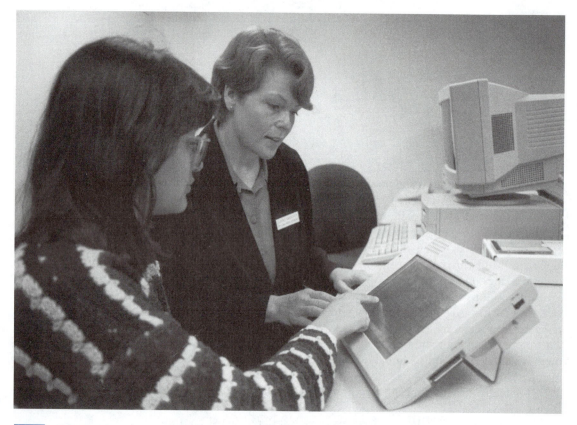

FIGURE 12-5   A variety of instruments and software packages are available for augmentative and alternative communication purposes *(Van Riper Clinic, Western Michigan University)*

4. What is meant by the term "dyskinesia," and what older term is this replacing in the classification of cerebral palsies?

5. Explain, as you would to the family of an individual with an acquired motor speech disorder, what is meant by "dysarthria."

6. What are the traditional six types of dysarthria, and how can we differentiate dysarthria from apraxia?

7. What aspects of speech can be affected by dysarthria?

8. For what do the initials AAC stand for, and what are three examples of AAC systems or strategies?

9. What types of clients are potential candidates for using AAC?

10. An interdisciplinary team working with children who have cerebral palsy is likely to have representation from what professions?

ENDNOTES

[1]For a review of the current trends regarding the cause and prevalence of cerebral palsy, see Pharoah et al. (1987).

[2]The two books by Marie Killilea (1952, 1963) present a moving portrait of parental dedication and the indomitable spirit of a cerebral-palsied child. See also books by Miers (1966), Blank (1966), Segal (1966), and Shelley and Shelley (1985), and the controversial play by Nichols (1967).

[3]Two references that will help you explore this topic are Morris (1982) and Logemann (1983).

[4]Crickmay (1966) presents a clear picture of this kind of treatment.

[5]Two approaches utilizing modern technology, biofeedback (Flodmark, 1986) and electrical implantation (Wolfe, Ratushik, and Penn, 1981) may turn out to be of benefit in the treatment of cerebral palsy.

[6]We are confident that technology will continue to produce new inexpensive, miniaturized communication aids. To keep up with new developments, consult the periodical *AAC: Augmentative and Alternative Communication.*

REFERENCES

Beukelman, D., and Mirenda, P. (1992). *Augmentative and Alternative Communication: Management of severe communication disorders in children and adults.*

Billeaud, F. (1993). *Communication disorders in infants and toddlers: Assessment and intervention.* Stoneham, MA: Butterworth-Heinemann.

Blackstone, S. (1986). *Augmentative communication: An introduction.* Rockville, MD: American Speech-Language-Hearing Association.

Blank, J. (1966). *19 steps up the mountain.* New York: Jove.

Blondis, T., Roizen, N., Snow, J., and Accardo, P. (1993). Developmental disabilities: A continuum. *Clinical Pediatrics,* 32(8), 492–498.

Crickmay, M. (1966). *Speech therapy and the Bobath approach to cerebral palsy.* Springfield, IL: Charles C. Thomas.

Darley, F., Aronson, A., and Brown, J. (1975). *Motor speech disorders.* Philadelphia: Saunders.

Duffy, J. (1995). *Motor Speech Disorders: Substrates, differential diagnosis, and management.* St. Louis, MO: Mosby-Year Book.

Emerick, L., and Haynes, W. (1986). *Diagnosis and evaluation in speech pathology* (3rd ed.). Englewood Cliffs, NJ: Prentice Hall.

Fishman, I. (1987). *Electronic communication aids: Selection and use.* San Diego, CA: College-Hill Press.

Flodmark, A. (1986). Augmented auditory feedback as an aid in gait training of cerebral-palsied children. *Developmental Medicine and Child Neurology,* 28, 147–155.

Hardy, J. (1994). Cerebral palsy. In G. Shames, E. Wiig, and W. Secord (eds.), *Human communication disorders: An introduction.* New York: Macmillan College Publishing Company.

Haynes, W., Pindzola, R., and Emerick, L. (1992). *Diagnosis and evaluation in speech pathology,* (4th ed.). Englewood Cliffs, NJ: Prentice Hall.

Jewell, G. (1994). *Geri.* New York: William Morrow and Company.

Johns, D. (ed.). (1985). *Clinical management of neurogenic communicative disorders.* Boston, MA: College-Hill Press.

Killilea, M. (1952). *Karen.* Englewood Cliffs, NJ: Prentice Hall.

Killilea, M. (1963). *With love from Karen*. Englewood Cliffs, NJ: Prentice Hall.

Logemann, J., Chair. (1987). Ad hoc committee on dysphasia report. *Journal of the American Speech and Hearing Association, 29*, 57–58.

Logemann, J. (1983). *Evaluation and treatment of swallowing disorders*. San Diego, CA: College-Hill Press.

Marinelli, R., and Orto, A. (eds.). (1984). *Psychological and social impact of physical disability* (2nd ed.). New York: Springer-Verlag.

Miers, E. (1966). *The trouble bush*. Chicago: Rand McNally.

Mirenda, P., and Mathy, P. (1989). Augmentative and alternative communication applications for persons with severe congenital communication disorders: An introduction. *AAC: Augmentative and Alternative Communication, 5*(1), 3–13.

Morris, S. (1982). *The normal acquisition of oral feeding skills: Implications for assessment and treatment*. New York: Therapeutic Media.

Nichols, P. (1967). *Joe Egg*. New York: Grove Press.

Pharoah, P., et al. (1987). Trends in birth prevalence of cerebral palsy. *Archives of Disease in Childhood, 62*, 379–384.

Rollin, W. (1987). *The psychology of communication disorders in individuals and their families*. Englewood Cliffs, NJ: Prentice Hall.

Segal, M. (1966). *Run away, little girl*. New York: Random House.

Shelley, H., and Shelley, M. (1985). *Love is two plastic straws*. Columbus, OH.

Sparks, S. (1984). *Birth defects and speech-language disorders*. San Diego, CA: College-Hill Press.

Tarnowski, K., and Drabman, R. (1986). Increasing the communicator usage skills of a cerebral-palsied adolescent. *Journal of Pediatric Psychology, 11*, 573–581.

Thompson, G., Rubin, I., and Bilenker, R. (eds.). (1983) *Comprehensive management of cerebral palsy*. New York: Grune and Stratton.

Wertz, R. (1985). Neuropathologies of speech and language: An introduction to patient management. In D. Johns (ed.), *Clinical management of neurogenic communicative disorders*. Boston, MA: College-Hill Press.

Wolfe, V., Ratusnik, D., and Penn, R. (1981). Long-term effects on speech of chronic cerebellar stimulation in cerebral palsy. *Journal of Speech and Hearing Disorders, 46*, 286–290.

SUPPLEMENTARY READINGS

Blackman, J. (ed.) (1990). *Medical aspects of developmental disabilities in children birth to three* (2nd ed.). Rockville, MD: Aspen.

Clark, C. (1981). Learning words using traditional orthography and the symbols of Rebus, Bliss and Carrier. *Journal of Speech and Hearing Disorders, 46*, 191–196.

Healy, A. (1990). Cerebral palsy. In J. Blackman (ed.), *Medical aspects of developmental disabilities in children birth to three* (2nd ed.). Rockville, MD: Aspen.

Sparks, S., Clark, M., Erickson, R., and Oas, D. (1990). *Infants at risk for communication disorders: The professional's role with the newborn*. Tucson, AZ: Communication Skill Builders.

Hearing and Hearing Impairment

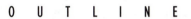

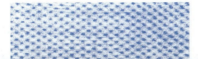

While all of our senses are extremely important to us, hearing is clearly the most critical for the development and maintenance of normal human functioning. Even Helen Keller, who could neither hear nor see, emphasized its importance, noting unequivocally that if she were able to choose to have either vision or hearing, she would choose to hear. People whose hearing is seriously impaired, by and large, are easily able to understand her choice. They, too, are acutely aware of how handicapping the loss of hearing can be.

Those of us who possess and take for granted the ability to hear normally, especially if we've had no family members or close acquaintances with impaired hearing, may have had little occasion to consider the exceptional significance of the auditory sense. The acquisition and monitoring of speech, the detection of potential danger, the perception of comfort conveyed by a friendly voice, the elemental feeling simply of existing in a living universe—all depend upon the auditory modality.

Thus far we have been considering communication problems associated with the formulation and sending of messages. But communication is a two-way street; spoken messages must also be received if communication is to occur. We have seen that some children with language difficulties have a history of hearing loss and that clients of any age with articulation or voice problems, whether functional or organic, may also have hearing difficulties that contribute to their disabilities. Moreover, we know that the prevalence of hearing loss will continue to rise as our population ages.

If you plan to become a speech-language pathologist, you will also have additional coursework that focuses on hearing and hearing impairment in much greater detail than we have included in this introductory overview. If you should decide to become an audiologist, of course, your highly specialized courses and practica will soon lead you to a much broader and deeper exploration of these very complex topics. But even if you do not expect to join either of these professions, you need at least to have a cursory understanding of the basic information in this chapter to be able to understand, and perhaps to serve in some other way, the many persons you will encounter who have some degree of hearing impairment.

THE HEARING MECHANISM

Although we shall not review the hearing mechanism[1] in detail, we will briefly discuss its three major parts: the outer ear, the middle ear, and the inner ear (Figure 13-1).

Auricle.
The visible outer ear.

The Outer Ear

When we ordinarily think of the ear we think of its visible portion, the **auricle** or *pinna*. Some of us can wiggle our auricles or pinnae. A few per-

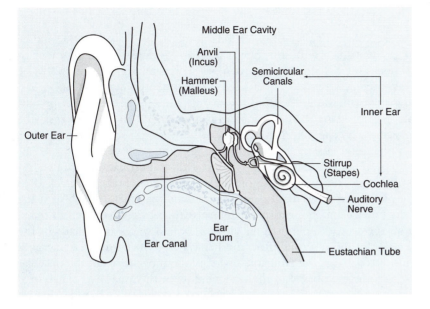

Middle Ear Cavity

Anvil
(Incus)

Hammer
(Malleus)

Semicircular
Canals

Inner Ear

Outer Ear

Stirrup
(Stapes)

Cochlea

Auditory
Nerve

Ear
Drum

Ear Canal

Eustachian Tube

FIGURE 13-1
Cross section of
the ear (*Courtesy of
Michigan Board of Health*)

sons are born without them and yet may have adequate hearing because
the ear you see makes only a minor contribution to hearing in humans. In
some animals, however, the external ears can be raised and pointed to help
in the location of sounds. Human auricles vary widely in size and shape so
much that some European police regularly use ear prints as well as fingerprints for identification. But even if your ears were cut off, their removal would result in a loss of hearing sensitivity of only about 5 or 6
decibels, not enough to make any real difference, and cupping your hand
to your ear increases your hearing sensitivity by the same negligible
amount. Turning your head toward the sound source helps somewhat in
locating it because of the head shadow effect (the ear away from the sound
source receives less energy).

Besides the auricle, the **outer ear** includes the *external auditory canal,*
a short passageway leading to the eardrum (**tympanic membrane**), When
sound waves are conveyed down this short funnel they cause the tympanic
membrane to vibrate in synchronization with the sound. On the inner surface of the canal there are small hairs, called cilia, and the ceruminous
glands, which secrete *cerumen,* the yellow wax you doubtless have noticed
from time to time. Both the cilia and the wax help to protect the tympanic
membrane from the dirt, insects, and foreign objects that far too often find
their way into the canal. The inner portion of the canal is bony and becomes
narrowed just in front of the eardrum, and it is there that foreign objects
tend to lodge. Help your children learn to keep things out of their ears.

Outer ear.
The auricles (pinnae)
and external ear canal.

Tympanic membrane.
The eardrum.

Cerumen.
Substance secreted by
external ear; earwax.

The Middle Ear

The second major part of our auditory mechanism is called the middle ear or tympanic cavity. Imagine it as a tiny irregularly shaped room or chamber about the size of a garden pea with a ceiling, a floor, and walls. The tympanic membrane is situated on the side wall of this chamber and it separates the outer ear from the middle ear. It is conical in shape, not flat, the tip of the shallow cone facing inward. When the otologist (the physician who specializes in diseases of the ear) inspects the ear, he sees only the outer surface of this tympanic membrane, and if normal, it appears pearly gray and tightly drawn and without perforations or other abnormalities. The rear surface of the tympanic membrane is attached to one of a set of three tiny bones, the **malleus** (hammer), which with the **incus** (anvil), and **stapes** (stirrup), forms an *ossicular chain*, which transforms the acoustic energy in the airborne sound waves as reflected by the vibration of the eardrum into a mechanical type of energy. This energy is transmitted across the tympanic cavity by the movements of the ossicular chain to the membrane of the oval window of the inner ear.[2] There it is transformed into liquid waves that trigger the nervous impulses that go to the brain.

Another important structure that we find within the middle ear is the opening to the *eustachian tube*. The eustachian tube forms a back-door connection between the middle ear and the **nasopharynx.** Its function is to aerate the middle ear so that the air pressure behind the drum equals that in front of it, an arrangement that lets it vibrate freely. We experience a feeling of fullness in our ears when we climb a mountain or make a rapid plane descent. This condition is due to differences in outside and inside air pressure and is relieved by yawning or swallowing, since during these activities the eustachian tube is then opened, allowing air to pass into the middle ear.

Although the eustachian tube performs this useful function, it is also the avenue for many infections that travel upward from the throat into the middle ear cavity and result in earaches. Finally, in the middle ear there are the tendons of two muscles, the tensor tympani and the stapedius, which tighten the eardrum immediately when very loud sounds occur, thus protecting our hearing from damage.

The Inner Ear

The third major part of the auditory mechanism is called the **inner ear,** also known as the labyrinth because of its many intricate chambers and canals. It contains three *semicircular canals* that help us to balance ourselves, a snail-shell-shaped structure called the *cochlea*, which contains the nerve endings of the eighth cranial nerve essential for the transmission of auditory information to the brain, and the *vestibule*, which connects the

Malleus.
The bone of the middle ear that rests against the eardrum.

Incus.
The second of three tiny bones in the middle ear.

Stapes.
The innermost bone of the middle ear.

Nasopharynx.
That part of the throat, pharnyx, above the level of the base of the uvula.

Inner ear.
Comprised of the cochlea, the semicircular canals, and the vestibule; important in balance as well as hearing.

cochlea with the semicircular canals. Since one of the tiny bones of the ossicular chain within the middle ear fits into an opening of the vestibule known as the *oval window,* its vibrations create movements in the inner-ear fluid; these fluid waves excite specialized nerve endings called *hair cells* in the cochlea; and the nervous impulses so produced then travel to the auditory cortex via the eighth (*acoustic* or *auditory*) cranial nerve to produce the sensations we call hearing.

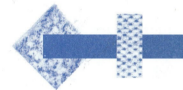

THE DETECTION AND EVALUATION OF HEARING LOSS

Although hearing loss affects nearly 30 million people in this country—more people than are affected by any other chronic health condition—impaired hearing too often is not easily recognized. Even instances of severe impairment are sometimes overlooked. Consequently, the person with impaired hearing may not receive appropriate or timely attention. This is especially unfortunate, because early intervention can help to reduce the impact of a hearing loss and prevent its worsening.

We will be more likely to know when a hearing loss might be suspected (in ourselves as well as in someone else) if we are aware of the variety of effects that may be associated with a hearing problem. The following list of indicators, adapted from those compiled by Bate and Davis (1985), can help us to know when a hearing loss may be present.

1. Complains of **tinnitus** (head noises or ringing in the ears) or stuffiness in the ears.
2. Has tenderness, itching, heat, or pain about the ear.
3. Has moisture or discharge in the ear canal or outer portion of the ear.
4. Experiences vertigo (dizziness).
5. Shows any sudden change in attitude or response, especially after an illness.
6. Shows inattention and frequent failure to respond to questions.
7. Frequently requests to have words, instructions, or assignments repeated.
8. Has difficulty hearing or understanding conversation in a group, as shown by frowning, straining, leaning forward when the person is addressed, or by misunderstandings of what was said.
9. Holds head in peculiar position, such as turning one ear toward the speaker or tilting the head while listening.
10. Has difficulty in locating the direction from which a sound comes and/or slow to respond to which person is talking.

Tinnitus.
Ringing noises in the ear.

11. Shows defects of speech, such as faulty articulation, mispronunciation of simple words, monotonous or abnormally pitched voice, abnormally loud or abnormally soft voice.
12. Shows signs of weariness or fatigue early in the day, or exhaustion at the end of the day.
13. Has emotional instability, unexplained irritability, timidity, marked introversion, supersensitivity, or withdrawal tendencies.
14. Waits for others to react. Follows the actions of others, taking cues from what others are doing, such as laughing, getting out books, materials, and following instructions.
15. Shows academic achievement below average, but IQ above average.
16. Seems to lose interest easily, especially when having to listen.
17. Appears to engage in frequent daydreaming.
18. Looks at other children's papers or work (school child).
19. Ignores or misunderstands announcements over loudspeaker systems.
20. Performs poorly on tasks requiring hearing only, such as tape recorded messages, telephone messages.
21. Appears to hear or understand when he or she really wants to, that is, seems to hear well when interest level is high.
22. Has deficient vocabulary.
23. Has deficient written work, as manifested by incomplete sentences, dropped endings of words, telegraphic style, and omitted articles.
24. Complains about, or is distracted by, background noise or other interfering noise. May be unable to ignore some competing noise.
25. Reports own voice "sounds funny."
26. Has difficulty following verbal instructions.
27. Turns TV volume too loud for others.
28. Has increased difficulty understanding persons with foreign accents or unfamiliar dialects.
29. Has difficulty hearing or understanding plays, lectures, and sermons.
30. Unable to hear as well when not facing the person speaking.
31. States that words seem clearer when spoken slowly than when spoken loudly.
32. Shows late development of speech and language in young child.
33. Fails to be awakened or quieted by sound of parent's voice (baby).
34. Fails to turn eyes and/or head in direction of sound (baby) (Figure 13-2).
35. Has history of hearing loss in family members.

When one or more of the foregoing signs are regularly noted, referral should be made to an audiologist or to an otologist so the individual's hearing can be evaluated. As we shall see later, certain conditions also are known to predispose infants to hearing loss, and in many communities provision is made for the early detection of such problems. Additionally, for legal as well as other reasons, adults who are at risk for hearing problems (for example, because of their frequent exposure to high noise levels) sometimes also are scheduled routinely for regular hearing evaluations.

In any event, when a hearing loss exists its degree and nature generally are evaluated by using two primary procedures, *pure tone* **audiometry** and *speech audiometry.* In both types of testing certain stimuli (tones at several frequencies or test words and phrases) are systematically presented to one or both ears of the client at varying intensity levels so that the threshold of hearing can be ascertained. In other words, the examiner seeks to discover how much the test stimuli must be amplified before the client can hear or recognize them. We include also brief descriptions of *acoustic immittance* testing and of *electrophysiological* procedures that do not require the volun-

Audiometry.
The measurement of hearing; includes pure tone testing and speech reception testing as well as a wide variety of specialized procedures.

 FIGURE 13-2   Estimations of a toddler's free-field hearing acuity may be obtained by observing her response (e.g., head turning) to varying levels of loudness when sounds are presented by loudspeaker (*Van Riper Clinic, Western Michigan University*)

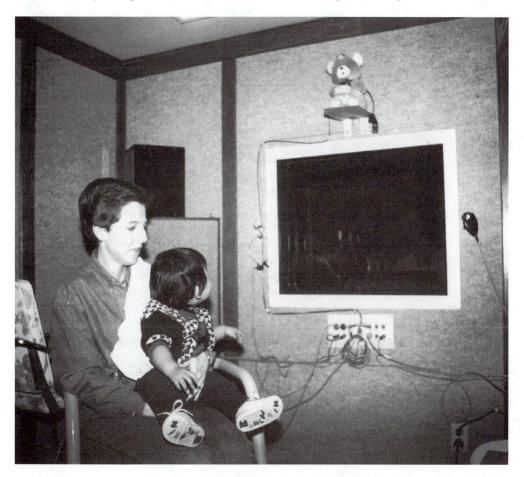

tary participation of the client and that help in determining what portion of the auditory mechanism is defective.

Pure Tone Audiometry

The pure tone audiometer is a carefully calibrated instrument that can generate and amplify tones of fixed frequency. Since hearing sensitivity varies over the range of audible frequencies, the audiometer can produce test tones ranging from the very low-pitched frequency level of 125 Hz through 250 (middle C), 500, 1000, 2000, 3000, 6000 Hz frequency levels to a final testing at the high-pitched sound of 8000 Hz. Using just one tone at a time, and feeding it into only one ear, the audiologist gradually increases its intensity in small steps until the client signals (usually by pressing a button to turn on a light or by raising his hand).

The following instructions to a client whose hearing is being tested by pure tone audiometry may make the procedure clearer.[3]

> I want to see how well you are able to hear several test tones (examiner lets the junior high school student hear 500, 1000, 2000 Hz at a loud level *before* putting on the earphones). That is what they sound like, but they will be much softer. Now, when I put the earphones on you, I will let you hear the test tone for 1 or 2 seconds at a comfortable listening level. The tone will be in only *one* earphone—we will start with your right ear since you feel you hear equally well in either ear. When you hear the tone, raise your hand. Keep your hand raised until the test tone stops and then lower it *immediately*. Once you get the feel for the task, I will make the tone very soft, and then make it louder or softer as you signal me. We will do each test tone in the same way. Do you understand? Remember, now, raise your hand *only* while you hear the tone, and then lower it right away when the tone stops.

Normally, we hear other people talking by means of air conduction, whereby the sound travels through the outer and middle ear and into the inner ear. When *we* speak, we hear ourselves by air conduction and also by **bone conduction.** In bone-conduction hearing, the stimulus is conveyed directly to the inner ear by the vibrations of the bones of the skull. It is because we normally hear ourselves by both air and bone conduction when we speak that many people are quite amazed to hear how their voices sound the first time they hear a tape recording of themselves. The reason they sound so different is that they are hearing themselves strictly by air conduction for the first time.

Bone conduction.
The transmission of sound waves directly to the cochlea by the bones of the skull.

In examining hearing, the audiologist tests both by air conduction and by bone conduction. The air-conduction testing is accomplished through earphones, whereas bone conduction is tested by bypassing the outer and middle ears and testing directly with a bone vibrator placed at some point on the skull. Formerly, the mastoid was the usual choice, but other placements, such as the forehead, now are used as the site for the vibrator.

The results obtained during this testing are expressed as audiograms such as those shown in Figure 13-3. On an **audiogram** the upper (zero) horizontal line represents the reference **intensity** level at which an average normal ear would detect a tone at each frequency (indicated by vertical lines). In the first audiogram, for example, a normal threshold was established for bone-conducted tones in both ears. Parallel lines below the zero line show relative intensity levels, or Hearing Level (HL). Again on our first audiogram, we see that this examinee did not respond to a 250 Hz air-conducted tone at any intensity level less than 45 dB HL in either ear. By inspecting the audiogram we can see how much (and what kind) of a hearing loss the client shows for each of the frequencies being tested. Shortly we shall return to a discussion of these types of hearing loss.

Speech Audiometry

Although the pure tone audiometer can provide a fairly accurate evaluation of hearing loss, the hearing-handicapped individual's main disability lies in his comprehension of speech. Accordingly, speech audiometers and testing procedures have been devised to determine how loud simple speech must be before the person can understand it. Speech audiometry, therefore, uses standardized sets of test words for this purpose. Among these are the lists of two-syllable words called *spondee* words. They are used to determine the *SRT* or *Speech Recognition Threshold* (also called the *ST* or *Spondee Threshold*), defined as the hearing level at which the client can repeat half of the series of words correctly. The more hard of hearing the person is, the more the words must be amplified before he gets half of them correct. These test words may come from the live voice of the audiologist in another soundproof room or from a recording. Either way they are delivered via earphones or through a loudspeaker.

Besides determining the speech recognition threshold, speech audiometry may include other testing procedures to discover, for example, the person's tolerance of amplified speech. In other words, the audiologist tries to find the intensity level at which the client feels too much discomfort, a factor important in the fitting of hearing aids. Since the hard-of-hearing person can often hear speech and yet, because a hearing disorder may interfere with intelligibility, not be able to understand speech, *word recognition,* or *speech discrimination,* testing is also administered to most clients. (As a matter of fact, one sign of an eighth cranial nerve lesion can be a deterioration of speech discrimination that is disproportionately great relative to any actual loss of hearing acuity.) The stimuli used in word recognition testing consist of lists of monosyllabic words, some of which may be phonetically balanced (PB) lists. Responses are scored in terms of the percentage of words heard correctly, as shown by the client's ability to repeat them or write them on a test sheet. This

Audiogram.
Graphic record of hearing test results showing hearing levels in dB at various frequencies.

Intensity.
The power or pressure magnitude of sound; loudness.

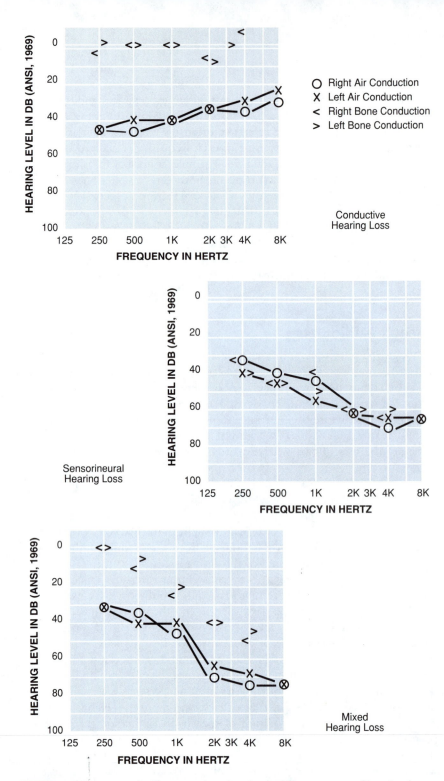

FIGURE 13-3 Audiograms showing three different types of hearing loss. (*ANSI refers to the American National Standards Institute reference zero for pure tone audiometers*)

procedure is used to determine how well the person understands speech under optimum listening conditions, as well as under other commonly encountered circumstances—such as when speech is present at an average conversational level (about 45 dB HL) and at faint speech levels (about 25 dB HL).

Acoustic Immittance Testing

A comprehensive hearing evaluation typically also involves *immittance testing* (also known as *otoadmittance*, or *aural acoustic immittance*, or *impedance* audiometry), which includes *tympanometry* and **acoustic reflex** measurement (Figure 13-4). In tympanometry, movements of the eardrum are measured while air pressure in the external auditory canal is being increased and decreased. The presence of fluid in the middle ear

> **Acoustic reflex.** Automatic contraction of the middle ear musculature in response to loud sound; a protective reaction.

FIGURE 13-4   Normal compliance of the right eardrum has been revealed by tympanometry results (*Van Riper Clinic, Western Michigan University*)

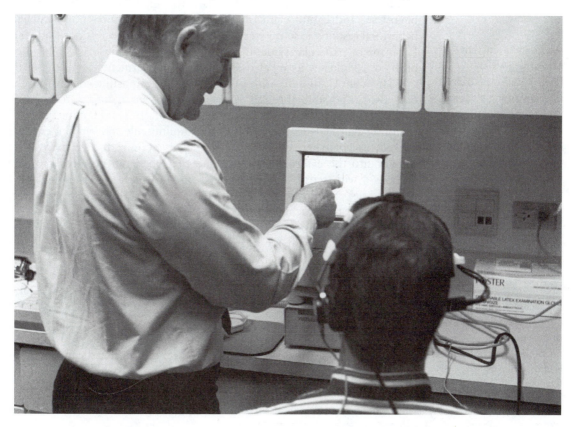

usually affects this test, as does blockage of the eustachian tube. Tympanometry evaluates middle ear function and can identify the need for medical attention even when hearing is not (or is not yet) seriously impaired. Acoustic reflex testing measures the responsivity of the stapedius and tensor tympani muscles to loud noise, thereby also providing information about middle ear function and, in some instances, about functioning of the eighth nerve and lower brainstem.[4]

Electrophysiological Measures

Although not done routinely in hearing evaluations, it is possible to examine some of the ways in which a person's auditory system is functioning (or not functioning) by observing brain wave activity in response to acoustic stimuli. In *auditory evoked response* (AER) or **auditory brainstem response** (ABR) testing, repetitive clicks at varied intensities are used to evoke electrical activity in the auditory portion of the eighth nerve and **brainstem** (Figure 13-5). These tiny waveforms, sensed by electrodes placed on the head, are processed by computer and compared to those of normal-hearing subjects. Delayed, absent, or abnormal waveforms then are differentially interpreted with regard to functioning of the cochlea, brainstem, and eighth cranial nerve. ABR testing requires no voluntary behavioral responses, so it is very useful with difficult-to-test populations. It can be of particular value in assessing infants (within hours following birth) or toddlers who are at risk for hearing impairment.

The identification of some hearing losses by evaluating cochlear function also is possible through *otoacoustic emissions testing*. Otoacoustic emissions (OAE) are sounds generated by expansions and contractions of the outer hair cells in the cochlea. These minuscule movements can be evoked, except when the cells are damaged, by introducing controlled sounds into the external ear canal, and they then can be measured (as "echoes") with sensitive computerized instrumentation. Assuming normal middle ear function, evoked OAE can help distinguish between cochlear and retrocochlear involvement in cases of **sensorineural hearing loss**.

Finally, we should mention *electronystagmography* (ENG), a battery of tests used, often by audiologists, to assess balance function. ENG actually monitors eye movements under a variety of stimulus conditions. Our brains normally use information from the inner ear, the eyes, and bodily muscles and joints to control balance. Balance problems may cause abnormal eye movements when the eyes and ears are stimulated in certain ways; and in ENG procedures, eye movements picked up by electrodes near the eyes and on the forehead can be computer analyzed and compared to norms in order to evaluate balance function.

Auditory brainstem response (ABR).
Procedure for detecting and measuring electrical activity in the brain in response to stimulation of the ear with sound; does not require voluntary response from examinee.

Brainstem.
The midbrain; pons and medulla oblongata.

Sensorineural hearing loss.
Impairment due to abnormality or disease of the inner ear or the cochlear portion of the auditory nerve.

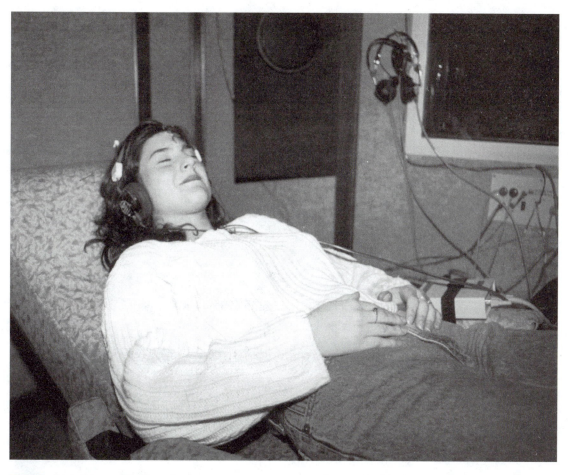

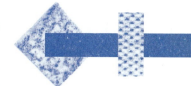

FIGURE 13-5   Auditory brainstem response testing is done with the client completely quiet and relaxed (*Van Riper Clinic, Western Michigan University*)

TYPES OF HEARING LOSS

When testing reveals a loss of hearing sensitivity by air conduction and bone-conduction thresholds are normal, then the hearing loss is classified as *conductive*. A typical audiogram for a conductive hearing loss was shown in Figure 13-3. Conductive hearing loss can be identified by the normal air-conduction threshold and by the obvious discrepancy between air- and bone-conduction thresholds, an *air-bone gap*. Rarely is the loss of hearing acuity more than 60 dB, and, once the individual's threshold for sound detection is crossed, he generally hears equally well at all higher intensity levels. In conductive hearing loss, the impairment is simply a reduction in *loudness* because the inner ear is normal and the breakdown lies in either the outer or middle portions of the hearing mechanism. The problem is with the conduction of sound to the inner ear.

When a loss of hearing is found by both air conduction and bone conduction and the bone-conduction thresholds are essentially at the same level as the air-conduction thresholds, the loss is classified as *sensorineural*. A typical audiogram for a sensorineural hearing loss was also shown in Figure 13-3. In this instance, the outer and middle ears are normal, and the breakdown is in the cochlear sense organ itself, or in the auditory nerve or brainstem. The problem is with the "perception" of sound in the inner ear or beyond. Now, in addition to a reduction in loudness, the individual has trouble with *clarity;* in fact, persons with sensorineural hearing loss often report that they can hear people talking but cannot understand what they are saying.

A third major classification of hearing loss (see Figure 13-3) is termed a *mixed type* of loss. As the term implies, this type of loss is a combination of a conductive and a sensorineural type loss. There is a loss of hearing by both air conduction and bone conduction, but the loss by bone conduction is not as great as the loss by air conduction, thus producing an air-bone gap at certain test frequencies. With this type of loss the bone-conduction thresholds show the presence of sensorineural loss, but, since air-conduction thresholds are much worse, there is also a conductive component to the hearing loss. This type of loss could result from any number of factors.

Conductive Impairments

The Outer Ear.
Hearing loss can, of course, occur at any time. Losses occurring before birth are said to be *congenital*. One kind of congenital hearing loss involving the outer ear is **atresia** of the external ear canal. Atresia means that a natural canal has been blocked. When this blocking occurs in the ear canal, it results in a conductive-type hearing loss. Atresia of the ear canal is usually not found as an isolated defect, but usually in conjunction with a small or deformed auricle or with middle-ear abnormalities.

Among persons with Down's syndrome, a population served quite regularly by some speech-language pathologists, it is not uncommon to observe outer ear anomalies, including small auricles and narrow ear canals, as well as excessive cerumen accumulation and frequent episodes of otitis externa. Such factors, of course, impact less on hearing than do their middle ear problems and the cochlear and nervous system disturbances that also are associated with the syndrome. Nevertheless, the external ear difficulties can at least further complicate an audiologist's efforts

Atresia.
The blockage of an opening or a canal.

to provide effective personal amplification instruments for individuals with Down's syndrome (Buchanan, Harding, and Hudner, 1991).

Another congenital condition resulting in a conductive hearing loss is the Treacher-Collins syndrome. This syndrome is marked by deformities of the facial bones resulting in a small receding lower jaw and eyes that are slanted downward in an antimongoloid fashion at the lateral corners. The auricles are deformed, and usually both external auditory canals and eardrums are missing bilaterally, along with ossicular chain deformities.

> Vivian, age five, was born with Treacher-Collins syndrome. There was malformation of both auricles, along with complete atresia of the left ear canal and marked stenosis (narrowing or stricture) of the right ear canal. Audiological evaluation revealed normal, bilateral inner-ear function with a moderate to severe loss by air conduction in the right ear. The left ear was not tested by air conduction. A sound field (loudspeaker) speech recognition threshold of 55 dB was obtained, and understanding of speech was normal when it was presented at a sufficient loudness level to overcome the conductive barrier. Further testing revealed that Vivian is delayed in her language development and has markedly defective articulation.

> Remedial procedures included a hearing aid fitted to her right ear. In addition, Vivian was placed in a school where she could receive an intensive program of academic instruction and remedial assistance in speech, language, and auditory training. Later, corrective surgery would be performed in an attempt to alleviate her conductive hearing loss.

Hearing losses occurring at any time after birth are referred to as acquired losses. One of the common acquired losses involving the outer ear is that of simple blockage of the ear canal by foreign objects or impacted wax. Children have been known to put into their ears such things as beans, crayons, small ball bearings, wads of paper, and just about anything else small enough to fit into their ear canals. Foreign objects cause a mild conductive loss if the blockage is complete. They are readily visible on otoscopic examination and should be extracted by the otologist.

The most common blockage is a result of impacted wax. Well-meaning mothers can cause this type of loss by cleaning their children's ears with cotton swabs. Since the cotton tip just fits the ear canal, it cannot get behind the wax and instead forces it back and may impact it against the tympanic membrane. One otologist, an acquaintance of the authors, is vehement in his objection to mothers using cotton swabs to clean their children's ears. He maintains that it is unnecessary to clean wax from the ears, since old accumulations will dry up and fall out naturally if left alone.

Impacted wax should be removed by the otologist since there is always danger of perforating the tympanic membrane unless it is done by a skilled person and with proper instruments such as a cerumen spoon. Often it is necessary to soften the wax with some type of softening agent before the wax can be removed. After the wax is softened, the ear is syringed and the wax flushed out. Syringing of the ear must also be done carefully, since a forceful stream of water directed at the tympanic membrane could rupture it. For this reason, the water is usually directed at the canal walls, so that only reflected water hits the membrane. Although impacted wax results in only a mild hearing loss, it often causes a youngster to have difficulty in school. This is the child who may become what the teachers refer to as a "behavior problem." Any child who does not seem to pay attention in school or suddenly changes in alertness should be suspected of having a hearing loss.

There are a number of other problems involving the outer ear that come under the broad title of *external otitis.* These would include seborrheic dermatitis, eczema, and other inflammatory conditions. The hearing loss resulting from these conditions resembles the loss from simple blockage of the ear canal. These conditions can result in a swelling of the external ear canal so that it is closed or nearly closed, or the collection of scaly debris in the canal. These types of conditions are treated medically and may involve other areas of the body as well as the ear canal and auricle.

A common type of otitis externa is called otomycosis or "swimmers' ears," since it is often found in people who are frequent swimmers. It consists of a fungus growth in the external canal, resulting in irritation and itching. Secondary infection can be set up by scratching in attempts to relieve the itching. The following case is an example of this type of ear problem.

> J. V., age forty-three, complained of some loss of hearing, but his chief complaint was the itching in his left ear canal. He attributed the itching to an accumulation of wax. In attempts to rid his left ear canal of what he thought was an accumulation of wax, J. V. poured hydrogen peroxide into it since this can be used to soften wax. This procedure resulted in a pain deep in the left ear and left him dizzy and nauseous.

> Audiological evaluation showed evidence of air-bone gaps in the low frequencies, indicating the presence of a conductive hearing loss. In addition, a mild high-frequency sensorineural hearing loss was present bilaterally. Physical examination of the left ear revealed a fungoid external otitis and a perforated tympanic membrane (Figure 13-6). Thus, the pain experienced upon application of the hydrogen peroxide was due to the fact that the peroxide was getting into the middle ear through the perforation. By carrying the bacteria from the ear canal with it, a middle-ear infection could have resulted. J. V. was referred for otologic treatment, and medication was prescribed to eliminate the fungus and to relieve the itching in his ear canal.

The foregoing case points up the danger of self-treatment combined with ignorance. Since Mr. J. V.'s hearing loss in the high frequencies was mild, further rehabilitation was deemed unnecessary.

The Middle Ear.   Congenital malformations can also be found in the middle ear. These take the form of deformed or broken ossicular chains, missing ossicles, replacement of the tympanic membrane by a primitive

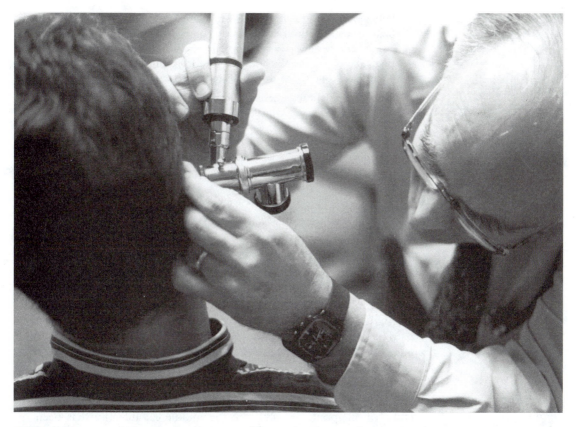

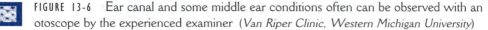 **FIGURE 13-6**   Ear canal and some middle ear conditions often can be observed with an otoscope by the experienced examiner (*Van Riper Clinic, Western Michigan University*)

bony plate, and fixation of the stapes in the oval window. As indicated earlier, these abnormalities are usually found with congenital atresia of the outer ear, but they can also be restricted to the middle ear itself. The following is a case of congenital middle-ear deformities resulting in a conductive-type hearing loss:

> T. W., a university student eighteen years old, was seen for an audiological evaluation, which showed the presence of a severe, bilateral, conductive hearing loss. Case history information revealed that T. W. had a bilateral, congenital middle-ear problem for which surgery was being contemplated. Both outer ears were normal, and she wore a binaural hearing aid built into glasses. With this type of amplification, speech reception thresholds and understanding of speech were well within the normal range. The left corner of her mouth was pulled to the side slightly, indicating a possible paresis, and she had a distorted /s/ sound.

Subsequent surgery on the left ear revealed a normal tympanic membrane but a defective ossicular chain consisting of a deformed incus and a rudimentary stapes. In addition, the oval window could not be identified. The operation was not successful from the audiologic standpoint because air-conduction thresholds in the left ear were not improved.

Since she was already wearing a binaural hearing aid, from which she appeared to obtain substantial benefit, T. W. was enrolled in therapy for correction of her defective /s/ sound and strengthening of muscular control around the mouth area. Within two semesters she was dismissed from therapy, but she continued to receive periodic hearing evaluations. She is scheduled for further ear surgery, which, it is hoped, will prove to be more successful.

Acquired middle-ear problems resulting in conductive hearing loss can result from many causes. One very common problem associated with this type of hearing loss is caused by a ruptured eardrum. The tympanic membrane can be penetrated by any number of sharp objects. In attempts to relieve itching or to dig out the wax from the ear canal people use hairpins or paper clips, and any slip can result in the penetration of the tympanic membrane. Sharp objects should never be introduced into the external ear canal. The tympanic membrane can also be ruptured by a sharp blow across the ears and is one of many very good reasons why children should not be struck on or about the head.

The eardrum can also be perforated from within by the building up of fluid in the middle ear. The size and location of the perforation will indicate how serious the problem is. Fortunately, small perforations will tend to heal spontaneously once the middle-ear infection has been removed. Other persistent perforations may indicate the presence of a more serious problem.

Otitis Media.   An inflammation or infection of the middle ear, *otitis media*, was responsible for nearly 25 million visits to medical offices by children in 1990, making this the leading problem for which children were seen by physicians (Stool, 1993). It also is one of the leading causes of hearing loss. Although the hearing loss can be mild and fluctuating, many clinicians (physicians, speech pathologists, and audiologists alike) are convinced that—because it begins to occur in children at a young age—speech and language development can be adversely affected by otitis media. Adults also suffer otitis media, usually acute and often painful, but more about that later.

Eustachian tube malfunctions, such as those caused by enlarged adenoids or by allergies, can set the stage for otitis media. Exposure to cigarette smoke is a suspected causal agent, as well, and any upper respiratory infection also can cause the eustachian tube to become swollen and unable to open properly. Since the middle ear is pressure-equalized through the eustachian tube, its blockage can cause a negative middle ear pressure (vacuum) to develop. This results in the eardrum bulging inward. It also results in the secretion of watery fluid from the mucous lining of the middle ear into the middle ear cavity itself. With the eardrum retracted, ossicular mobility is impeded and a conductive hearing loss appears. This condition is known as *serous otitis media*, or as OME, *otitis media with effusion*. Serous refers to the fluid that may partially or completely fill, or *effuse* into the middle ear cavity. Technically, when there is infection in the middle ear, with or without fluid, the term *acute otitis media* may be applied.

Although it now is believed that OME often subsides on its own over a period of three to six months, in the past it has been fairly standard practice to begin treatment with antibiotics immediately upon diagnosis. Additionally or alternatively, the child's adenoid and tonsil tissue has been surgically removed and the tympanic membrane has been lanced (with or without the insertion of small polyethylene tubes to keep the middle ear open to outside air) and fluid suctioned from the middle ear.

Under certain circumstances, or for older children, any one or more of these procedures still may be both appropriate and necessary for a specific child—especially if adenoids actually are diseased, for example, or if the child has Down's syndrome, a cleft palate, or other complicating condition.

Such coexisting conditions are not usually an issue, however, and the U.S. Public Health Service has suggested uniform guidelines for conservative treatment of OME in *otherwise healthy children up to the age of three*. In brief, the PHS guidelines encourage a three-month period of close observation by the physician, during which time antibiotic therapy *might* be considered. Counseling about environmental risk factors (e.g., smoke) also is advised.

Only when OME has continued for three to six months and the toddler has a bilateral hearing level of 20 dB or worse do the guidelines indicate that bilateral **myringotomy** with tube placement should be considered. Tonsillectomy or adenoidectomy and steroid or antihistamine therapy are not among the procedures recommended at any stage for otherwise healthy very young children. The Public Health Service acknowledges, of course, that the guidelines are only general guidelines and that the medical judgment of the physician must prevail in individual cases.[5]

The following youngster is not unlike others who may be seen in the schools by the speech-language pathologist.

David, age seven, had been enrolled in speech therapy for correction of an articulation problem. After about two months of therapy, it was decided to have his hearing evaluated. It was readily apparent that David was a mouth breather, and when asked to close his mouth and breathe through his nose, he was unable to do so because of congestion. Oral examination revealed extremely large **tonsils.**

Audiological evaluation showed a mild, bilateral, conductive type of hearing loss. The child did not complain of pain in his ears. Treatment called

Myringotomy.
Surgical perforation of the eardrum, usually accompanied by insertion of pressure-equalizing tube; used in treatment of persistent otitis media.

Tonsils.
Lymphoid tissue at back edges of oral cavity; also known as palatine tonsils.

for a T & A and myringotomy as well as investigation of a possible allergic condition that might account for the chronic nasal congestion.

Following the T & A the child's congestion diminished, and he actually became much more understandable. The denasality in his speech disappeared. Hearing returned to the normal range. Further speech therapy could then be expected to correct his misarticulations.

Acute otitis media is the problem that is usually experienced by a child or adult as a result of an upper respiratory infection such as a cold or an allergy attack. Coughing, sneezing, or blowing the nose forces secretions containing bacteria through the eustachian tube into the middle ear. Infants and children are particularly susceptible to this type of infection because their eustachian tubes tend to lie on a horizontal plane. In the adult this relationship changes, the tube becoming more vertical, and thus it is more difficult for infected material to be forced into the middle ear. Acute otitis media is accompanied by the earache familiar to all of us. The fluid in the ear may initially be clear but it soon changes to pus, and the pressure of this fluid causes the eardrum to bulge outwardly to produce pain.

If the condition is caught in time, medical treatment with antibiotics may be all that is needed. Once the infection has cleared up, the debris will be absorbed. However, it is interesting to note that some otologists feel that their work has increased because of antibiotics. The drug clears up the infection, but fluid may be left in the middle ear. If left there over a period of time, the fluid can turn into a thick, mucous, sludgelike material resulting in even greater loss of hearing. This condition, sometimes referred to as "glue ear," probably is more commonly seen in children than in adults, since fluid in the adult middle ear often resolves with medical treatment (Silverstein, Wolfson, and Rosenberg, 1992, pp. 14–15).

Chronic otitis media is a condition in which infection of the middle ear continues over a long period of time. It is not a recurring infection, but one that never completely clears. This could happen, perhaps, because a child's OME never was diagnosed. Or perhaps serous otitis media or acute otitis media was accurately diagnosed, whether in a child or adult, but appropriate follow-up treatment did not take place. In such instances there can be an accumulation of fluid in the middle ear that gradually erodes the ossicular chain. The combination of these factors may result in a severe conductive hearing loss. If the mastoid process becomes infected and the infection is allowed to persist, it could result in an infection of the brain.

G. O., age forty-nine, suffered from chronic otitis media for years. The infection was not properly controlled and resulted in infection of the mastoid bones. Eventually the infection traveled to the brain and resulted in some tissue damage. G. O. is now subject to epileptic like seizures and is under constant medication for control of them. In addition, he has a severe conductive hearing loss due to the erosion of his middle-ear structures.

Discharge from the ear or complaints of earaches from children should never be ignored. The speech pathologist and audiologist in the public schools can do much to help teachers and parents understand conductive hearing losses, refer children for proper medical treatment, help the otologist with follow-up, and provide the child with the extra help she may need until an infection can be cleared up.

Otosclerosis.   Another condition of the middle ear that accounts for a great number of conductive hearing losses in adults is *otosclerosis.* In otosclerosis the hearing loss is the result of a formation of spongy bone that displaces normal bone and fixates the footplate of the stapes in the oval window of the cochlea. The fixation impedes transmission of sound from the eardrum to the inner ear. The exact cause of this sclerotic process is not known, but otosclerosis is known to be an inherited condition. It is more common in females than males and is usually first noticed during the late teens or early twenties. The hearing loss often worsens during pregnancy, perhaps because hormonal changes in the woman's body enhance the spongy bone growth. In some persons with otosclerosis the progressive middle ear deterioration can be compounded by related damage to the cochlea, causing a sensorineural hearing loss to become a permanent component of the problem.

Individuals with otosclerosis tend to have increasing difficulty understanding speech at conversational levels as the disease progresses, so they may experience repeated and ever greater frustration in their efforts to communicate. Not surprisingly, they may begin to withdraw and to show other signs of social and/or emotional indifference. As with other hearing problems, the effects often extend beyond the patient. Friends, workplace associates, and particularly members of the patient's family are not exempt from negative impacts of the hearing loss.

No drugs are effective for treating otosclerosis, but surgical treatment nearly always is very successful. In a procedure called *stapedectomy* the fixated stapes is replaced by a small prosthetic device, with resultant remobilization of the ossicular chain and correction (or marked improvement) of the conductive loss. A variation, *laser stapedotomy,* also achieves this goal. Any sensorineural component will remain, of course, which is one reason the surgery may not restore completely normal hearing. Even then, however, the hearing usually is substantially improved.

Sensorineural Impairments

Congenital sensorineural hearing loss can result from genetic factors or from other circumstances that impact the pregnant woman and her fetus, and our information about both of these types of causes has been expanding rapidly in recent years. We have learned, for example, that some 200 possible types of inherited hearing loss exist, although hereditary

Otosclerosis. Pathologic condition in which the footplate of the stapes becomes rigidly affixed to the oval window and is thus unable to transmit mechanical vibrations from the eardrum to the cochlea; common cause of hearing impairment in adults.

Toxoplasmosis.
Disease caused by parasites in the bloodstream; prenatal infection may cause death or severe brain damage.

Hyperbilirubinemia.
Excessive amounts of bile substance in the blood; can produce jaundiced appearance and is among the factors indicating an infant may be at risk for hearing loss and other problems.

Apgar score.
Rating of newborn's physical condition based upon observations of heart rate, respiration, skin color, muscle tone, and reflexes.

Ventilation.
A process using a mechanical apparatus designed to maintain or assist respiration in patients unable to breathe or able to breathe only weakly due to respiratory paralysis or other medical problems.

Syndrome.
Collection of signs and symptoms that together characterize a disease or other abnormal condition.

losses may not be present at birth (one such instance being otosclerosis, as we've just seen). But still only the tip of the iceberg has begun to be exposed, especially with regard to genetics.[6]

In any event, because hearing losses present at birth are largely of the sensorineural type, and since half or more of all newborn and infant hearing impairment is believed to be genetically based, we should take a moment or two now to look at early onset.

It is estimated that the prevalence of hearing loss in newborns and infants is 1.5 to 6.0 of every 1,000 live births (American Speech-Language-Hearing Association, 1994) and that the hearing of one of every 750 newborn infants is severely to profoundly impaired. All too often, however, early-onset hearing impairment (including very serious hearing loss) has gone undetected for months and sometimes years, even though "high risk registries" have been established to facilitate early detection.

Congenital hearing loss can also occur as a result of illnesses, drugs, and accidents sustained by the mother during pregnancy. The prediction that hearing loss may be present can be made also on the basis of some identifiable characteristics of the neonate, but most such observations of mother and infant necessarily have focused on circumstances that are more easily demonstrated than are any but the more obvious genetic factors.

The 1994 Position Statement of the Joint Committee on Infant Hearing cites the following "indicators associated with sensorineural and/or conductive hearing loss" (American Speech-Language-Hearing Association, 1994).

> *For use with neonates (birth through age 28 days) when universal screening is not available.* 1. Family history of hereditary childhood sensorineural hearing loss. 2. In utero infection, such as cytomegalovirus, rubella, syphilis, herpes, and **toxoplasmosis.** 3. Craniofacial anomalies, including those with morphological abnormalities of the pinna and ear canal. 4. Birth weight less than 1,500 grams (3.3 lbs). 5. **Hyperbilirubinemia** at a serum level requiring exchange transfusion. 6. Ototoxic medications, including but not limited to the aminoglycosides, used in multiple courses or in combination with loop diuretics. 7. Bacterial meningitis. 8. **Apgar scores** of 0–4 at 1 minute or 0–6 at 5 minutes. 9. Mechanical **ventilation** lasting 5 days or longer. 10. Stigmata or other findings associated with a **syndrome** known to include a sensorineural and/or conductive hearing loss.

Audiological evaluation is recommended for any newborn manifesting a risk factor, as well as for infants age 29 days through 2 years "when certain health conditions develop that require rescreening" or "who require periodic monitoring of hearing" and for whom additional indicators are listed.

Note that these indicators are intended to assist in early identification "when universal screening is not available." Screening refers to *hearing screening;* universal means screening that is conducted systematically on *all* newborns. This is not yet a standard practice, but hopefully it soon will be. Even then, some newborns will slip through with undetected hearing loss, but universal screening can vastly enhance our efforts—especially when genetic factors are operative—to ensure that early intervention services are provided for the families of hearing-impaired infants. The importance of early detection and diagnosis is obvious when we realize that medical and educational intervention should be initiated by the age of six months if optimal results are to be obtained. Less obvious, perhaps, but equally important are the implications of early detection for purposes of possible genetic counseling for the parents of an infant with inherited hearing impairment.

Before ending our look at early onset issues we must return briefly to nongenetic concerns. As we do so, though, we also remind ourselves that genetic and environmental factors can interact in ways that are not clearly understood and that can cause (or not cause) hearing loss and other problems that may be even more complex than those related to the action of either factor alone. Multiple factors present in either the environmental or the genetic arena or in both will further complicate individual cases.

As reflected in the indicators noted above, it is clear that some congenital hearing losses are related to illnesses or infections suffered by the mother during pregnancy and that her use of certain drugs—prescription or over-the-counter, legal or illegal—also may cause these and many other problems.

We will not try here to pursue these matters much further, but it is important to note that the timing and circumstance of such events are critical in determining the nature of their effects. A particular infection may be very harmful to the fetus during the first trimester of pregnancy, for example, and less dangerous at a later stage. Or it may affect the fetus differently at different stages. Similarly, ingestion of certain substances might have different but equally serious effects, depending on timing and amounts.

We are well aware that alcohol and smoking are to be avoided, and the problems of Fetal Alcohol Syndrome have become relatively well known. We are becoming more fully aware of the consequences observed in children born to cocaine-addicted mothers. Ototoxic medications such as streptomycin are especially dangerous during pregnancy, but it may be less well known that even common aspirin can affect hearing. It is probably a good rule for a pregnant woman not to take any type of drug that is not specifically prescribed by her physician and even then reluctantly.

Years ago one of the greatest causes of congenital hearing loss was maternal rubella (German measles) occurring during pregnancy. Usually a rather mild disease in the child or adult, rubella is extremely dangerous to a fetus during the early months of pregnancy. However, the implementation of a broad immunization program in the 1970s has almost completely eliminated rubella risks. Unfortunately, a sinister replacement has appeared.

Cytomegalovirus (CMV) infection in utero now has become a major cause of nonhereditary congenital hearing loss, and it is expected that even those infected infants who show no symptoms at birth may later develop sensorineural hearing losses and a variety of neurological problems similar to those seen in children who at birth do show such overt CMV symptoms as rash, enlarged liver and spleen, reduced head size, jaundice, and low birth weight (Johnson, Williamson, and Chmiel, 1991). CMV is a member of the herpes virus group and is said to infect most of us at some time during our lives, but usually with few or no symptoms or with mild symptoms somewhat like those associated with mononucleosis. This seemingly harmless virus can pass through the placenta, however, and cause serious damage to the fetus, or a neonate can become infected during vaginal delivery (Crawford and Studebaker, 1990). The lack of striking symptoms in adults makes CMV difficult to detect in infants who have no overt symptoms at birth but who nevertheless have contracted the virus, so the story of CMV and hearing likely will continue to be revealed in greater detail as infected children mature in coming years.

Later Onset.   Having survived intrauterine life and birth trauma, the human being is still subject to a great many events that can cause hearing loss. We will limit our comments to just a few of the more common causes, but we would refer you to sources such as Martin (1994) and Newby and Popelka (1992) for more comprehensive information.

Effects of Drugs on Hearing.   Just as drugs taken by the mother can be harmful to the fetus, so too can various drugs be ototoxic to the individual, often causing irreversible hearing impairment. Some people, of course, are simply allergic to specific drugs. For instance, some people cannot take penicillin, since they are prone to allergic reactions that can range from mild to fatal. Such reactions aside, dihydrostreptomycin, neomycin, kanamycin, streptomycin, and other of the aminoglycoside antibiotics can be extremely ototoxic to most of us, perhaps more so when injected directly into the bloodstream. A patient's hearing should be monitored while on these drugs, and any changes in hearing level should signal that the treatment must be reconsidered (and usually stopped, especially if there is any history of kidney problems). Even aspirin in large doses may prove to be ototoxic in susceptible individuals, although aspirin-induced losses may be only temporary.

In Figure 13-7 we see an audiogram obtained on one individual with a drug-induced bilateral sensorineural loss, a loss that markedly reduced his ability to understand speech even when it was presented at intensity levels well above normal conversational levels. His hearing loss might have been avoided or held to a milder degree had monitoring audiometry been performed while he was on streptomycin.

Certain diuretics used to control water retention or high blood pressure also have ototoxic effects and are used with great care when a hear-

Cytomegalovirus (CMV).
Type of herpes virus; can be asymptomatic in adults; congenitally, CMV is a major cause of sensorineural hearing impairment in children.

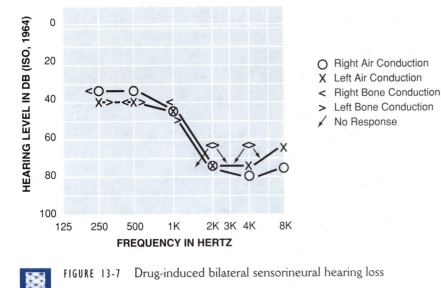

FIGURE 13-7   Drug-induced bilateral sensorineural hearing loss

ing loss already exists or, again, when renal disease is present. At times, of course, the benefits associated with a particular ototoxic drug may be seen as far outweighing the risks. This can be the case, for example, in cancer chemotherapy using cisplatinum where no alternative may be available in seeking to save the patient's life. Even then, however, regular monitoring of hearing can play an important role in serving the long-term needs, even short-term circumstances, of patients and their families.

Although perhaps not technically regarded as drugs, alcohol, caffeine, and nicotine should be mentioned here. There is virtually no disagreement among the experts that these substances can have adverse physical effects throughout the body, including the ear. They also may interact with other ototoxic agents to increase their ototoxicity, or vice versa. Needless to say, the ear also is not exempt from the negative bodily effects of various illegal substances.

Infectious Disease.   Childhood diseases that many people think have no serious consequences nevertheless can cause hearing loss. Mumps, measles, chicken pox, scarlet fever, diphtheria, and whooping cough can attack the end organ of hearing and cause sensorineural hearing loss. Fortunately, it is now no longer inevitable that a child undergo these diseases, since vaccines are available to immunize children against measles, rubella, and mumps.

Hearing loss resulting from these diseases is usually bilateral, except for mumps. Mumps is the most common cause of unilateral hearing loss, and the loss is usually total. The following case illustrates hearing loss from mumps.

John, age seven, is presently enrolled in therapy for an articulation problem that consists mainly of substitutions of one sound for another. At the age of five, he came down with a case of mumps that resulted in a profound loss of hearing in his right ear. His left ear is normal. His audiogram is typical of unilateral deafness due to this disease.

In this youngster's case it would have been a mistake to think that his articulation problem was in any way related to his hearing loss. People with unilateral hearing are able to function fairly normally, although the sense of direction of sound may be somewhat impaired. With a child, however, even this tends to be something they are able to compensate for. In John's case, the important thing was to prevent any damage to his good ear either by illness or accident. His parents were advised of the importance of trying to help John avoid exposure to loud noise and of watching for any sign of change in his hearing. They also were urged to take him to the doctor as soon as possible if they ever suspected that John was having an ear infection. His teachers in school were told of his loss, and he was given preferential seating. Naturally, his clinician makes sure during speech therapy that he is working from his unimpaired side.

Acute bacterial meningitis also is able to cause hearing loss, in some cases profound loss, as well as loss of vision, and other types of neurological damage. Permanent bilateral sensorineural hearing impairments are, in fact, a fairly common sequel to bacterial meningitis, and hearing always should be tested prior to hospital discharge in order to ensure that the post-meningitic patient receives any auditory rehabilitation help that may be needed. The disease can occur at any age, but the vast majority of those who contract it are children younger than five years. At this early age, even children who escape with only relatively minor neurological aftereffects nevertheless may encounter difficulties that can significantly interfere with developmental learning and motor skills. On a positive note, however, inoculations to protect against Haemophilus influenza type B—the most common precursor of meningitis in preschoolers—can substantially reduce its incidence. Hopefully, the availability of this vaccine will result in fewer infants and youth falling victim to the disabling sequelae of meningitis.

Finally, given the prevalence of AIDS here and around the world, we should note that sudden sensorineural hearing loss is one of the many complications that the AIDS patient may suffer. And a mild hearing loss can be one of a very few neurological signs that appear, before AIDS is diagnosed, in males who are serologically positive for human immunodeficiency virus (HIV) infection.

Effects of Noise.   Prolonged exposure to excessively loud noise commonly leads to bilateral sensorineural hearing losses. Workers in noisy factories, farmers spending hours on loud tractors, people using power grass mowers or other power tools, even the Eskimo who has abandoned his dogsled for a snowmobile, all are at risk for noise-induced hearing loss if no precautions (such as wearing ear protectors) have been taken to reduce the noise levels to which they are subjected.[7]

> J. V., age forty-seven, stated that he was no longer able to hear birds sing or the tick of his watch. He complained of a "high-pitched ringing" in both ears. He also complained of difficulty hearing speech in group situations or in the presence of background noise. J. V. had worked in a drop forge for twenty-three years and was exposed to extremely loud noise for most of the working day. He had spent the last twelve years operating a huge hammer used to flatten steel bars. A subsequent hearing evaluation revealed the high-frequency, sensorineural hearing loss shown in Figure 13-8.

> J. V. was fitted with a hearing aid that gave a high-frequency emphasis and a special earmold that further emphasized the higher frequencies. Since he had worked in an environment that made normal communication almost impossible, he already had become rather adept at speechreading. He was advised to wear earprotective devices while working to prevent any further damage to his ears.

 FIGURE 13-8   Noise-induced hearing loss

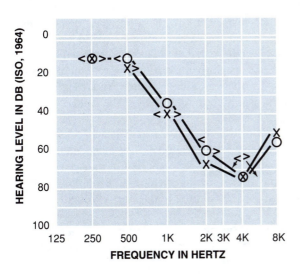

A sound pressure level (SPL) of 80–85 decibels is sometimes mentioned as the level that cannot be exceeded safely, and the Occupational Safety and Health Administration has determined that exposure to 85 dB for eight hours may cause ear damage. At greater levels, damage can occur in a much shorter time, perhaps in as little as 30 minutes if the level is sufficiently loud.

But there are wide differences in susceptibility to the effects of noise. Some of us may experience hearing loss at lower levels, while others conceivably might be unaffected at slightly higher levels (at least in the short term). Also, there are factors that alter an individual's susceptibility, such as alcohol and tobacco use while in the presence of loud noise, or the person's own past history of exposure. Clearly, it would be wise to err on the conservative side in avoiding risk, and one guideline that may be helpful actually is a "rule of arm": When noise is loud enough to interfere with normal conversational speech at arm's length distance it is potentially damaging.

Noise damage causes hearing loss first in the higher frequencies, often beginning with a characteristic "dip" on the audiogram in the region of 4000–6000 Hz. The loss occurs because excessive noise actually destroys hair cells in the cochlea (see Figure 13-9).

Another danger to the ears is found in frequent long exposures to loud music. Simply listening to powerfully amplified hard rock in a live concert can cause at least the temporary worsening of hearing thresholds. No doubt the same is true when a "boom box" cranked to maximum volume rides on the shoulder within inches from a youngster's ear; and it is well known that the earphones used with sound systems, even of the small walkman type, are easily capable of delivering excessive sound pressure levels directly to the eardrum.

Musicians who themselves are working in very close proximity to powerful on-stage amplifiers also are known to suffer temporary threshold shifts that, when experienced regularly, lead to permanent and often quite serious hearing impairment. For that matter, it has been reported that even symphony orchestra performers can incur permanent hearing loss that appears related to their music, especially since significantly poorer hearing has been measured in the left than in the right ear among violinists.

Perhaps it is not too surprising that permanent hearing loss is a familiar consequence experienced by professional rock performers or that the same fate can await even some professional classical musicians. But at least one study in Japan has suggested that beginning evidence of noise-induced hearing loss can be detected among brass band members as young as at the junior high level.

The onset of noise-induced hearing impairment is gradual, and many musicians do not become aware of the worsening problem until far too

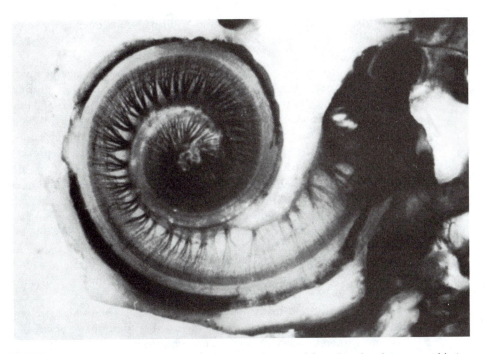

FIGURE 13-9   Noise-induced inner ear damage. Note that the degenerated hair cells in the basal portion of the cochlea (larger part, pictured to the right) have nearly disappeared. This is where the high-frequency receptors are located. (From H. Engstrom and B. Engstrom. Structural changes in the cochlea following overstimulation by noise. *Acta Otolaryngologica, Supplement,* 360, 1979, 75–79. Used by permission.)

late. In San Francisco an organization known as H. E. A. R. (Hearing Education and Awareness for Rockers) exists for the specific purpose of increasing the awareness of risk and reducing the incidence of this problem through informational and hearing testing programs for musicians and fans alike. And, now that it is possible to order specially designed ear plugs that reduce the overall loudness without distorting the high or the low frequencies, some musicians are more inclined to use ear protection devices.

Prolonged exposure to noise can also cause other physical impairments, including low fetal birth weight, ulcers, and cardiovascular disorders. Evidence is also abundant that high-volume sound, even when of a type that may not be inherently objectionable, can be very distressing for a variety of reasons to individuals (and, for that matter, to entire neighborhoods) and that noise pollution can indeed be psychologically debilitating. A great deal more remains to be learned about the effects of noise, so it is fortunate that this becomes a focus of particular interest for some of our audiology colleagues.

Presbycusis.   The hearing loss that people incur with advancing age is called **presbycusis.** It is the most common kind of sensorineural hearing loss. The incidence of presbycusis seems to be increasing, understandably when one considers that people live much longer than they used to and that we now have a substantial percentage of senior citizens in this country. The loss of hearing by presbycusis is a rather slow, insidious process and probably starts early in life, although the symptoms of hearing loss are usually not manifested until the person is over sixty years of age, and men are more severely affected than women. The higher sound frequencies are affected first, and as the disorder gradually progresses, the person has trouble in hearing lower-frequency sounds as well. Comprehension of speech may be affected to a much greater degree than would be expected from thresholds on a pure tone audiogram. Even in the presence of a mild loss in pure tone thresholds, the person may have extreme difficulty understanding speech.

Consequently, and making matters even worse, when older persons have auditory difficulties, they may be regarded as somewhat "senile" because of the inappropriate responses and confusions which can occur. Too often, then, older peoples'

> sense of aloneness and abandonment may be significantly increased by impaired hearing, especially (when they reside in nursing homes), and may account for considerable despair and depression . . .(It is not hard to) understand the confusion, apprehension, and fear an older hearing-impaired person must experience as a hospital patient trying to determine what is going on; or the frustration of half-heard movies, plays, and lectures; the disappointment of not being able to have the full worship experience at church or synagogue; the embarrassment and problems resulting from missed announcements from a public address or paging system in an airport . . . the problems that arise at home when food boils over, bathtubs overflow, and timers, alarm clocks, doorbells, and telephones are not heard; the insecure feelings of not hearing storms,. . . prowlers, tornado warnings, grandchildren crying. . . . It is difficult enough to deal with such problems in a friendly and understanding environment, but too often the older person encounters a somewhat hostile environment lacking in understanding and patience (Bate, 1985, p. 196).

Presbycusis.
The hearing loss characteristic of old age.

Cerebral cortex.
Outer layer of gray matter over the cerebral hemispheres; responsible for higher level cognitive functions.

Obviously, the effects of presbycusis can be dramatic, disabling, and complex. Its causes are also complex. There is apparently a degeneration of structures not only in the inner ear, but along the central pathways and in the **cerebral cortex** of the brain. It has also been stated that the hearing loss is due to the wear and tear on the ear from everyday living in our noisy society; studies on primitive tribes do not reveal nearly the amount of loss with age that is seen in industrialized societies. It is likely that several subtypes of presbycusis exist (e.g., *mechanical, sensory, metabolic, neural,* and *central*), and that individual cases can reflect more than just one cause. And, of course, some people may be relatively un-affected by any of these causes and have relatively good hearing even into very old age. The following, however, illustrates problems typical of presbycusis.

> J. D., age sixty-seven, was referred for an audiological evaluation and hearing-aid evaluation and selection following otologic consultation for his hearing problem. He was originally examined by the otologist upon the insistence of his daughter with whom he had been living since the death of his wife two years previously. The otologist diagnosed his dis-order as presbycusis.

> J. D. stated that he had noticed a decrease in hearing sensitivity for a number of years but that it had become much worse during the past two years. He complained of difficulty hearing the radio and television, and he had to have the volume turned up beyond the comfort level of other family members. Consequently, he had gradually lost interest in watch-ing television. Conversation was also difficult for him to follow, and he found himself more and more frequently having to ask what was said. He felt that if other family members would not mumble or speak so fast he would be able to hear them without difficulty.

> An interview with J. D.'s daughter revealed that she had become con-cerned for her father since he was showing an increasing tendency to iso-late himself from other people. She also felt guilty. She worked outside the home and was usually tired in the evening. Talking with her father was a strain. She had to speak louder and often repeat what she said. This was annoying to her, so she found herself avoiding conversation with her father. It was at this point that she decided to seek professional advice and thought that perhaps a hearing aid might help him.

> Audiological evaluation revealed the moderate, bilateral, sensorineural hearing loss shown in Figure 13-10. Fortunately, J. D.'s understanding of speech, when it was presented at a fairly loud level, was good. A sub-sequent hearing-aid evaluation indicated that he received substantial benefit from wearing amplification.

The foregoing case, although it has its unique aspects, is typical not only of the hearing loss, but also of the family dynamics that are often in-volved. A hearing aid was not the total answer to this man's problem. He needed to have a greater understanding of his problem and so did the other family members. Rehabilitation in this type of case should involve family counseling so that its members can do their share in improving communications. For example, we often find improvement in communi-cation by pointing out to the family that shouting at the hard-of-hearing person does no good, and that instead they should talk more slowly and distinctly. It is also important that the family realize the advantages and disadvantages of hearing aids and how they operate.

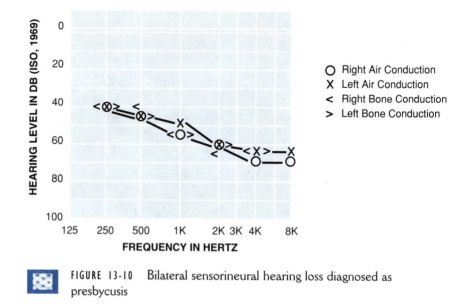

FIGURE 13-10   Bilateral sensorineural hearing loss diagnosed as presbycusis

Ménière's Disease.   The most debilitating symptom of this disease is the recurring sudden vertigo attack, lasting from a few minutes to several hours, that can make it impossible for the individual to maintain balance, whether walking, simply standing, or even sitting. Usually only one ear is affected, and the associated hearing loss initially may be mild and intermittent. As the disease progresses, the hearing loss becomes greater. Other features that identify Ménière's disease are constant ringing in the ear and a sensation of pressure or fullness. The disorder is known to be due to excess fluid pressure in the inner ear, and diuretics as well as dietary sodium restrictions have been known to help; but medical treatment is generally ineffective. Under certain circumstances, however, surgery is undertaken to relieve the buildup of inner ear pressure; and in extreme cases when virtually no hearing remains in the affected ear, surgical destruction of the inner ear may be the procedure of choice.

Central Auditory Processing Problems.   The terms *central deafness, auditory comprehension deficit, word deafness* (and probably many others) have been used to describe this type of impairment. Some problem in the auditory pathways of the brainstem or the auditory cortex itself causes the person to have difficulty using incoming stimuli meaningfully. Even though the pure tone audiogram may be normal, and even though speech is heard at normal hearing levels, the afflicted person has difficulty understanding speech. A similar disorder is called *auditory agnosia*. As we have seen in our chapter on aphasia, in auditory agnosia the person hears but is unable to recognize meaningful sounds, a condition that often accompanies receptive aphasia and greatly complicates therapy. When a central processing problem occurs in the child before the development of speech, it can be difficult to distinguish it from a peripheral hearing loss, and its interference with speech and language development may be substantial. Needless to say, the child who has central processing problems also can be significantly impeded in learning, particularly in areas such as spelling and reading. A great deal remains to be learned about these processing difficulties, but we do know that this child will need much support and understanding from his family. The assistance of the classroom teacher, as well as of the speech pathologist and the audiologist, also will be essential if he is to be able to compensate for the social and educational barriers erected by this little-understood problem.

Hearing Impairment. Many persons use the term "deafness" to refer to any degree of hearing impairment. They say, for instance, that they are "just a little deaf in one ear." What they mean, of course, is that they have some amount of unilateral hearing loss. Again, if they say "The man is a deaf-mute," they probably make two mistakes: first, believing that he is without any hearing at all (which is very rare), and second, that he cannot produce any sound at all (which is completely false). Nearly all persons do have some hearing, even if their hearing is almost nonexistent. Individuals classified as deaf usually can be shown to have some hearing at some level of sound intensity at some frequency or frequencies. How much use can be made of this hearing is another matter, however, and the answer to this question determines whether an individual is regarded as deaf or as hearing impaired.

"Persons who are hearing impaired do not readily fit neatly into the categories of hard-of-hearing or deaf. Thus the adverbs *audiometrically* and *functionally* . . . become essential when describing hearing impairment" (Sanders, 1993). The first term, Sanders explains, refers only to audiometric measures; the latter term takes into account how the individual functions and also acknowledges that the same individual may behave differently under differing conditions. It should be noted, too, that the age at which a hearing loss is incurred will be an important determinant of resultant effects on function. Thus, when we categorize we must do so with caution and with the reminder once again that the *person*, not the impairment or degree of impairment, must remain the focus of our attention and concern.

And there are many such persons. We are not sure exactly how many have hearing impairments, but it is generally agreed that in 1991 approximately 28 million of all people in the United States had some degree of hearing loss, as estimated by the National Institute on Deafness and other Communication Disorders (NIDCD). Some two million people are estimated to be deaf or severely hearing impaired. It is probable that as many as 5 percent of children from birth to 18 years have impaired hearing (not including many of those who have fluctuating or mild losses related to otitis media), that the incidence of hearing loss in special education students is higher than in the general school population, and that noise-induced sensorineural losses among secondary students are becoming more common (American Speech-Language-Hearing Association, 1993). Among adults, it is estimated by the NIDCD that presbycusis is experienced by 30 percent of those in the 65-to-74-year age group and by over 50 percent of those over 75 years of age.

The Deaf.   An audiometric cutoff point that distinguishes the profoundly deaf from the hard of hearing is a loss of 90 dB or more at several frequencies (250 to 2000 Hz). Even though these persons occasionally may be able to hear a few extremely loud sounds they cannot rely on their hearing for communicative purposes, even with amplification. They live in a very silent world. Based upon the time of their hearing loss, they are divided into two groups, the *congenitally deaf* and the deafened (*adventitiously deaf*). The latter were born with normal hearing but later lost their sense of hearing through illness or accident. One reason for the distinction is that if the hearing loss occurs after children have learned to talk (as was true of Heather Whitestone, Miss America 1995), the communication, social, and educational issues they face will differ markedly from those of congenitally deaf children.

The Hard of Hearing.   As in the case of persons who are deaf, the time at which a lesser degree of hearing impairment begins also will affect various of its consequences for the individual. The degree of hearing loss is usually classified as *mild* (a loss of 20 to 40 dB), *moderate* (40 to 55 dB), and *marked* (55 to 70 dB). Persons with mild hearing losses usually have fairly normal speech and can understand normal conversation if the other speaker is not too far away, but they may have trouble hearing the teacher in school or others who speak faintly or indistinctly (see Table 13.1). Persons with moderate hearing losses can understand you only if you talk to them loudly. They have difficulty participating in group discussions or hearing you in the presence of noise. Their language and vocabulary may be limited and they may show their hearing loss by their articulation errors and voice deviations. The severely impaired often resemble the deaf. They may be barely able to hear the sound of a very loud voice from about a foot away, but they probably cannot understand what is said. Even with powerful amplification they tend to have trouble distinguishing the con-

⊞ TABLE 13.1 Levels of Hearing Impairment*

Degree of Impairment	Threshold Level	Ability to Understand Speech
None	-20–20 dB	No difficulty
Mild	20–40 dB	Difficulty with soft speech
Moderate	40–55 dB	Frequent difficulty with normal speech
Marked	55–70 dB	Frequent difficulty with loud speech
Severe	70–90 dB	Understands only shouted or amplified speech
Extreme	90 dB	Cannot understand even amplified speech

*Any assessment of the degree of impairment must also include the *client's* perception of her communicative ability. See M. Demorest and S. Erdman, Development of the communication profile for the hearing impaired, *Journal of Speech and Hearing Disorders*, 1986, 52: 129–143.

sonant sounds. Their comprehension, language, voice, and articulation problems can be so extensive that the severely impaired are often called the "borderline deaf."

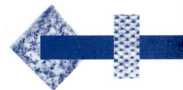

HEARING REHABILITATION

As in the case of many communication disorders, the most effective rehabilitation of individuals with impaired hearing takes place when skilled and knowledgeable specialists work cooperatively together and with the individual and her or his family. Many professionals, including neonatology nurses, pediatricians, classroom and special education teachers and consultants, speech pathologists, interpreters, vocational counselors, genetics counselors, and perhaps psychologists and social workers may be involved at various times, depending upon the individual's initial and evolving needs. Primary roles typically will be played by *audiologists* and by *otologists* (also known as otorhinolaryngologists or, more simply, as ENT physicians).

The otologist is concerned with the medical aspects of hearing impairment. He or she is, first, a physician who is concerned with the total well-being of a patient and, second, a specialist in the area of pathological hearing. The otologist is interested in determining if a hearing loss is present and in differentiating between conductive and sensorineural impairments. She may use various tuning fork tests or perform an audiometric evaluation or check the functioning of the **vestibular system** by means of **caloric tests** since ear problems often manifest themselves through spells of dizziness or vertigo. Also at her disposal is the information that can be gained by laboratory procedures such as X rays, CAT scans, blood tests, bacteriological tests, neurological examinations, and so on. In addition to the specialized techniques used to determine the medical status of a patient's ears, the otologist treats aural pathologies. This treatment may take the form of prescribing medication such as antibiotics for a middle-ear infection, or it may entail some type of ear surgery.

The audiologist's chief role is one of rehabilitation.[8] At least in our present context, this includes detecting hearing losses and referring patients for otologic consultation. It also includes conducting and interpreting specialized tests that may help to determine the site of damage to the hearing system, thus aiding the otologist in making a differential diagnosis. The audiologist is also often able to obtain information about the hearing function of very young children and difficult-to-test individuals. In any event, the habilitation and rehabilitation aspects of hearing impairment are essential domains of the audiologist (see Sanders, 1993).

The audiologist is able to plan the therapy and other assistance needed to help the hearing-impaired person cope with everyday communicative demands. Aural rehabilitation has been defined as

> rehabilitation of the . . . individual through the procedures . . . of speechreading training, speech-hearing training (auditory/listening training), related skills training, speech training, manual communication training, hearing aid orientation and guidance, and family/significant other counseling, so as to enable the individual to function meaningfully with *a minimum of handicap* (Bate, 1987).

Any one person may not need all of these services, but we usually find that auditory training and speechreading form a core of therapy for many people with hearing impairments.

Auditory Training

Auditory training teaches the hearing-impaired person to make the best possible use of residual hearing (Figure 13-11). Even among those individuals classified as profoundly deaf, there is usually some residual hearing for low-frequency sounds. Hard-of-hearing persons often have a great deal of residual hearing that encompasses a relatively broad frequency range, but they may not be making full use of the hearing they possess. Auditory training is training in listening. Listening skills can be improved by training not only in the hearing impaired but even among normally hearing children and adults. To cite a simple example—a person learning to play the guitar usually has a difficult time tuning it since this requires

Vestibular sytem.
Portion of the inner ear that controls balance.

Caloric test.
Water is inserted in the ear canal to induce nystagmus (repetitive eye movements) as a test of vestibular function and balance.

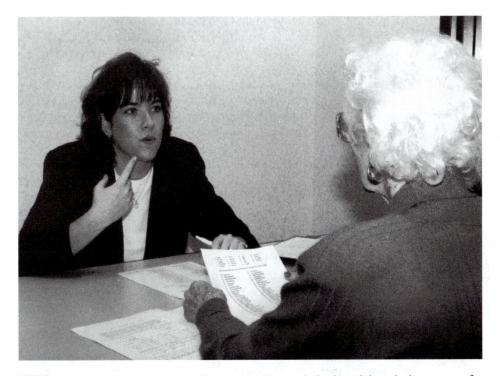

 FIGURE 13-11   Aural rehabilitation training can help the adult make better use of residual hearing (*Van Riper Clinic, Western Michigan University*)

the ability to tell when two strings sound exactly alike when they are held in a certain manner by one hand and plucked with the other. With a bit of persistent practice, the person is usually able to tune the guitar quite readily, becoming able to hear even a slight discrepancy between the tones and to make the proper adjustment. We don't usually refer to this discriminatory process as auditory training, but that is exactly what it is; and it illustrates the point that the discriminating ability of the ear can be improved.

Auditory training must vary according to the age of the person, the age of the onset of hearing loss, and with severity of the loss. It need not be as intensive with adults who have previously had normal communication skills as it would be with a child who must learn to send and receive verbal messages despite a hearing loss. With children, auditory training may start at the level of gross sound discrimination. At this level the child is first taught to differentiate bells from whistles or whistles from horns by the noises they make. Identification training is begun by using only two objects at one time, and then gradually other noisemakers are added. This type of training is continued until the child is quite aware of the importance of sound in making the identification, and until he can make correct differentiations consistently without the aid of visual clues.

From this stage we progress to what is often referred to as "gross speech discriminations." Depending on the skill of the child, the discrimination of speech sounds can begin by first distinguishing between such words as "ball" and "car" and then proceeding to the more difficult contrasts of "bell" and "ball." In the latter instance, although the discrimination is finer, we would still consider this gross speech discrimination since the distinctive differences are produced by dissimilar vowels. Finer speech discriminations are called for when two words such as "same" and "came" are contrasted because consonants do not have as much acoustic power or duration as do the vowels. The acoustic differences between them are even less detectable when such words as "same" and "shame" are contrasted. This pair of words would be particularly difficult for persons having a high-frequency hearing loss because much of the energy necessary for the intelligibility of [s] and [sh] is found in the frequency range of greatest loss. Nevertheless, through skillful auditory training most persons can make real gains.

After he is proficient in making discriminations of single words, the hard-of-hearing person should go on to sentences and paragraphs. Many clinicians feel that therapy should begin with the larger wholes and then work toward the finer discriminations in single words, the argument being that there are more helpful clues in a sentence. Single unrelated words are harder to identify than sentence strings. Therefore, key words are often used, and the patient is asked to repeat the sentence or write down what he hears. To be correct, he must hear the key words in the sentences. Paragraphs can also be prepared that concern subjects or activities suitable for children or adults. After reading the paragraph, the clinician can ask prepared questions to determine how well the person was able to follow running speech. Since many hard-of-hearing persons have difficulty understanding speech in group situations or in the presence of a background noise, all of the above levels can be repeated by introducing varying levels of background noise. The clinician can make tape recordings of various types of noise or the babble of conversation and present this noise at gradually increasing intensity levels until the patient has increased his discrimination proficiency.

Speechreading.
Perceiving the spoken word visually by observing the speaker's facial expressions, gestures, lip movements, also called *lipreading*.

Speechreading

The term ***speechreading*** has now generally displaced the older term *lipreading*, doubtless because there is much more involved in comprehension through visual cues than in just watching lips. Facial expressions, head movements, gestures—all of these can furnish important clues as to what is being said. Even normally hearing people use visual clues to a greater extent than they realize.

Numerous approaches in teaching speechreading have been advocated, but basically they can be divided into two broad categories: the analytic and the synthetic approaches. The analytic approaches stress careful analysis of phonetic elements, whereas the synthetic approaches advocate grasping the "whole" rather than one part at a time. Few audiologists adopt only one of these approaches since research does not seem to show that any one method is any better than the others. The better contributions of each method can be adapted to specific individuals in therapy by educational and rehabilitative audiologists.

Whatever approach is used, there are certain principles that must be followed. The stimulus material must be presented in a *natural* manner much as it would be encountered in a normal communication situation. Whenever material is presented pantomimically (without voice), there is a tendency to exaggerate mouth movements. This is why we use a voice when stimulating the hard-of-hearing person in speechreading. However it is important, especially at the beginning of speechreading training, that the visual channel be emphasized as much as possible; for if the client can hear the clinician, he may be depending on his hearing too much and not obtaining enough practice in observing visual clues.

Beginning speechreading training for children should present the more visible speech sounds so that the child can experience some success right from the start. The child can be told how each sound is made, but care should be taken not to become too analytical.

It must be remembered that speechreading alone is not a perfect substitute for hearing since many sounds of English are just not visible. For this reason a combination approach of auditory training and speechreading is usually recommended. Also, a truly effective program of speechreading must be geared to the interest of the patients involved. With children, lessons can be made enjoyable and interesting if they revolve around things which children tend to love, such as animals or fairy tales. School subjects such as arithmetic, history, and language can be incorporated into speechreading lessons. These kinds of lessons also have the advantage of preparing the child for the vocabulary encountered in the regular classroom.

Initially, speechreading lessons may revolve around matching the movements of the articulators to the names of common objects. However, progress must be made toward the goal of grasping thoughts and concepts conveyed in more abstract language. Thus, speechreading progress is from the concrete to the more abstract. Where we begin depends a lot upon the age and severity of the hearing loss. Determining the needs of the individual is all-important in any good therapy.

The Deaf: Oral, Manual, or Total Communication.

Since you still are likely to encounter it if you work with handicapped children, we should at least mention the oral versus manual controversy that raged hotly just a few years ago and that yet may simmer in a few locales. *Oralists* insisted that a deaf child should be taught to speak and lipread, no matter how long it might take. Their approach would refuse to permit the child or the parents to use signs of any type. They reason that a reliance upon signing will not only impoverish the child's intellectual growth, it will also limit his social outlets to other deaf persons.

The *Manualists* argued that before children will reach out to learn oral language, they must become acquainted with the structure of language. Signs enable exploring the nature of language, they note, and afford a facile means of communication with others. The Manualists point out that the success rate of the Oralists' approach is low and that deaf children will use nonvocal means of communication with each other no matter how adults try to prevent it.

Decisions today tend to focus more on the needs and capabilities of the particular child and on the history and attitudes of the family than on theoretical controversies. *Total Communication* may be promoted, wherein children are encouraged and taught to use all systems, signs and the manual alphabet, amplification and auditory training, speechreading, and oral communication in whatever ways will best enable the individual child.

It would be appropriate here to note, however, that there are deaf people who regard deafness as a positive cultural marker. "What is wrong," they might ask of the Oralist, "with the child's social outlets being limited to other deaf persons?" They feel that striving to use oral communication and otherwise trying to function easily in the normal-hearing community has contributed to others viewing them as inferior and inadequate. They believe that deaf children should use signing without apology and should be helped to develop a sense of pride in belonging to the deaf community. They no doubt would dismiss vigorously Helen Keller's comment that we cited at the beginning of this chapter; and, however we might feel about this deaf **culture** view, it is important to understand that it often is strongly held. Parents, as well as professionals working with deaf children, may find it helpful to consult references which address some of these issues in greater depth.

Culture.
Shared collection of socially transmitted attitudes, beliefs, behavioral characteristics, institutions; not synonymous with race or ethnic group.

Hearing Aids

Many people with sensorineural hearing losses derive substantial benefit from hearing aids. The number of hearing aids used by people with conductive losses is decreasing, on the other hand, because modern surgical techniques are increasingly able to restore their hearing thresholds to levels where amplification is not needed.

Hearing aids have undergone many changes in recent years, and they continue to be improved as advances in technology become incorporated in their design. Certain basic principles and major components, however, are common to all hearing aids. The instrument must have a *microphone* that picks up sound and converts the acoustic signal to electrical energy. The intensity of this electrical signal is increased by an *amplifier,* and the magnified electrical energy is then fed into a miniature loudspeaker, or *receiver,* where it is converted back to sound waves and delivered to the ear. The intensity of the sound wave reaching the ear, usually by way of an individually fitted custom *earmold,* now is greater than it was when originally picked up by the microphone. Beyond these component parts, the hearing aid amplifier must have a source of power. Zinc air batteries are becoming the battery of choice, although the most powerful aids still may require a mercury battery.

Hearing aids can be classified into two types according to where they are worn: body aids or ear-level aids. And ear-level hearing aids, all of which are worn on the head, include a variety of subtypes.

Body hearing aids are larger and more powerful than ear-level aids, but their use today is largely limited to infants and toddlers. The microphone and amplifier unit of this type of aid is worn, as suggested by its name, somewhere on the front of the body. The amplified signal is sent by wire to the receiver, which, in turn, is connected to the earmold.

Ear-level aids take advantage of the benefits associated with having the microphone located very near, sometimes in, the ear itself. Early versions, seldom encountered today, used instruments that were built into the frames of glasses. More current versions of this type of hearing aid include the *Behind-the-Ear* hearing aid, which is hooked behind the auricle with amplified sound being fed to the ear mold by a short piece of plastic tubing. An *In-the-Ear* hearing aid also is available that includes all components of the instrument in a custom-fitted casing that can be inserted into the ear just as an earmold would be. Finally, the *In-the-Canal* hearing aid, an even more miniaturized instrument, suitable for mild and moderate hearing impairments, can be custom molded so that the entire aid can be worn in the ear canal.

Hearing aids generally are able to selectively amplify and suppress sound at various frequencies, and some make provision for special settings to be used in particular situations (such as when using the telephone). Depending on the individual, amplification can be be either **monaural** or **binaural,** or monaural amplification can be modified so that some of the features of binaural hearing seem to be represented. Some aids use digitizing circuitry to enhance their fidelity, and some will automatically adjust to suppress low frequency noise when it becomes excessive. Others have been developed and are being refined that can be preprogrammed by computer to provide optimal amplification under a desired selection of different listening conditions.

Once an appropriate instrument has been obtained, the person with a hearing loss is in need of some hearing-aid orientation sessions. In these

Monaural.
Hearing with one ear.

Binaural.
Pertaining to both ears.

she learns how to care for and use her hearing aid. This would include such things as changing batteries, cleaning the earmold, adjusting the volume control, and so on. She must also come to realize right from the beginning that she is not getting her ears back. For one thing, the quality of sound reproduction is not very good because a hearing aid is essentially a low-fidelity instrument, and hearing-aid users often expect too much from their instruments. We must help such a person understand that a hearing aid is not usually the total answer to her problem.

Difficult listening situations such as those involving groups or background noise will also be difficult when wearing a hearing aid. In fact, in some situations the hearing aid may even add to the confusion. Then, too, the hearing aid may seem so unnatural to the person that he may tend to reject it too hastily. One reason for this is that with the instrument, he is now hearing sounds he has never heard or hasn't heard for a long time, and so he feels bombarded by noise. This is especially true of the adult who has gradually lost part of his hearing over a period of time. Just as a person with normal hearing has to adapt to noise and to direct his attention to what he desires to hear, the hard-of-hearing person must also learn to ignore extraneous noises and to devote his attention to what is being said.

At times a child or adult may complain that his hearing aid squeals whenever he turns the volume control up to where he is getting effective amplification. This squealing or whistling sound probably is due to some of the amplified sound returning to the pickup microphone. This feedback noise can result from sound leaking out around an improperly fitting earmold, perhaps because the earmold was not fitted properly in the first place. Or the size of the ear canal itself may have changed—due to growth in a child, or even due to the wearer having lost weight. Wax impacted in the ear canal can cause this problem, as can changes in the weather, and sometimes the whistling occurs because of an internal problem in the aid, rather than because of earmold leakage.

The first few weeks of using a hearing aid will probably be the most difficult for the hard-of-hearing person. However, if he is helped to understand more about his particular problem, can manipulate the controls of the aid, and understands that the hearing aid is only as good as the effort he puts forth in learning to use it, he is well on his way to becoming an effective and satisfied hearing-aid user.

Vibrotactile Devices

These devices (one example is seen in Figure 13-12) convert sound energy into vibrations that the hearing-impaired person can feel. Much in the manner of a conventional hearing aid, a microphone is used to pick up speech and other sounds. The signal is then sent, in the form of electrical impulses, to an amplifier that magnifies the signal and sends it to one or more vibrators (rather than to a miniaturized loudspeaker). In our pic-

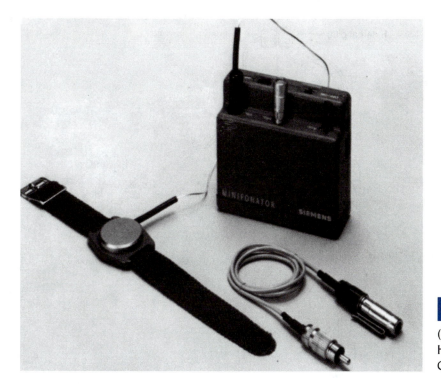

FIGURE 13-12
Vibrotactile aid
(Courtesy of Siemens
Hearing Instrument
Company, Inc.)

tured instrument the vibrator is worn on the wrist, one location that is particularly sensitive to the feeling of vibrations. Other such devices use filters to send different frequency bands of the amplified signal to different locations on the body so that the user may be able to learn to distinguish among various types of environmental and speech sounds, sometimes with remarkable accuracy.

Implantable Devices

For individuals who are deaf or profoundly hearing impaired, recent years have seen the development and continuous refinement of miniature prostheses that replace or bypass the dysfunctional cochlea. The *cochlear implant,* surgically implanted in the cochlea, contains electrodes capable of stimulating the auditory nerve. Sounds picked up by a microphone, worn near an ear, are amplified and filtered by a sophisticated sound processor and then transmitted to the implanted electrodes (Figure 13-13).

In carefully selected patients, this surgery—followed by systematic training in use of the device—has enjoyed considerable success, and it is estimated that over 10,000 individuals are now benefitting from cochlear implants.

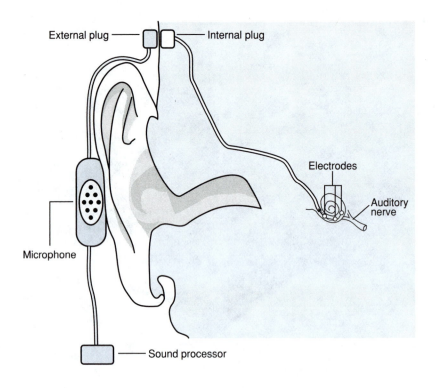

FIGURE 13-13
Cochlear implant

An even more recent arrival on the scene, the *auditory brainstem implant,* would seem to hold substantial promise for patients in whom the auditory nerve itself has been severed or is otherwise dysfunctional. Similar in principle to the cochlear implant, in this procedure the electrodes deliver processed electrical stimulation directly to the auditory brainstem.

Although you may feel that we have overloaded you with information in this chapter, we have truly only skimmed the surface of what you will learn about hearing and hearing disorders if you plan to become an audiologist or a speech-language pathologist. Nevertheless, the topics we've reviewed should prepare you to better understand, and perhaps to better serve, the many people with hearing impairments you will meet in years to come. And you may be better prepared to cope effectively with the hearing loss you yourself are likely to experience in the longer term.

STUDY QUESTIONS

1. Describe the structure and function of the middle ear and the ossicular chain.

2. What is the eustachian tube, where is it located, and what important role(s) does it play?

3. What are the basic anatomic components of the inner ear?

4. What are six indicators of possible hearing loss that may not, in and of themselves, immediately lead someone to suspect a hearing problem?

5. Why may dizziness be related to a possible hearing problem?

6. How would you describe, to a friend who has been scheduled for a hearing evaluation, what he or she should expect to experience during pure tone audiometry?

7. For what purposes is *acoustic immittance testing* included in a comprehensive hearing evaluation?

8. What is the difference between a conductive hearing loss and a sensorineural hearing loss?

9. What is *otitis media,* and why does this condition in a young child cause particular concern for the speech-language pathologist as well as for the audiologist and the otologist?

10. What evidence exists that exposure to noise may lead to permanent hearing loss?

11. Explain, as you would to your grandmother, what is meant by *presbycusis,* and tell her something about its symptoms.

12. What are the basic components of a hearing aid, and what types of hearing aids are generally in use today?

ENDNOTES

[1]Comprehensive presentations of anatomy and physiology of the hearing mechanism may be found in many sources, including Martin (1994), Newby and Popelka (1992), or Perkins and Kent (1986).

[2]Note in Figure 13-1 the lever arrangement of these small ossicles (the stapes is about the size of a grain of rice) that concentrates vibratory energy received at the eardrum.

[3]Behavioral conditioning, rather than a procedure such as this, often is used very successfully to discern responses in young children.

[4]Detailed discussions of immittance testing and of various of the electrophysiological procedures that follow are presented by Martin (1994), Newby and Popelka (1992), and Silverstein, Wolfson, and Rosenberg (1992).

[5]Further information about OME and its management may be obtained from the AHCPR Publications Clearing House, P. O. Box 8547, Silver Springs, MD 20907.

[6]Certain syndromes are known to include sensorineural hearing loss (e.g., Waardenburg and Usher's, which have received particular attention, but others such as Pendred's, Ullrich-Turner, Townes-Brocks, and Coffin-Lowry also are implicated); and many neurodegenerative disorders also are associated with hearing

loss (e.g., neurofibromatosis, myoclonic epilepsy, Friedreich's ataxia, Huntington's chorea, Werdnig-Hoffman disease, Tay-Sach's disease, infantile Gaucher's disease, Niemann-Pick disease, Charcot-Marie-Tooth disease, or any infantile demyelinating neuropathy). To explore genetic matters a bit further, see Arnos, Israel, and Cunningham (1991); also see Hereditary and other childhood auditory deficits (1995).

[7]Newby and Popelka (1992), in their chapter on "Industrial Audiology" provide an excellent overview of the effects of noise.

[8]This in no way minimizes the importance of such activities as research, consulting with industry, and the like. We would note also that some audiologists become highly specialized (for example, in dispensing hearing aids) and seldom, if ever, provide traditional aural rehabilitation services. See Chapter 14 and also the ASHA "Scope of Practice" statement reproduced in Appendix C.

REFERENCES

American Speech-Language-Hearing Association. (1993). Guidelines for audiology services in the schools. *Asha, 35,* 24–32.

American Speech-Language-Hearing Association. (1994). Joint Committee on Infant Hearing 1994 Position Statement. *Asha, 36,* 38–41.

Arnos, K., Israel, J., and Cunningham, M. (1991). *SHHH Journal,* March/April, 28–32.

Bate, H. (1985). Aural rehabilitation of the older adult. *Seminars in Hearing,* 6(2), 193–205.

Bate, H. (1987). *To clients in the Western Michigan University Aural Rehabilitation Program.* Kalamazoo, MI: Western Michigan University.

Bate, H., and Davis, A. (1985). *Hearing impairment in the greater Kalamazoo area: A guide to information and services.* Kalamazoo, MI: The Constance Brown Hearing and Speech Center.

Buchanan, L., Harding, K., and Hudner, C. (1991). Hearing disorder management in Down syndrome patients. *Hearing Instruments,* 42(11), 12–15.

Crawford, M., and Studebaker, G. (1990). Cytomegalovirus: A disease of hearing. *The Hearing Journal,* 43(1), 25–30.

Demorest, M., and Erdman, S. (1986). Development of the communication profile for the hearing impaired. *Journal of Speech and Hearing Disorders,* 52, 129–143.

Engstrom, H., and Engstrom, B. (1979). Structural changes in the cochlea following overstimulation by noise. *Acta Otolaryngologica, Supplement,* 360, 75–79.

Hereditary and other childhood auditory deficits. (1995). *Journal of the American Academy of Audiology,* 6.

Howes, H. (1979). Civilization takes its toll on Eskimo hearing. *Audecibel,* 29, 139–142.

Johnson, K., Williamson, D., and Chmiel, R. (1991). Management of hearing disorder resulting from cytomegalovirus. *Hearing Instruments,* 42(11), 20–22.

Martin, F. (1994). *Introduction to audiology* (5th ed.). Englewood Cliffs, NJ: Prentice Hall.

Newby, H., and Popelka, G. (1992). *Audiology* (6th ed.). Englewood Cliffs, NJ: Prentice Hall.

Sanders, D. (1993). *Management of hearing handicap: Infants to elderly* (3rd ed.). Englewood Cliffs, NJ: Prentice Hall.

Silverstein, H., Wolfson, R., and Rosenberg, B. (1992). Diagnosis and management of hearing loss. *Clinical Symposia,* 44(3). New York: CIBA-GEIGY Corporation.

Stool, S. (1993). Chronic otitis media: speech and language implications. *Van Riper Lectures.* Presentation made in Kalamazoo, MI: Western Michigan University.

SUPPLEMENTARY READINGS

American Speech-Language-Hearing Association. (1990). Guidelines for screening for hearing impairment and middle-ear disorders. *Asha*, 32(Suppl 2), 17–24.

Hall, J., and Chase, P. (1993). Answers to ten common clinical questions about otoacoustic emissions today. *The Hearing Journal*, 46(1), 29–34.

National Deafness and Other Communication Disorders Advisory Board. (1992). *Research in human communication*. (NIH Publication No. 93–3562). Annual Report. Bethesda, MD: National Institute on Deafness and Other Communication Disorders.

Perkins, W., and Kent, R. (1986). *Functional anatomy of speech, language, and hearing*. San Diego, CA: College-Hill Press.

Roeser, R., and Downs, M. (1995). *Auditory disorders in school children*. New York: Thieme Medical Publishers, Inc.

The Center for Hearing Loss in Children, Boys Town National Research Hospital, 555 North 30th Street, Omaha, NE 68131 (402/498–6319) This center, funded by NIDCD, publishes and disseminates a very informative and clearly written "Public Information Series" that covers a wide variety of topics in easily understood terms.

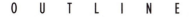

Chapter 14

The Speech and Hearing Professions

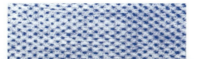

At the beginning of this book we invited the reader to watch a few speech-language pathologists and audiologists as they went about their appointed rounds serving children and adults with communication disorders. We sought to present verbal portraits of real human beings as they struggled with speech, language, or hearing disabilities. In subsequent chapters we looked briefly at normal communication processes, and we have reviewed some of the major types of communication disorders. So by now you should have acquired a relatively broad (but far from complete) picture of the professions of audiology and speech-language pathology and of the problems with which they must cope.

Perhaps you are intrigued enough to think about entering one or the other of these two fields of study, or maybe you have decided at least to explore them more closely as you consider various vocational options. But even those of you who are headed in other directions should know more about the speech and hearing professions, if only in order to be able to refer someone with a communication disorder to an appropriately qualified professional. A competent clinician often can be of great help to you or your family or to some of the individuals you may serve in your own profession.

In this chapter you will learn a bit about the history of speech-language pathology and audiology[1] and something more about the present status of the two professions. And, while crystal balls are notoriously fallible, we'll nevertheless dust off ours and identify some possible future trends.

ORIGINS OF THE SPEECH AND HEARING PROFESSIONS

Early Precursors

When we were tadpoles and you were a fish in Paleozoic time, there were no speech or hearing clinicians, although disorders of speech and hearing have been noted even in the earliest historical accounts. A piece of clay found in Assyria bears the hieroglyphics of a woeful stutterer. They tore out the tongues of liars in ancient China. Demosthenes not only stuttered but could not say his /r/ sounds. The Bible tells of lisps and hearing losses and of people losing entirely their ability to speak. The Greeks and Romans as well as some Christian popes castrated young boys so that they would continue to sing soprano. Deaf mutes, the congenitally "deaf and dumb," were treated by the ancients as mental incompetents who were totally unable to learn. Old skulls of the Incas showed they had severe mastoid infections and cleft palates. Ever since humans invented speech, some persons have suffered from speech and hearing problems.

And some of these people had clinicians—of a sort. Demosthenes was trained by the actor Satyrus to shout against the waves of the sea with pebbles in his mouth, to put heavy lead plates on his chest, and to run up the mountain while talking. The Oracle of Delphi told a Greek named Battos, who according to Herodotus had a shrill and stammering voice, to get the hell out of Greece, to exile himself in Libya and never come back. This is a therapy that many clinicians still would like to offer at times to certain clients.

Aristotle said that many voice disorders were caused by shouting too loudly after a full meal and prescribed silence. Celsus, classic physician to the Roman world during the first century A.D., wrote: "When the tongue is paralyzed, either from a vice of the organ, or as a consequence of other diseases, and when the patient cannot articulate, gargles should be administered. He should drink water, and the head, neck, and parts below the chin be well rubbed." Near the end of the seventh century a Bishop John of York is reported to have cured a young deaf boy of **mutism.** After making the sign of the cross on the boy's tongue, the Bishop instructed him in the mouth movements for various sounds and words. His success was regarded as a heavenly miracle; but in this approach we see intimations of the **motokinesthetic** method, which enjoyed popularity early in our own century. Nor is it difficult to find traces of other of these early remedies in modern clinical practice.

The Middle Ages and Beyond

Abu Ali Hussain Avicenna, about a thousand years after Christ, was a court philosopher and physician in Arabia who described many speech disorders, attributing them to lesions of the brain or of the nerves. He believed that stammering was caused by spasm of the epiglottis. Yet another physician during the Middle Ages recommended that stutterers be given large doses of croton oil, a very potent laxative. Probably this made them afraid to force or struggle!

It was to be a few hundred years before much progress would be made in the understanding of hearing or speech processes. During the century following the discovery of America, an Italian anatomist, Eustachius, first described in detail the auditory tube that continues to bear his name. In that same century, a Spanish monk, Pedro Ponce de Leon, taught some deaf children not only to read and write, but also to read lips; and a few decades later, in 1616, Giovanni Bonofacio wrote a book on sign language for the deaf. Until this period, little evidence is found of anyone believing that deaf individuals were able to be educated.

Mutism.
Without speech. Voluntary mutism: refusal to speak.

Motokinesthetic method.
A methods for teaching sounds and words in which the therapist directs the movements of the tongue, jaw, and lips by touch and manipulation.

In England at about the same time, Francis Bacon offered an interesting cure for stammering, which he felt was due to a tongue that was too cold. He suggested warming it with wine. And those who followed his advice probably gained some fluency temporarily. Early in the 1700s Moses Mendelssohn, a great Jewish philosopher who stuttered himself, theorized that stuttering was the product of conflicting needs to speak and to refrain from speaking because of fear or other emotion. His view of stuttering as an approach-avoidance conflict anticipated the work of Joseph Sheehan two hundred years later. In the field of hearing, the first public school for the deaf was opened in Paris in 1775, nearly fifty years before Thomas Gallaudet (after whom Gallaudet College for the deaf in Washington is now named) established the first such school in the United States in Hartford, Connecticut.

The Early Nineteenth Century

In the early 1800s, a Dr. Yates in New York invented what came to be known as "The American Method" for curing stuttering. The secret method consisted of holding the tip of the tongue elevated toward the palate and wearing a cotton pad under the tongue to help keep it elevated. This century was also marked by efforts to cure stuttering by surgery. Dieffenbach, a German physician, sliced across the base of the tongue and later also took a wedge out of its middle in order to prevent lingual spasms. The method spread like wildfire because of the reported cures, and stutterers were butchered all over the world until the fashion ran its course and died out.

It was also during the nineteenth century, though, that speech and hearing processes and disorders first began to be studied systematically and various methods of treatment explored—mostly in Germany, Austria, England, France, and the United States. Arnott, an Englishman, felt that the basic problem in stuttering was a laryngeal spasm, with inability to produce voice at will. And around the time of our Civil War, Herman Klencke in Germany was among the first to describe the anxieties and fear of the stutterer and to suggest, among other things, that rate control could overcome the fear.

Much of the early work focused on stuttering, but there was growing interest in other areas as well. Medical descriptions of wooden and bone "plugs," carved for closing clefts in the hard palate, were published as early as 1823. Alfonso Corti was studying the inner ear and described in 1836 the organ that contains the sensory cells essential to hearing **(Organ of Corti)**. In 1854 a singing teacher in France, Manuel Garcia, discovered how to use a mirror to illuminate and observe the vocal folds, a technique that soon thereafter was employed by the Austrian physicians Turck and Czermak to examine pathologies of the larynx. At about the same time, along with studying how the ossicular chain carries vibrations

Organ of Corti.
Organ in the cochlea containing sensory hairs that transform mechanical movements into electrical impulses capable of stimulating the auditory nerve; the "organ of hearing."

to the inner ear, Helmholtz was formulating his "resonance theory" of hearing.

In the early 1800s the phrenologist Franz Gall was busy relating behaviors and character traits to conformation of the skull, ideas that gave rise to speculations about the causes of aphasia. Then in 1861 the neurologist Paul Broca, whose name still is attached to an area of the cortex, presented his argument for the concept of cerebral localization, leading a procession of writers such as Wernicke and Jackson on that subject. Also in the 1860s, Theodor Billroth performed the first surgical amputation of a larynx and enlisted one of his pupils, Karl Gussenbauer, to construct the first artificial larynxes.

Alexander Graham Bell, whose father had developed the "Visible Speech" symbol system for teaching deaf students to produce speech sounds, began to train teachers of the deaf in Boston in 1872 and became a professor at Boston University in 1873. His understanding of vocal anatomy and speech sound production, combined with his interest in electricity, drove the ongoing laboratory experiments that led to his invention of the telephone in 1875. In 1890 he founded the American Association to Promote the Teaching of Speech to the Deaf, known today as the Alexander Graham Bell Association for the Deaf. Bell is said to have observed in later years that he would rather be remembered as a teacher of the deaf than as inventor of the telephone. Perhaps, as others of us might understand, he had come to be annoyed when interrupted too often by a ringing phone!

Another very famous inventor, a contemporary of A. G. Bell, also should be mentioned here. Thomas Alva Edison seldom appears in accounts of our origins, though occasional reference is seen to his progressive hearing loss. However, from Edison's work—in particular his inventions of the phonograph and incandescent electric lighting, and his later contributions to motion picture photography—invaluable tools evolved for research and clinical work in speech and hearing.

The Early Twentieth Century

At the turn of the century a few speech clinics already existed in Austria, Denmark, and Germany. Also in Europe, a new medical specialty called "phoniatrics" was emerging for the treatment of speech and voice disorders. Meanwhile, in the United States, "institutes" for the treatment of speech defects, such as the Lewis, the Millard, and the Bogue commercial schools, thrived in the early 1900s. Each one guaranteed a cure for an exorbitant fee, and each insisted that the applicant swear an oath of secrecy never to divulge the method. All types of speech disorders received the same treatment: a period of silence, breathing exercises, phonetic drills, chanting to a time beat, speaking in unison with others or with arm swings. Your senior author attended one of these institutes in 1922 along with some 64 patients of all ages from all over the world. All of the "cured" stutterers, he later learned, had relapsed within a year. He himself had relapsed on the train on his way home.

More positive developments also were underway, however, here as well as in Europe. Carl Emil Seashore, director of the Psychological Laboratory at the University of Iowa, was studying the psychology of music, conducting basic voice research, and continuing his development of the audiometer, an instrument he had worked on as a graduate student at Yale University with E.W. Scripture. In 1914, Emil Froeschels focused the efforts of his Viennese clinic on the treatment of speech disorders stemming from head wounds—World War I was beginning— and voice problems "caused by neuroses." In Chicago and in Detroit "speech correction teachers" were employed by the public schools as early as 1910, with Boston soon to follow. A few physicians and psychologists started to create small speech clinics in universities. The first of these was established in 1914 by Smiley Blanton at the University of Wisconsin, the same institution that soon (in 1921) would award to Sara M. Stinchfield the first doctoral degree ever earned in speech correction. At this time we still could count only a handful of workers in the field of speech pathology, though there were comparatively many teachers of the deaf, who were among the predecessors of the field of audiology. It was in 1928 that Georg von Békésy began the long series of cochlear studies that led to his receipt, in 1961, of the Nobel prize in medicine for his contributions to our understanding of the ear and hearing.

The More Recent Past

Many accounts trace the formal beginnings of speech-language pathology in the United States to the 1920s. In 1925 Seashore sponsored a meeting in Iowa City, convened by Lee Edward Travis, among a handful of people who represented various disciplines but who shared a common interest in the study and treatment of speech disorders. It is of interest to note that a year earlier, in Vienna, Froeschels had gathered together a group of some 65 phoniatrists and other physicians, logopedists (non-physician speech therapists), and academicians to form the organization that today is known as the *International Association of Logopedics and Phoniatrics* (IALP). Here in our country, the Iowa City conference led later in 1925 to formation of the *American Academy of Speech Correction*, known today as the *American Speech-Language-Hearing Association*, with Robert West of the University of Wisconsin as its first president.

The original members brought to the academy a wide variety of professional perspectives. Among them, for example, were Max Goldstein, the otolaryngologist who founded the Central Institute for the Deaf in

St. Louis, and Pauline Camp from Wisconsin, the first state director of a public school speech correction program, as well as Mabel Gifford, who directed the state public school program in California. One charter member was a public school speech correctionist, one a speech correctionist in a school for the blind, another was principal of the School for the Deaf in Hawaii, and yet another was a graduate student of West's. There were two more physicians, a number of university faculty members, and others. Perhaps in part because of this diversity, a broad foundation was laid, and the subsequent evolution of this organization largely paralleled and often led the ongoing development of the speech and hearing professions.

The academy's name was changed in 1927 to the *American Society for the Study of Disorders of Speech* and then to the *American Speech Correction Association* in 1934, and it had begun in 1936 to publish the *Journal of Speech Disorders*. From a total of 22 members in 1926, membership had grown fifteen years later to a total of 374, when the United States became engaged in World War II. These 374 members included not only your senior author, but some of his contemporaries who already were becoming leaders in the new profession. Among them was Wendell Johnson, whose prolific work—both in stuttering and in general semantics—would soon gain wide acclaim and would contribute enormously to the eventual recognition and acceptance of speech pathology in academic, professional, and governmental arenas.

During and after the war, treatment and rehabilitation for veterans and then for other disabled persons became high priority concerns among Americans. Considerable growth and technical progress occurred in various of the helping and special service professions, including speech and hearing. Seashore had trained C. Bunch in 1920 as a "psychologist of otology" who then devoted years to the development of hearing testing methods; and Scott Reger, also a Seashore student, had been working with clinical audiometry since 1931. But it was not until the mid-1940s that audiology began actually to emerge as a clearly defined area of professional practice.

Raymond Carhart and Norton Canfield generally are credited with promoting the term "audiology" in 1945 as a name for the study of hearing and hearing disorders. Like many other of the early audiologists, Carhart was a speech pathologist who, because of the war, became involved in aural rehabilitation work for the army; and Canfield was an otology consultant for the government at the same time. At any rate, although christened belatedly, the profession derived from many decades of productive effort by clinicians, scientists, educators, and engineers.[2]

College coursework in audiology began to appear in the 1940s, and university speech clinics became speech *and hearing* clinics. Increasing numbers of students, practitioners and researchers focused their attention on hearing and hearing disorders, and in 1947 the *American Speech Correction Association* was renamed the *American Speech and Hearing Association*. The following year its journal was retitled the *Journal of Speech and Hearing Disorders.*

Growth of the organization and of the professions has been steady and, at times, exceptionally rapid over the years that followed. In 1958 the Association opened its first National Office in Washington, DC, and hired an audiologist, Kenneth O. Johnson, its first full-time paid employee, as executive secretary. That same year brought publication of the first volume of the *Journal of Speech and Hearing Research,* and the monthly periodical *Asha* made its initial appearance.

In 1969 ASHA created a Legislative Council, comprised of elected representatives from every state and from the international membership, to serve as the governing body of the Association. It was 1969 also when Florida became the first state to establish a law requiring the licensure of speech pathologists and audiologists. By now the total ASHA membership had grown to just over 12,000, but doubtless there were at least another three or four thousand non-ASHA-members who were actively working in the field.

The Current Scene

By the 1970s increasing numbers of speech clinicians in the schools were recognizing the underlying language problems represented in their caseloads, especially among youngsters who also had learning disabilities. Their professional focus broadened and, reflecting this "new" perspective (although, of course, speech pathologists long had been recognized as the providers of language therapy for persons with aphasia, delayed speech development, severe hearing loss, and so on), we became speech-language pathologists and our national organization underwent its most recent (and perhaps its final) name change. In 1978 it became the *American Speech-Language-Hearing Association* but retained its by then familiar and established acronym, ASHA.

From its 1978 membership of 30,000, ASHA has grown to over 83,000 in 1995, of whom about 12,000 are audiologists. And, although it is impossible to know exactly the number of practitioners, researchers, and academicians who are not affiliated with ASHA, some observers in the past have estimated that ASHA represents 60 to 70 percent of the speech-language pathology and audiology national workforce. Whatever the actual number may be, it is substantial (and probably well over 100,000). As you might expect, the variety of settings in which these thousands of professionals work, and the diversity and complexity of the roles they fill, have expanded as dramatically as have their numbers over the past fifty years.

ORGANIZATIONS AND STANDARDS

American Speech-Language-Hearing Association

Although most of the speech-language pathologists and audiologists in the United States are affiliated with ASHA, the ASHA membership is not limited to clinical practitioners, nor is it limited to U.S. citizens. It includes language, speech, and hearing research scientists, university faculty members, program administrators, government officials, and others who share a common interest in human communication and its disorders.

A few ASHA members reside in other countries, including Australia, Canada, England, Germany, Greece, Israel, Japan, Mexico, New Zealand, Saudi Arabia, South Africa, Switzerland, Taiwan, the Scandinavian countries, several South American nations, and others. And ASHA itself is now one of 50 organizations from over 30 countries that are affiliates of the *International Association of Logopedics and Phoniatrics*. IALP, as you will recall, is the organization that was formed by Froeschels in Vienna just before ASHA was born in Iowa City.

The purposes toward which the considerable resources of ASHA are directed today may appear incredibly ambitious; but, in reality, they (appropriately) do not differ substantially from the aims of our founders. As set forth in the Bylaws of the Association, the seven basic purposes of ASHA remain compelling and relevant:

1. To encourage basic scientific study of the processes of individual human communication with special reference to speech, language, and hearing.
2. To promote appropriate academic and clinical preparation of individuals entering the discipline of human communication sciences and disorders and promote the maintenance of current knowledge and skills of those within the discipline.
3. To promote investigation and prevention of disorders of human communication.
4. To foster improvement of clinical services and procedures concerning such disorders.
5. To stimulate exchange of information among persons and organizations thus engaged, and to disseminate such information.
6. To advocate the rights and interests of persons with communication disorders.
7. To promote the individual and collective professional interests of the members of the Association.

The National Office of the organization is located in Rockville, Maryland, and has over 100 paid employees who, along with member volunteers, legislative councilors, and elected office holders, are engaged in carrying on the business of the Association. Among the many activities in which it is engaged, ASHA now publishes a host of monographs and special reports, some of which are consumer-oriented, and some of which target legislators and governmental agencies. The Association also publishes four scholarly journals in addition to the monthly periodical, *Asha* (eleven issues per year): *Journal of Speech and Hearing Research*, six per year; *Language, Speech and Hearing Services in Schools*, four each year; and, three times each year, *American Journal of Speech-Language Pathology*, and *American Journal of Audiology*.

Some 10,000 or more members and guests attend its Annual Convention, and many more participate in various of the other continuing education programs sponsored or approved by ASHA. Most importantly, according to some members, the Association has developed and actively administers standards programs for (1) certifying the competence of individual clinicians, (2) accrediting graduate programs that prepare entry-level clinicians, and (3) accrediting facilities that provide clinical services to the public.

Satisfaction of ASHA standards for academic and practicum preparation (in an accredited graduate program) by individual students, together with successful completion of a Clinical Fellowship Year and a passing performance on the National Examination in Speech-Language Pathology (or in Audiology) culminates in the receipt of the Certificate of Clinical Competence, either in speech-language pathology (CCC-SLP) or in audiology (CCC-A). Detailed outlines of the respective requirements can be found in Clinical Certification Board (1994).

We should note that ASHA has established a number of Special Interest Divisions (SIDs) in an effort to better accommodate the professional diversity of its members. At the present time there are thirteen such divisions, and any member may join one or more of these SIDs: *Language Learning and Education; Neurophysiology and Neurogenic Disorders; Voice and Voice Disorders; Fluency; Speech Science and Orofacial Disorders; Hearing Disorders; Aural Rehabilitation; Hearing Conservation; Hearing in Childhood; Administration; Augmentative and Alternative Communication; Swallowing and Swallowing Disorders;* and *Communication Disorders and Sciences in Linguistically Diverse Populations*. Moreover, mechanisms now are evolving whereby individual practitioners with sufficient experience and expertise, and who already hold the CCC, will be able to qualify for "specialty recognition" in particular disorder areas.

American Academy of Audiology

Another professional organization in our country that has experienced significant growth in the past few years is the *American Academy of Audiology* (AAA). Founded in 1988 "for the purpose of promoting the

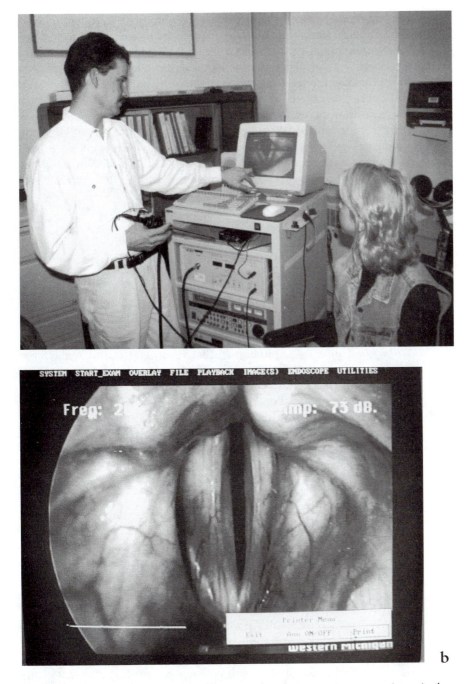

FIGURE 14-1   (A) Graduate students gain hands-on practicum experience in the Voice Laboratory, where (B) videotaped laryngeal images can contribute to an understanding of voice disorders. (*Photos by Cameron Photography, Phoenix, Arizona*)

public good by fostering the growth, development, recognition, and status of the profession of Audiology and its members" (American Academy of Audiology, 1992), the AAA maintains a national office in Arlington, Virginia. According to its mission statement, the Academy seeks to serve the special interests and needs of audiologists ". . . through professional development, education, research, and increased public awareness of hearing disorders and audiologic services." Like ASHA (see Appendix A) and any professional organization, the AAA has developed and promulgates a Code of Ethics (see Appendix B), which is intended basically to protect the welfare of those persons served professionally by its members.

Other Organizations

Depending upon their work settings, interests, and responsibilities, speech-language-hearing professionals often are members of such organizations as the *Acoustical Society of America,* the *Council of Exceptional Children,* the *Alexander Graham Bell Association for the Deaf,* the *United States Society for Augmentative and Alternative Communication,* the *National Black Association for Speech, Language and Hearing,* the *Academy of Dispensing Audiologists,* the *Society of Hospital Directors of Communicative Disorders Programs,* or others—and there are dozens. Undergraduate and graduate students preparing to enter the professions are able to become members of the *National Student Speech-Language-Hearing Association* (NSSLHA); and, in fact, this organization is entitled to two voting positions on the ASHA Legislative Council. Some 17,000 students were members in 1994, and local chapters of NSSLHA are found on many university campuses. If there is one on yours, you may find it a good source of professional insights (and a good way to expand your social circle!).

Every state in the country has a state speech-language-hearing association, many of which are relatively large and very active. Some publish their own journals, some maintain placement-employment services, and virtually all hold annual conferences. In some instances, two or three adjacent states join together for the purpose of holding conferences. Finally, you also may expect to find local professional organizations, especially in larger metropolitan areas.

In Appendix D you will find addresses and telephone numbers for a sampling of these organizations as well as for a few of the many consumer and support groups that relate to communication sciences and disorders. Often you will find such contacts can provide a wealth of information on highly specialized topics. They also provide advice, and sometimes even financial assistance, for people who wish to establish local support groups.

SOME LEGAL AND ETHICAL CONSIDERATIONS

We've mentioned the national program of clinical certification that has been administered in its present general form by ASHA since 1965. And CCC is a minimum expectation of many employers of clinicians. It is important to recognize, however, that seeking national certification is voluntary and that the CCC has no *legal* status. In forty-four states the practice of speech-language pathology and/or audiology is *legally regulated by licensure laws*. One state (Alaska) licenses audiology but not speech-language pathology, and one (New Hampshire) licenses speech-language pathology but not audiology. The remaining forty-two states regulate (Minnesota, by "registration" rather than licensure) both professions, and six regulate nether.

The requirements for licensure generally follow closely the ASHA requirements for certification, but this is not always true, and there are several other types of differences in licensure law from state to state. Some have reciprocity provisions so that a licenseholder from another state may automatically qualify for licensure; others have no such provision. Some require licensure for work in *any* employment setting, others may exempt certain practitioners from licensure requirements. For example, clinicians employed by public school systems may not be *required* to hold licenses (although, of course, they are not prevented from obtaining licenses if they wish and if they meet the requirements of the state's licensure law). Some state laws allow the audiologist to dispense hearing aids, others do not. Characteristics of state licensure laws (1995) will give you, at a glance, a feel for the variabilities involved. If you hope to practice in a state that has licensure, it will be wise for you to become thoroughly familiar—as early as possible—with any particular requirements you may need to satisfy while you are in graduate or undergraduate school.

We should acknowledge that there are a few states that do not have licensure laws, or where exemption from licensure is available, that also have no requirement that clinicians hold the master's degree—even though for thirty years there has been national recognition of the master's degree as the *minimum* level of preparation for entering our fields. In some states that require the master's degree, employers have been known nevertheless to hire bachelor's level graduates as clinicians. Technically, such practices may not be *illegal* in the strictest sense. However, we know that undergraduate preparation is insufficient, and we believe it is clearly *unethical* to offer "service" by unqualified personnel to trusting clients and their families. Nevertheless, because of the shortage of qualified clinicians, and because many employers are expected—with inadequate budgets—to provide services for communication disorders, we may continue to see this behavior. We hope that you will not be party to such shenanigans, even if you agree (and we certainly do) that "cost containment" is an imperative for the health and human service professions. And, by the way, what principles and rules do you find in the Code of Ethics of ASHA and the Code of Ethics of AAA that address this type of situation? Are there ways that expenses can be minimized while still holding paramount the welfare of our clients?

Federal Laws

As much as we might believe that government sometimes can become too pervasive or intrusive in our daily lives (especially at tax time), we also recognize that certain federal legislation has provided impetus for positive change. The same can be said for some state laws (at least in some states). However, our brief focus here is on just a few national initiatives that seem to have enhanced the delivery of services to individuals who have speech, language, or hearing problems. It is worth noting that whenever a federal and state law conflict, federal law must be followed unless the state law sets the higher standard. For the most part, the following federal laws are among those of particular relevance to our professions.

Social Security Act of 1965. This act established federally funded Medicare for the elderly and disabled, including Part B (supplementary and voluntary), which made outpatient rehabilitation more readily available. It also established Medicaid for women and children on welfare and for the elderly poor, blind, and disabled. (Although Medicaid is administered at the state level, Medicaid funding actually comes from federal grants to the states.)

Public Law 90-538 (1968). This legislation established model programs via the Handicapped Children's Early Education Program (HCEEP) to demonstrate the feasibility of providing special education and related services to young children with disabilities. Small grant incentives were provided to states for each preschool child who received services of the type being given to school-aged children.

Federal Rehabilitation Act of 1973, Section 504. Under this law any agency receiving any type of federal assistance was forbidden to refuse services or employment to a qualified handicapped person because of the handicap.

Public Law 94-142 (1975). The Education of the Handicapped Act guaranteed that disabled children and youth from 5 to 21 years of age would receive free and appropriate public education in the "least restrictive environment," including special education and related services.

Public Law 98-199 (1983).   A state planning grant program was established under HCEEP providing grants to states for planning, developing, and implementing services for children from birth through age five.

Public Law 99-457 (1986).   These amendments to PL 94-142 established multidisciplinary programming for infants and toddlers with disabilities and their families and required the development of Individualized Family Service Plans. The law also mandated provision of services to all preschool children ages 3 to 5 (to begin in 1991) and required coordination, monitoring, and evaluation of service delivery by a designated case manager.

Individuals with Disabilities Education Act (IDEA) of 1990.   This act reauthorized the 1975 Education of the Handicapped Act and altered the language used in referring to its beneficiaries.

Public Law 101-336 (1990).   Known as the Americans with Disabilities Act, PL 101-336 assures that persons with disabilities receive protections in the private sector similar to—but more encyclopedic than—those provided in the public sector by the 1973 Federal Rehabilitation Act. Among other things, the ADA requires "reasonable accommodation" of disabilities in the workplace and the removal of architectural and communication barriers, including the provision of relay stations for users of telecommunication devices for the deaf (TDDs). This legislation is far too comprehensive for us to review adequately here; but we would urge any reader, regardless of career intentions, to peruse the very readable digest written by Fox-Grimm (1991). The ADA will impact broadly on our entire society, and we all will do well to be familiar with it, personally as well as professionally.

CAREER OPTIONS

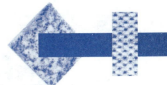

The roles, responsibilities, and prerogatives of speech, language, and hearing professionals today would astound our founding fathers and mothers, foresighted though they were. As you will see in Appendix C, the ASHA approved scopes of practice for audiologists and speech-language pathologists are broad indeed. Among the purposes served by the Scope of Practice document is the education of other professionals and the public regarding the preparation and credentialing of clinicians and regarding the variabilities that exist among and between practitioners in speech-language and hearing. You will find Appendix C of particular interest if you plan to join us, but bear in mind that even during your remaining years in school it is very likely that new and broadened scopes of practice will evolve continuously.

Members of the speech and hearing professions are to be found working in college and university clinics, hospitals, extended care and home health facilities, governmental agencies, research laboratories, private and public schools, physicians' offices, private practices, rehabilitation centers, and even in business and industry.

Recent data indicate that about 80 percent of all certified ASHA members are involved *primarily* in the direct provision of clinical services (although 90 percent provide such services). Among speech pathologists, about 55 percent are employed in schools; among audiologists, about 13 percent. Some 45 percent of audiologists work in nonresidential health-care facilities, 20 percent in hospitals. Among speech pathologists the comparable figures are 10 percent and 16 percent, respectively. Few (about 0.7 percent) are unemployed, other than by personal choice, and they are among the health and human service professionals expected to enjoy increasing demand as we move into the 21st century.

 FIGURE 14-2   Learning one form of manual communication (*Van Riper Clinic, Western Michigan University*)

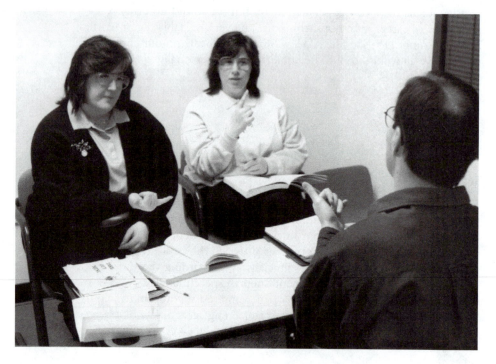

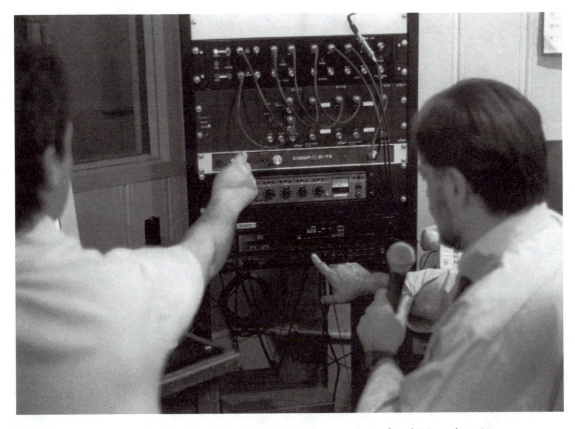

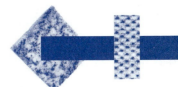
FIGURE 14-3   The scientific study of speech requires an array of sophisticated equipment (*Speech Acoustics Laboratory, Western Michigan University*)

FUTURE TRENDS

We are confident that the speech and hearing professions will continue to thrive, although there will be challenges to face and problems to resolve. We've already mentioned cost containment as a fundamental thrust that no doubt will bring about changes in some of the ways some clinical services now are delivered. We expect to see much greater utilization of support personnel for more routine tasks not requiring extensive educational preparation, and it may well be that fully qualified speech and hearing clinicians will spend greater portions of their time in collaborative consultation with other professionals who can assist in the therapy

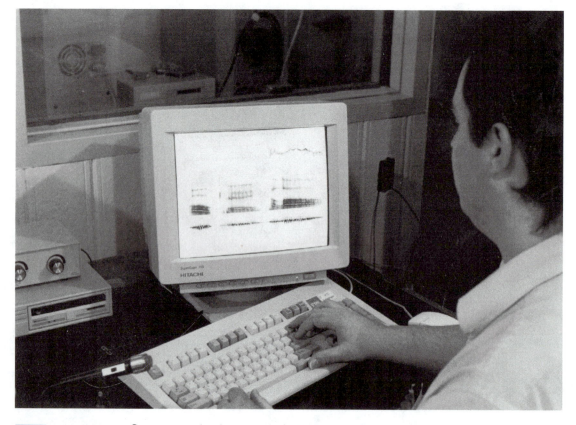

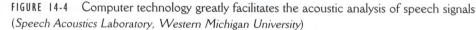

FIGURE 14-4   Computer technology greatly facilitates the acoustic analysis of speech signals (*Speech Acoustics Laboratory, Western Michigan University*)

process. It remains to be seen whether current movements toward specialization or toward the doctorate as the minimum entry level preparation will be seen as viable and as serving the public interest in times of fiscal constraint.

There will be continued call for "multi-skilled" workers who can shift from role to role, presumably providing a variety of rehabilitation services more economically than otherwise would be possible. We'll also see greater participation on multidisciplinary teams that seldom may meet face to face but whose assessments and recommendations will be coordinated somehow by a case manager. Health care in general will be revisited (and re-revisited) by our government, and we will be expected to demonstrate very convincingly not only the efficacy but the cost effectiveness of our clinical services.

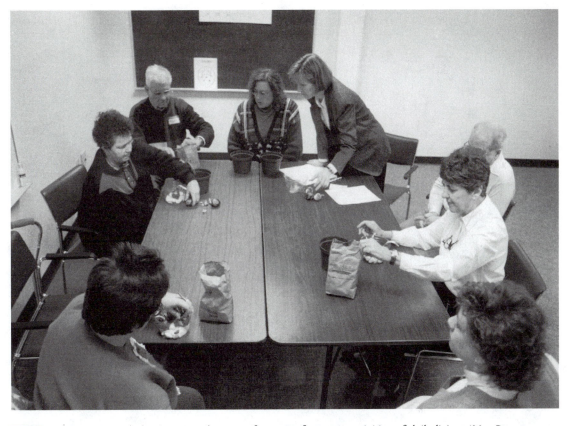

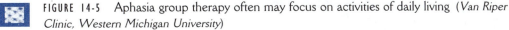

FIGURE 14-5   Aphasia group therapy often may focus on activities of daily living (*Van Riper Clinic, Western Michigan University*)

Unfortunately, and we hope we're wrong about this, the cost containment pressures of the future may further divert our attention and our resources from the critical need to maintain and further enhance the research and science bases of our professions. This we must avoid if we genuinely are to hold paramount the welfare of the clients we serve. Without a solid and expanding knowledge base we are ill-equipped to improve clinical services or to work effectively toward the prevention of communication disorders. We dare not allow these professions, so long in the making, to be transformed to mere occupations or skilled trades.

Among the more knowable aspects of the future, it is very clear, as we've mentioned many times in this book, that our country's population demographics are changing. We are becoming more culturally and racially diverse, and we are getting older. We have little question, however, that

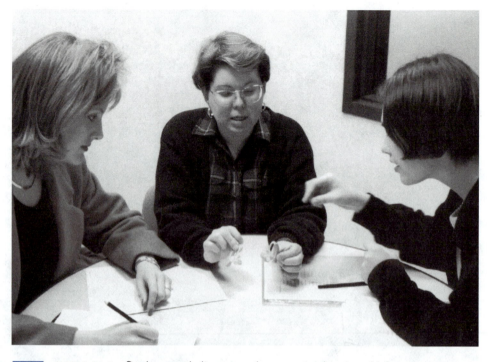

 FIGURE 14-6   Students and clients together examine hearing aid features (*Van Riper Clinic, Western Michigan University*)

the speech and hearing professions have the will and the means to respond appropriately and effectively to the challenges posed by demography. The members of our professions are robust and creative, and they will rise to any reasonable challenge.

Most students enter a career in speech pathology because they want to help others, because they are compassionate, and certainly their ability to help communicatively deprived persons solve their problems is one of their major satisfactions. We need meaningfulness in our lives. Having status and power and material possessions and belly pleasures are not enough to constitute a good life. Surely there should be something more. Most clinicians find that extra something in their fellow humans, in seeing some twisted life become untangled as the result of their efforts.

But there are other satisfactions as well. For one thing, the work itself is usually pleasant work. Our clients come to us feeling that speaking is unpleasant, that communication is full of threat. They are often hesitant to enter a close relationship. Accordingly, one of our first tasks is to change these attitudes; we must make conversing pleasant rather than punishing. With little children much of our work is done through play, and even with adults our interaction is usually flavored with humor and

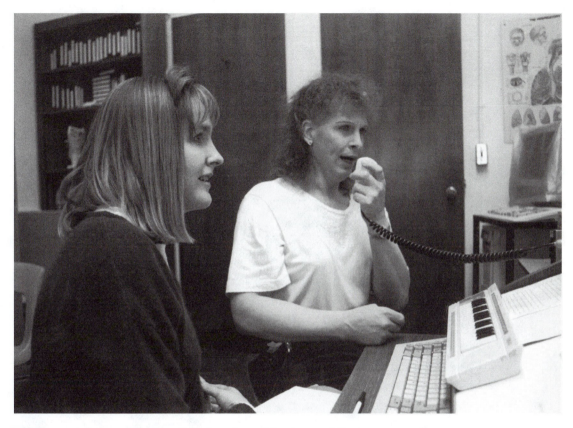

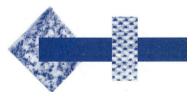 FIGURE 14-7   The visual display of vocal fundamental frequency on a computer screen can help the client and the clinician to monitor and control pitch of the voice (*Van Riper Clinic, Western Michigan University*)

comradeship. The best clinicians we have known have shared several traits in common: They cared deeply about others and they were very sensitive to human needs and feelings. They were genuine, open, and reasonably well adjusted.

SOME CONCLUDING COMMENTS

Especially for readers who are thinking of careers in speech-language pathology or audiology, we'd like to conclude by indulging in some philosophy about the professions—both for your sake and, just as importantly, for the sake of the clients who one day will rely on your knowledge, skill, and commitment.

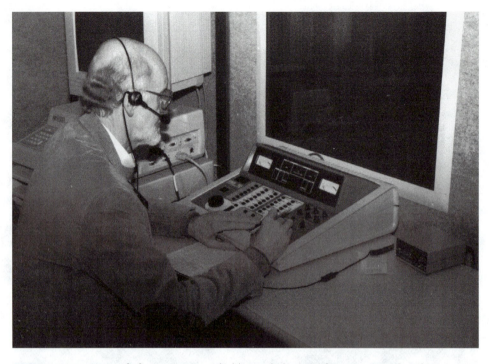

FIGURE 14-8 Information provided by audiologists often is essential to the differential diagnosis of hearing losses (*Van Riper Clinic, Western Michigan University*)

Each of us has a choice.

And the choice begins to take shape *now*—in undergraduate school, or perhaps it began even earlier.

We can choose to be technicians who simply apply the skills of our "trade" to the tasks of testing, evaluating, diagnosing, and treating communication disorders. Without any question, we can do these things on a mechanical and routine basis, day after day, and we can collect our paychecks—all without serious commitment and certainly with little thought or insight except, perhaps, thoughts about how to better market our "business."

Some students probably will consciously choose to be technicians. And they even may be satisfied with this choice, at least for awhile, since technicians certainly are employable, and often at attractive salaries.

Some also may become technicians "by default" simply because they lack the desire, the ability, the maturity, or the knowledge to be anything more; but, hopefully, very few of our readers belong in such categories.

Another choice, and one that can be far more rewarding, is to choose to become truly a professional—one whose focus of concern is the *person* with a communication disorder; one who is committed to helping people overcome their problems; and one who recognizes that knowledge, understanding, and sensitivity are as essential to clinical competence as are any of the myriad technical skills that also must be acquired.

What will be *your* choice?

Aspiring professionals are rather easily recognized, even as students. They tend to take their studies seriously, perhaps because they know intuitively that serving people requires immense knowledge and serious commitment, as well as a portion of selflessness. Their attitudes toward learning and toward their own development and growth reflect a mature understanding that the future holds a multitude of challenges demands, and opportunities that cannot be fully anticipated in the present. They also recognize that true professionals must be prepared to contribute to their professions and to the greater good of humanity at large.

To be a successful and effective professional contributor—either as an audiologist or as a speech-language pathologist—the practitioner must possess an information base that includes, but also goes beyond, the knowledge required to help people overcome communication disorders. It must rest on a broad liberal and liberating education. And then, like other health and human service professions, we must be aware of the ethical principles and the political-legislative-economic-social forces that impact upon and continue to reshape systems for the delivery of our clinical services.

Without such understandings the clinician is relegated to the role of technician to work under the direction of some other autonomous profession, and his or her clients will not be very well served in the longer term. Poorly informed clinicians are unable to contribute to the advancement of their professions or to the general enhancement of services for communicatively impaired persons. Technicians, for the most part, are not likely to be bothered by such concerns. We seek to educate professionals. We even dare hope that some students who otherwise may have chosen the technician role might be persuaded to rethink their decisions and to consider aiming for the professional role.

STUDY QUESTIONS

1. Name four people other than A. G. Bell and T. Edison who, prior to 1900, contributed to our understanding of speech and/or hearing processes. For what contribution(s) is each known?
2. By what means has stuttering been treated over the years?

3. How did the work of Alexander Graham Bell and the inventions of Thomas Alva Edison help "pave the way" for the modern speech and hearing scientist?

4. What professions and work settings were represented among the original members of the *American Academy of Speech Correction*?

5. What particular impacts did World War II have on the developing fields of speech pathology and audiology?

6. What is a *phoniatrist*, and how does a phoniatrist differ from a *logopedist*? From a *laryngologist*?

7. When did hearing and audiology become official "members of the family" of speech pathology, and who were the leading figures in this expansion of the professions?

8. With what national organization are most audiologists are speech-language pathologists affiliated, what are the purposes of that organization, and what publications does it issue on a regular basis?

9. Does your state license audiologists and/or speech-language pathologists? If so, outline the basic features of the state's licensure law; if not, interview one or two practitioners and be able to outline an explanation for the lack of such a law.

10. How does the Code of Ethics of ASHA differ from that of AAA?

11. Does your hometown have a support group for laryngectomees?

12. In what ways does a *professional* differ from a *tradesperson*, a *businessperson*, or a *technician*?

ENDNOTES

[1]In this recounting of origins we have drawn upon the personal recollections of the senior author, upon some archival materials (e.g., Van Riper, 1970), and upon some other writers. For ease of readability we've not included specific references here, but additional and more detailed accounts can be found in the following of our sources: Moeller (1976), Newby (1972), Paden (1974), Perelló (1976), and Silverman (1960). The June/July 1989 *Asha* also contains an interesting series of historical perspectives by various writers under "Roots of the Profession and the Association," pp. 69–86. A very detailed account of very early history also may be found in O'Neill (1980).

[2]Beyond the persons we've mentioned, scores of individuals played important roles in the initial shaping of audiology. Those whose contributions seem to have been particularly influential include Hallowell Davis, Max Goldstein, Victor Goodhill, William Hardy, Ira Hirsh, Jacqueline Keaster, Dean Lierle, Helmer Myklebust, Hayes Newby, Miriam Pauls, Earl Schubert, George Shambaugh, and S. Richard Silverman.

REFERENCES

American Academy of Audiology. (Amended 10/92). *Bylaws of the American Academy of Audiology.*

Clinical Certification Board. (1994). Standards and implementations for the certificates of clinical competence. *Asha, 36,* 71–78.

Fox-Grimm, M. (1991). Americans with Disabilities Act. *Asha, 33,* 41–45.

Moeller, D. (1975). *Speech pathology and audiology: Iowa origins of a discipline.* Iowa City, IA: The University of Iowa.

Newby, H. (1972). *Audiology* (3rd ed.). Englewood Cliffs, NJ: Prentice Hall.

O'Neill, Y. (1980). *Speech and speech disorders in western thought before 1600.* Westport, CT: Greenwood Press.

Paden, E. (1970). *A history of the American Speech and Hearing Association: 1925–1958.* Washington, DC: American Speech and Hearing Association.

Perelló, J. (1976). *The History of the International Association of Logopedics and Phoniatrics.* Barcelona, Spain: Editorial Augusta, S.A.

Roots of the profession and the Association. (1989). *Asha, 31,* 69–86.

Silverman, S. (1960). From Aristotle to Bell. In H. Davis and S. Silverman (eds.), *Hearing and deafness,* (rev. ed.). New York: Holt, Rinehart and Winston.

Van Riper, C. (1970). A brief history of our profession: Excerpts from a tape prepared for my students when I go deer hunting. *WMU Journal of Speech Therapy,* 7(3), 1–5.

SUPPLEMENTARY READINGS

American Speech-Language-Hearing Association. (1990). *Reflections on ethics: A compilation of articles inspired by the May 1990 ASHA ethics colloquium.* Rockville, MD: American Speech-Language-Hearing Association.

American Speech-Language-Hearing Association. (1994). The role of research and the state of research training within communication sciences and disorders. *Asha,* 36 (March, Suppl 12) 21–23.

American Speech-Language-Hearing Association. (1994). Model bill of rights for people receiving audiology or speech-language pathology services. *Asha,* 36, (Mar), 70.

American Speech-Language-Hearing Association. (1994). Plan for specialty recognition. *Asha,* 36 (Jan), 53–59.

Council of Graduate Programs in Communication Sciences and Disorders. (1993) *1992–93 National Survey.* Minneapolis, MN: Author.

Erickson, R. (1983). What should be the content and objectives of undergraduate education in communication disorders? In N. Rees, and T. Snope (eds.), *Proceedings of the 1983 National Conference on Undergraduate, Graduate, and Continuing Education,* ASHA Reports 13. Rockville, MD: American Speech-Language-Hearing Association.

Flower, R. (1984). *Delivery of speech-language pathology and audiology services.* Baltimore: Williams and Wilkins.

Silverman, F. (1983). *Legal aspects of speech-language pathology and audiology: An overview of law for clinicians, researchers, and teachers.* Englewood Cliffs, NJ: Prentice Hall.

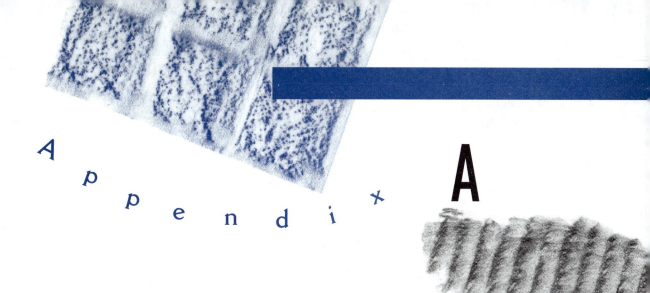

Appendix A

Code of Ethics
American Speech-
Language-Hearing
Association

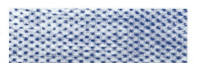

CODE OF ETHICS
Revised January 1, 1994
American Speech-Language-Hearing Association

Preamble

The preservation of the highest standards of integrity and ethical principles is vital to the responsible discharge of obligations in the professions of speech-language pathology and audiology. This Code of Ethics sets forth the fundamental principles and rules considered essential to this purpose.

Every individual who is (a) a member of the American Speech-Language-Hearing Association, whether certified or not, (b) a nonmember holding the Certificate of Clinical Competence from the Association, (c) an applicant for membership or certification, or (d) a Clinical Fellow seeking to fulfill standards for certification shall abide by this Code of Ethics.

Any action that violates the spirit and purpose of this Code shall be considered unethical. Failure to specify any particular responsibility or practice in this Code of Ethics shall not be construed as denial of the existence of such responsibilities or practices.

The fundamentals of ethical conduct are described by Principles of Ethics and by Rules of Ethics as they relate to responsibility to persons served, to the public, and to the professions of speech-language pathology and audiology.

Principles of Ethics, aspirational and inspirational in nature, form the underlying moral basis for the Code of Ethics. Individuals shall observe these principles as affirmative obligations under all conditions of professional activity.

Rules of Ethics are specific statements of minimally acceptable professional conduct or of prohibitions and are applicable to all individuals.

Principle of Ethics I

Individuals shall honor their responsibility to hold paramount the welfare of persons they serve professionally.

Rules of Ethics

A. Individuals shall provide all services competently.

B. Individuals shall use every resource, including referral when appropriate, to ensure that high-quality service is provided.

C. Individuals shall not discriminate in the delivery of professional services on the basis of race or ethnicity, gender, age, religion, national origin, sexual orientation, or disability.

D. Individuals shall fully inform the persons they serve of the nature and possible effects of services rendered and products dispensed.

E. Individuals shall evaluate the effectiveness of services rendered and of products dispensed and shall provide services or dispense products only when benefit can reasonably be expected.

F. Individuals shall not guarantee the results of any treatment or procedure, directly or by implication; however, they may make a reasonable statement of prognosis.

G. Individuals shall not evaluate or treat speech, language, or hearing disorders solely by correspondence.

H. Individuals shall maintain adequate records of professional services rendered and products dispensed and shall allow access to these records when appropriately authorized.

I. Individuals shall not reveal, without authorization, any professional or personal information about the person served professionally, unless required by law to do so, or unless doing so is necessary to protect the welfare of the person or of the community.

J. Individuals shall not charge for services not rendered, nor shall they misrepresent,* in any fashion, services rendered or products dispensed.

K. Individuals shall use persons in research or as subjects of teaching demonstrations only with their informed consent.

L. Individuals whose professional services are adversely affected by substance abuse or other health-related conditions shall seek professional assistance and, where appropriate, withdraw from the affected areas of practice.

Principle of Ethics II

Individuals shall honor their responsibility to achieve and maintain the highest level of professional competence.

Rules of Ethics

A. Individuals shall engage in the provision of clinical services only when they hold the appropriate Certificate of Clinical Competence or when they are in the certification process and are supervised by an individual who holds the appropriate Certificate of Clinical Competence.

B. Individuals shall engage in only those aspects of the professions that are within the scope of their competence, considering their level of education, training, and experience.

---

*For purposes of this Code of Ethics, misrepresentation includes any untrue statements or statements that are likely to mislead. Misrepresentation also includes the failure to state any information that is material and that ought, in fairness, to be considered.

C. Individuals shall continue their professional development throughout their careers.

D. Individuals shall delegate the provision of clinical services only to persons who are certified or to persons in the education or certification process who are appropriately supervised. The provision of support services may be delegated to persons who are neither certified nor in the certification process only when a certificate holder provides appropriate supervision.

E. Individuals shall prohibit any of their professional staff from providing services that exceed the staff member's competence, considering the staff member's level of education, training, and experience.

F. Individuals shall ensure that all equipment used in the provision of services is in proper working order and is properly calibrated.

Principle of Ethics III

Individuals shall honor their responsibility to the public by promoting public understanding of the professions, by supporting the development of services designed to fulfill the unmet needs of the public, and by providing accurate information in all communications involving any aspect of the professions.

Rules of Ethics

A. Individuals shall not misrepresent their credentials, competence, education, training, or experience.

B. Individuals shall not participate in professional activities that constitute a conflict of interest.

C. Individuals shall not misrepresent diagnostic information, services rendered, or products dispensed or engage in any scheme or artifice to defraud in connection with obtaining payment or reimbursement for such services or products.

D. Individuals' statements to the public shall provide accurate information about the nature and management of communication disorders, about the professions, and about professional services.

E. Individuals' statements to the public—advertising, announcing, and marketing their professional services, reporting research results, and promoting products—shall adhere to prevailing professional standards and shall not contain misrepresentations.

Principle of Ethics IV

Individuals shall honor their responsibilities to the professions and their relationships with colleagues, students, and members of allied professions. Individuals shall uphold the dignity and autonomy of the professions, maintain harmonious interprofessional and intraprofessional relationships, and accept the professions' self-imposed standards.

Rules of Ethics

A. Individuals shall prohibit anyone under their supervision from engaging in any practice that violates the Code of Ethics.

B. Individuals shall not engage in dishonesty, fraud, deceit, misrepresentation, or any form of conduct that adversely reflects on the professions or on the individual's fitness to serve persons professionally.

C. Individuals shall assign credit only to those who have contributed to a publication, presentation, or product. Credit shall be assigned in proportion to the contribution and only with the contributor's consent.

D. Individuals' statements to colleagues about professional services, research results, and products shall adhere to prevailing professional standards and shall contain no misrepresentations.

E. Individuals shall not provide professional services without exercising independent professional judgment, regardless of referral source or prescription.

F. Individuals shall not discriminate in their relationships with colleagues, students, and members of allied professions on the basis of race or ethnicity, gender, age, religion, national origin, sexual orientation, or disability.

G. Individuals who have reason to believe that the Code of Ethics has been violated shall inform the Ethical Practice Board.

H. Individuals shall cooperate fully with the Ethical Practice Board in its investigation and adjudication of matters related to this Code of Ethics.

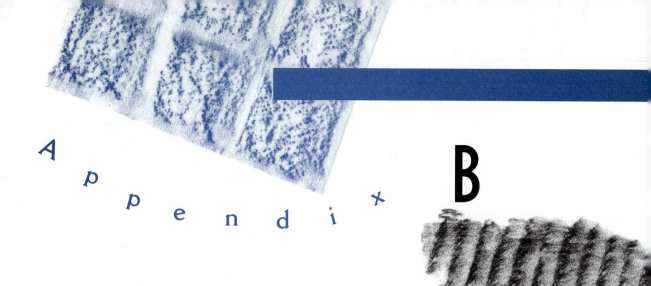

A p p e n d i x **B**

Code of Ethics
American
Academy of
Audiology

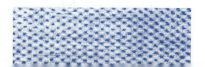

Preamble

The Code of Ethics of the American Academy of Audiology specifies professional standards that allow for the proper discharge of audiologists' responsibilities to those served and that protect the integrity of the profession. The Code of Ethics consists of two parts. The first part, the Statement of Principles and Rules, presents precepts that members of the Academy agree to uphold. The second part, the Procedures, provides the process that enables enforcement of the Principles and Rules.

Part I   Statement of Principles and Rules

Principle 1:   Members shall provide professional services with honesty and compassion and shall respect the dignity, worth, and rights of those served.

Rule 1a: Individuals shall not limit the delivery of professional services on any basis that is unjustifiable, or irrelevant to the need for the potential benefit from such services.

Principle 2:   Members shall maintain high standards of professional competence in rendering services, providing only those professional services for which they are qualified by education and experience.

Rule 2a: Individuals shall use available resources, including referrals to other specialists, and shall not accept benefits or items of personal value for receiving or making referrals.

Rule 2b: Individuals shall exercise all reasonable precautions to avoid injury to persons in the delivery of professional services.

Rule 2c: Individuals shall not provide services except in a professional relationship, and shall not discriminate in the provision of services to individuals on the basis of sex, race, religion, national origin, sexual orientation, or general health.

Rule 2d: Individuals shall provide appropriate supervision and assume full responsibility for services delegated to supportive personnel. Individuals shall not delegate any service requiring professional competence to persons unqualified.

Rule 2e: Individuals shall not permit personnel to engage in any practice that is a violation of the Code of Ethics.

Rule 2f: Individuals shall maintain professional competence, including participation in continuing education.

Principle 3: Members shall maintain the confidentiality of the information and records of those receiving services.

Rule 3a: Individuals shall not reveal to unauthorized persons any professional or personal information obtained from the person served professionally, unless required by law.

Principle 4: Members shall provide only services and products that are in the best interest of those served.

Rule 4a: Individuals shall not exploit persons in the delivery of professional services.

Rule 4b: Individuals shall not charge for services not rendered.

Rule 4c: Individuals shall not participate in activities that constitute a conflict of professional interest.

Rule 4d: Individuals shall not accept compensation for supervision or sponsorship beyond reimbursement of expenses.

Principle 5: Members shall provide accurate information about the nature and management of communicative disorders and about the services and products offered.

Rule 5a: Individuals shall provide persons served with the information a reasonable person would want to know about the nature and possible effects of services rendered, or products provided.

Rule 5b: Individuals may make a statement of prognosis, but shall not guarantee results, mislead, or misinform persons served.

Rule 5c : Individuals shall not carry out teaching or research activities in a manner that constitutes an invasion of privacy or that fails to inform persons fully about the nature and possible effects of these activities, affording all persons informed free choice of participation.

Rule 5d: Individuals shall maintain documentation of professional services rendered.

Principle 6: Members shall comply with the ethical standards of the Academy with regard to public statements.

Rule 6a: Individuals shall not misrepresent their educational degrees, training, credentials, or competence. Only degrees earned from regionally accredited institutions in which training was obtained in audiology, or a directly related discipline, may be used in public statements concerning professional services.

Rule 6b: Individuals' public statements about professional services and products shall not contain representations or claims that are false, misleading, or deceptive.

Principle 7:   Members shall honor their responsibilities to the public and to professional colleagues.

Rule 7a: Individuals shall not use professional or commercial affiliations in any way that would mislead or limit services to persons served professionally.

Rule 7b: Individuals shall inform colleagues and the public in a manner consistent with the highest professional standards about products and services they have developed.

Principle 8:   Members shall uphold the dignity of the profession and freely accept the Academy's self-imposed standards.

Rule 8a: Individuals shall not violate these Principles and Rules, nor attempt to circumvent them.

Rule 8b: Individuals shall not engage in dishonesty or illegal conduct that adversely reflects on the profession.

Rule 8c: Individuals shall inform the Ethical Practice Board when there are reasons to believe that a member of the Academy may have violated the Code of Ethics.

Rule 8d: Individuals shall cooperate with the Ethical Practice Board in any matter related to the Code of Ethics.

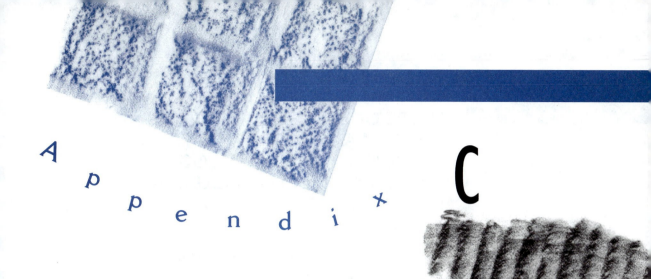

Scope of Practice, Speech-Language Pathology and Audiology American Speech-Language-Hearing Association

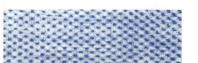

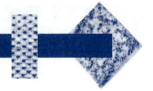

SCOPE OF PRACTICE, SPEECH-LANGUAGE PATHOLOGY AND AUDIOLOGY AMERICAN SPEECH-LANGUAGE-HEARING ASSOCIATION

Committee on Interprofessional Relationships
American Speech-Language-Hearing Association

The following document, prepared by the American Speech-Language-Hearing Association (ASHA) Committee on Interpersonal Relationships, was adopted as an official statement by the ASHA Legislative Council (LC 6-89) in November 1989.

Preamble

The purpose of this statement is to define the scope of practice of speech-language pathology and audiology in order to: (1) inform members of ASHA and certificate holders of the activities for which certification in the appropriate area is required in accordance with the ASHA Code of Ethics; and (2) educate health-care and education professionals, consumers, and members of the general public of the services offered by speech-language pathologists and audiologists as qualified providers.

The scope of practice defined here, and the areas specifically set forth, are part of an effort to establish the broad range of services offered within the profession. It is recognized, however, that levels of experience, skill, and proficiency with respect to the activities identified within the scope of practice will vary among the individual providers. Similarly, it is recognized that related fields and professions may have knowledge, skills, and experience that may be applied to some areas within the scope of practice. By defining the scope of practice of speech-language pathologists and audiologists, there is no intention to exclude members of other professions or related fields from rendering services in common practice areas for which they are competent by virtue of their respective disciplines.

Nothing in the scope of practice statement is intended to affect the licensure laws of the various states or the implementation or interpretation of such laws.

Finally, it is recognized that speech-language pathology and audiology are dynamic and continuously developing practice areas. In setting forth some specific areas as included within the scope of practice, there is no intention that the list be exhaustive or that other, new, or emerging areas be precluded from being considered as within the scope of practice.

Statement

Speech-language pathologists and audiologists hold either the master's or doctoral degree, the Certificate of Clinical Competence of the American Speech-Language-Hearing Association, and state license where applicable. These professionals identify, assess, and provide treatment for individuals of all ages with communication disorders. They manage and supervise programs and services related to human communication and its disorders. Speech-language pathologists and audiologists counsel individuals with disorders of communication, their families, caregivers, and other service providers relative to the disability present and its management. They provide consultation and make referrals. Facilitating the development and maintenance of human communication is the common goal of speech-language pathologists and audiologists.

The practice of speech-language pathology includes:

- screening, identifying, assessing and interpreting, diagnosing, rehabilitating, and preventing disorders of speech (e.g., articulation, fluency, voice) and language;
- screening, identifying, assessing and interpreting, diagnosing, and rehabilitating disorders of oral-pharyngeal function (e.g., dysphagia) and related disorders;
- screening, identifying, assessing and interpreting, diagnosing, and rehabilitating cognitive/communication disorders;
- assessing, selecting and developing augmentative and alternative communication systems and providing training in their use;
- providing aural rehabilitation and related counseling services to hearing impaired individuals and their families;
- enhancing speech-language proficiency and communication effectiveness (e.g., accent reduction); and
- screening of hearing and other factors for the purpose of speech-language evaluation and/or the initial identification of individuals with other communication disorders.

The practice of audiology includes:

- facilitating the conservation of auditory system function; developing and implementing environmental and occupational hearing conservation programs;
- screening, identifying, assessing and interpreting, diagnosing, preventing, and rehabilitating peripheral and central auditory system dysfunctions;

- providing and interpreting behavioral and (electro)physiological measurements of auditory and vestibular functions;
- selecting, fitting and dispensing of amplification, assistive listening and alerting devices and other systems (e.g., implantable devices) and providing training in their use;
- providing aural rehabilitation and related counseling services to hearing impaired individuals and their families; and
- screening of speech-language and other factors affecting communication function for the purposes of an audiologic evaluation and/ or initial identification of individuals with other communication disorders.

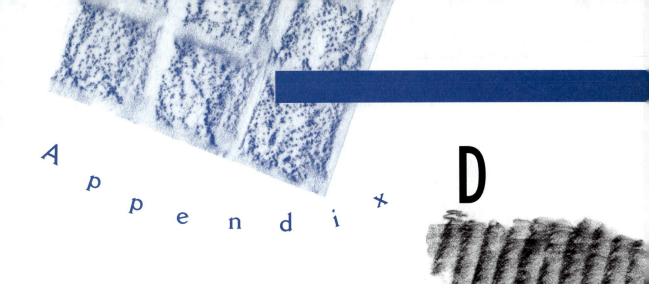

Organizations, Agencies, and Support Groups Related to Communication Sciences and Disorders

Alexander Graham Bell Association for the Deaf
Volta Bureau
3417 Volta Place, NW
Washington, DC 20007
202/337-5220
FAX: 202/337-8314

American Academy of Audiology
Suite 950
1735 North Lynn Street
Arlington, VA 22209
703/524-1923; 800-AAA-2336
FAX: 703/524-2303

American Cleft Palate-Craniofacial Association
1218 Grandviev Avenue
Pittsburgh, PA 15211
412/481-1376
CLEFTLINE for consumer requests: 800/24-CLEFT
FAX: 412/481-0847

American Occupational Therapy Association
1383 Piccard Drive, Suite 300
Rockville, MD 20850

American Society for Deaf Children
814 Thayer Avenue
Silver Spring, MD 20910
301/585-5400; 800/942-ASDC
FAX: 215/963-8700

American Speech-Language-Hearing Association
10801 Rockville Pike
Rockville, MD 20852-3279
301/897-5700; 800/638-TALK
FAX: 301/571-0457

Better Hearing Institute
P.O. Box 1840
Washington, DC 20013
703/642-0580
FAX: 703/750-9302

Center for Hearing Loss in Children
Boys Town National Research Hospital
555 North 30th Street
Omaha, NE 68131
402/498-6319

Council for Exceptional Children
1920 Association Blvd.
Reston, VA 22071

Council of Graduate Programs in Communication
    Sciences and Disorders
P.O. Box 26532
Minneapolis, MN 55426
612/920-0966
FAX: 612/920-6098

International Association of Laryngectomees
c/o American Cancer Society
1599 Clifton Road, NE
Atlanta, GA 30329-4251

John Tracy Clinic
806 West Adams Blvd.
Los Angeles, CA 90007
213/748-5481; 800/522-4582
TDD: 213/747-2924
FAX: 213/748-5481

March of Dimes
Birth Defects Foundation
1275 Mamaroneck Avenue
White Plains, NY 10605

National Center for Neurogenic
    Communication Disorders
The University of Arizona
Tucson, AZ 85721
602/621-2444; 800/926-2444

National Center for Voice and Speech
Wendell Johnson Speech and Hearing Center
The University of Iowa
Iowa City, IA 52242
319/335-6600

National Easter Seal Society
2023 W. Ogden Avenue
Chicago, IL 60068

National Information Center on Deafness
Gallaudet College
800 Florida Avenue NE
Washington, DC 20002

National Institute on Deafness and
Other Communication Disorders
National Institutes of Health
U.S. Department of Health and Human Services
Bethesda, MD

National Society for Children and Adults with Autism
Suite 1017
1234 Massachusetts Avenue NW
Washington, DC 20005

National Spasmodic Dysphonia Association
P.O. Box 203
Atwood, CA 92601
800/714-6732

National Stroke Association
Suite 1000
8480 East Orchard Road
Englewood, CO 80111
800/STROKES
FAX: 303/771-1886

Our Voice A newsletter for spasmodic dysphonia
patients and health professionals
365 West 25th Street, Suite 13E
New York, NY 10001-5816

Registry of Interpreters for the Deaf
Suite 310
8719 Colesville Road
Silver Spring, MD 20910
301/608-0050
FAX: 301/608-0508

Self Help for Hard of Hearing People (SHHH)
Suite 100
4848 Battery Lane
Bethesda, MD 20814

Speech Foundation of America
5139 Klingle Street, NW
Washington, DC 20016
202/363-3199; 800/992-9392
FAX: 901/452-3931

United Cerebral Palsy Association
Suite 141
425 I Street, NW
Washington, DC 29001

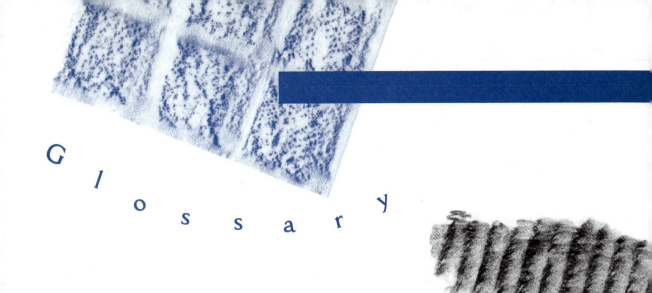

Glossary

Abduct. To move away from the midline.

Acalculia. Inability to do simple arithmetic problems due to brain injury.

Acoustic. Pertaining to sound.

Acoustic reflex. Automatic contraction of middle ear musculature in response to loud sound; a protective reaction.

Adduct. To move toward the midline.

Adenoids. Growths of lymphoid tissue on the back wall of the throat; also called pharyngeal tonsils.

Affricate. A consonantal sound beginning as a stop (plosive) but expelled as a fricative. The *ch* /ʧ/ and the *j* /ʤ/ sounds in the words *chain* and *jump* are affricates.

Agnosia. Inability to interpret the meanings of sensory stimulation due to brain injury; may be visual, auditory, or tactual.

Agraphia. Difficulty in writing due to brain damage.

Agrammatism. Form of aphasia in which grammar and syntax are unusually disturbed.

Alaryngeal. Without a larynx.

Alaryngeal speech. Speech in which a sound source other than the larynx is used in place of normal voicing.

Allophone. One of the variant forms of a phoneme.

Alveolar ridges. The ridges on the jawbones beneath the gums. An alveolar sound is one in which the tongue makes contact with the upper-gum ridge.

American Sign Language (ASL). Manual communication system used primarily by individuals who are congenitally deaf; ASL is recognized as a language in its own right, with rules for grammar and syntax.

Aneurysm. A swelling or dilation of an artery due to weakening of the wall of the blood vessel.

Anomaly. An anatomic deviation from normal structure or form.

Anomia. Inability to remember familiar words due to brain injury.

Anoxia. Oxygen defiency.

Aperiodic. Not regularly repetitive; a sound source vibrating aperiodically produces noise.

Apgar score. Rating of newborn's physical condition based upon observations of heart rate, respiration, skin color, muscle tone, and reflexes.

Aphasia. Impairment in the use of meaningful symbols due to brain injury.

Aphonia. Loss of voice; without phonation.

Approach-avoidance. Refers to conflicts produced when the person is beset by two opposing drives to do or not do something.

Approximation. Behavior that comes closer to a standard or goal.

Apraxia. Loss of ability to make voluntary movements such as producing speech sounds, while involuntary movements remain intact; caused by neurologic damage.

Articulation. The utterance of the individual speech sounds.

Artificial larynx. Electronic or pneumatic vibrator used by a laryngectomee to produce a voice-like sound for speech.

Aspirate. Breathy; the use of excessive initial airflow preceding phonation as in the *aspirate* attack.

Assimilation. A change in the characteristic of a speech sound due to the influence of adjacent sounds. In assimilation nasality, voiced sounds followed or preceded by a nasal consonant tend to be excessively nasalized.

Ataxia. Loss of ability to perform gross motor coordinations.

Athetosis. One of the forms of cerebral palsy characterized by writhing, shaking, involuntary movements of the head, limbs, or the body.

Atresia. The blockage of an opening or a canal.

Atrophy. A withering; a shrinking in size and decline in function of some bodily structure or organ.

Audiogram. Graphic record of hearing test results showing hearing levels in dB at various frequencies.

Audiometry. The measurement of hearing; includes pure tone testing and speech reception testing as well as a wide variety of specialized procedures.

Auditory brainstem response (ABR). Procedure for detecting and measuring electrical activity in the brain in response to stimulation of the ear with sound; does not require voluntary response from examinee.

Augmentative and Alternative Communication (AAC). The use of non-speech techniques and devices (e.g., picture boards, symbol systems, computerized speech) as a substitute or supplement for speech communication.

Aural. Pertaining to hearing.

Auricle. The visible outer ear.

Autism. Disorder resulting in a detachment from environmental surroundings; almost complete withdrawal from social interaction.

Avoidance. A device such as the use of a synonym or circumlocution to escape from having to speak a word upon which stuttering is anticipated.

Axon. Nerve fiber that conducts impulses away from the cell body.

Babbling. A continuous, free experimenting with speech sounds.

Baseline. An initial level of response prior to conditioning.

Bifid. Divided into two parts, as in a cleft or bifid uvula.

Bilabial. A sound produced with both lips as the main articulators.

Binaural. Pertaining to both ears.

Black English. Dialects of Standard American English often used by persons of African descent; also called Black English Vernacular (BEV).

Blissymbolics. A set of pictographs for the nonverbal person.

Bone conduction. The transmission of sound waves directly to the cochlea by the bones of the skull.

Brainstem. The midbrain; pons and medulla oblongata.

Bradylalia. Abnormally slow utterance.

Breathiness. Air wastage during phonation; voice quality heard when the vocal folds do not fully approximate during the vibratory cycle.

Caloric test. Water is inserted in the ear canal to induce nystagmus (repetitive eye movements) as a test of vestibular function and balance.

Cancellation. The voluntary repetition of a word on which stuttering has occurred.

Canonical. Canonical syllables have a vowel nucleus and consonant margins (CVC).

C.A.T. Children's Apperception Test, a projective test of personality.

Catastrophic response. A sudden extreme change in behavior by the aphasic characterized by irritability, flushing or fainting, withdrawal from random movements.

Catharsis. The discharge of pent-up feelings.

Central nervous system (CNS). The brain and spinal cord.

Cerebellum. Structure of the brain that regulates and coordinates complex motor activities.

Cerebral cortex. Outer layer of gray matter over the cerebral hemispheres; responsible for higher level cognitive functions.

Cerebral palsy. A group of disorders due to brain injury in which the motor coordinations are especially affected. Most common forms are athetosis, spasticity, and ataxia.

Cerebrovascular accident (CVA). Injury to blood vessels of the brain (see *Stroke*).

Cerebrum. Refers to the general structure of the brain.

Cerumen. Substance secreted by external ear; earwax.

Clavicular breathing. A form of shallow speech-breathing in which the shoulders move with short inhalations.

Closed head injury. Traumatic brain injury.

Cluttering. A disorder of time or rhythm characterized by unorganized, hasty spurts of speech often accompained by slurred articulation and breaks in fluency.

Coarticulation. Influence of adjacent phonemes on the articulation of a speech sound (also see *Assimilation*).

Cochlea. The spiral-shaped structure of the inner ear containing the end organs of the auditory nerve.

Cochlear implant. Surgically implanted device that directly stimulates the auditory nerve when an externally worn component receives sound input; used only with severely hearing impaired individuals who are unable to benefit from a hearing aid.

Code switching. Conscious shifting from one language or dialect to another, depending on speaking situation.

Cognate. Referring to pairs of sounds that are produced motorically in much the same way, one being voiced (**sonant**) and the other unvoiced (**surd**). Some cognates are /t/ and /d/, /s/ and /z/.

Cognition. Higher mental functions, thoughts, interpretations, ideas.

Compression. The phase during a vibratory cycle when molecules are pressed more closely together creating a region of high pressure.

Conductive hearing loss. Hearing impairment due to middle (or outer) ear problem; cochlea and auditory nerve are not involved.

Congenital. Present at the time of birth.

Contact ulcer. Small lesion on the posterior medial edge of the vocal fold; may be caused by reflux of stomach acids or abusive use of the voice.

Content words (Contentives). Words such as nouns and verbs that carry the major burden of meaningfulness.

Contingent reinforcement. Following as a consequence of some preceding behavior.

Continuant. A speech sound that can be prolonged without distortion, e.g., /s/ or /f/ or /u/.

Covert. Hidden; inner feelings, thoughts, reactions.

Culture. Shared collection of socially transmitted attitudes, beliefs, behavioral characteristics, institutions; not synonymous with race or ethnic group.

CV. A syllable containing the consonant-vowel sequence as in *see* or *toe* or *ka*.

CVC. A syllable containing the consonant-vowel-consonant sequence, as in the first syllable of the word *containing*.

Cytomegalovirus (CMV). Type of herpes virus; can be asymptomatic in adults; congenitally, CMV is a major cause of sensorineural hearing impairment in children.

Decibel (dB). A unit of loudness or sound intensity.

Deciduous teeth. The temporary or "baby" teeth of children.

Deep testing. The exploration of an individual's ability to articulate a large number of words, all of which include one specific sound, to discover those in which that sound is spoken correctly.

Delayed auditory feedback (DAF). The hearing of one's own voice delayed electronically by a fraction of a second.

Dementia. General mental deterioration.

Denasality. A lack of, or reduced, nasality.

Dendrite. Part of the neuron that transmits impulses toward the cell body.

Dental. Pertaining to the teeth. A dentalized *l* sound is made with the tongue tip on the upper teeth.

Desensitization. The toughening of a person to stress; increasing the person's ability to confront the problem with less anxiety, guilt, or hostility; a type of adaptation to stress therapy used for beginning stutterers.

Diadochokinesis. Rate of repetition of a spoken syllable.

Dialect. Regional, social, or cultural variation of a language.

Diaphragm. Sheet of muscle separating the thorax from the abdomen; contraction expands the thorax for inhalation of air.

Differential diagnosis. The process of distinguishing one disorder from another.

Diphthong. Phoneme produced by the blending of two vowel sounds into a single speech sound.

Diplophonia. Voice in which two separate tones are present simultaneously; associated with laryngeal pathology.

Discourse. Verbal exchange, as in conversation; may refer also to written verbal expression.

Displacement. The transfer of emotion from an original source to another stimulus.

Distinctive features. Acoustic and articulatory properties of phonemes.

Distortion. The misarticulation of a standard sound in which the latter is replaced by a sound not normally used in the language. A lateral lisp is a distortion.

Dysarthria. Group of motor speech impairments that stem from neuromotor damage; may disturb respiration, phonation, articulation, resonance, and prosody.

Dyslexia. Reading disability.

Dysphagia. Disorder of swallowing due to neck or mouth injury or to a neurological condition.

Dysphasia. The general term for aphasic problems.

Dysphemia. A poorly timed control mechanism for coordinating sequential utterance.

Dysphonia. Disorder of voice.

Dystonia. Abnormal muscle tonicity due to neurologic causes; may cause spasms or writhing movements.

Ear training. Therapy devoted to self-hearing of speech deviations and standard utterance.

Echolalia. The automatic involuntary repetition of heard phrases and sentences.

Echo speech. A technique in which the patient is trained to repeat instantly what he or she is hearing, following almost simultaneously the uttterance of another person. Also called "shadowing."

Edema. Swelling caused by accumulation of serous fluid.

Egocentric. Self-centered; pertaining to the self and its display.

Ego strength. Morale or self-confidence.

Electroencephalogram (EEG). Recording of electrical activity associated with brain waves; used in diagnosing neurological disorders.

Electrolarynx. Battery-operated device used by laryngectomees to produce sound as a replacement for lost voice.

Electromyography (EMG). Recording of electrical activity associated with muscle contraction.

Embolism. A clogging of a blood vessel as by a clot that moves.

Empathy. The conscious or unconscious imitation or identification of one person with the behavior or feelings of another.

Encephalitis. A disease characterized by inflammation or lesions of the brain.

Encoding. Process of converting an idea into an audible or visual signal.

Epiglottis. The shieldlike cartilage that hovers over the front of the larynx.

Epilepsy. A neurological disease characterized by convulsions and seizures.

Epithelium. Cellular tissue that forms a lining for body cavities and covers body surface.

Esophageal speech. Speech of laryngectomized persons produced by air pulses ejected from the esophagus.

Esophagus. The tube leading from the throat to the stomach.

Etiology. Causation.

Eunuchoid voice. A very high-pitched voice similar to that of a castrated male adult.

Eustachian tube. The passageway connecting the throat cavity with the middle ear.

Expressive aphasia. The difficulty in sending meaningful messages, as in the speaking, writing, or gesturing difficulties of the aphasic.

False vocal folds. Folds of tissue lying immediately above the true vocal folds; also known as *ventricular folds.*

Falsetto. The upper, high-pitched register of voice; produced with stretched, thinned vocal folds; also known as *loft register.*

Fauces. The rear side margins of the mouth cavity that separate the mouth from the pharynx; also called faucial pillars.

Feedback. The backflow of information concerning the output of a motor system. Auditory feedback refers to self-hearing; kinesthetic feedback to the self-perception of one's movements.

Fixation. In stuttering, the prolongation of a speech posture.

Flaccidity. State of passive relaxation, uncontracted, limp in appearance.

Fluency. Unhesitant speech.

Formant. Frequency range in which the acoustic energy of a speech signal is concentrated by vocal tract resonance.

Frenum. The white membrane below the tongue tip; also called *frenulum.*

Fricative. A speech sound produced by forcing the airstream through a constricted opening. The /f/ and /v/ sounds are fricatives. Sibilants are also fricatives.

Functional. Refers to a disorder that has no organic cause; may or may not be "psychogenic."

Function words (functors). Words that indicate action, arrangement, and relationship. Examples include prepositions, articles, adverbs, and conjunctions.

Fundamental frequency. Basic rate of vibration of a sound source; the physical correlate of pitch.

Generative (transformational) grammar. A system of rules for producing well-formed sentences of a language.

Gibbegedong. A velar-tongue click.

Glide. A class of speech sounds in which the characteristic feature is produced by shifting from one articulatory posture to another. Examples are the *y* /j/ in *you*, and the /w/ in *we*.

Glottal catch (or stop). A tiny cough-like sound produced by the sudden release of a pulse of voiced or unvoiced air from the vocal folds.

Glottal fry. A low-pitched ticker-like continuous clicking sound produced by the vocal folds; also known as *vocal fry* and as *pulse register*.

Glottis. The space between the vocal cords when they are not brought together.

Hard contacts. Hypertensed fixed articulatory postures assumed by stutterers in attempting feared words.

Harelip. A cleft of the upper lip (term is no longer used).

Harmonics. Vibrations that occur at whole number multiples of the fundamental frequency.

Harshness. Voice quality usually associated with excessive laryngeal tension.

Hematoma. Localized swelling filled with blood.

Hemianopsia. Blindness of one-half of the visual field.

Hemiplegia. Paralysis or neurological involvement of one side of the body.

Hemorrhage. Bleeding.

Hertz (Hz). Unit of measurement of rate of vibration of sound source; same as *cycles per second*.

Hierarchy. A series of items graded according to difficulty.

Hoarseness. Voice quality often defined as a combination of *breathiness* and *harshness*.

Hyperactivity. Excessive and often random movements as often shown by a brain-injured child.

Hyperbilirubinemia. Excessive amount of bile substance in the blood; can produce jaundiced appearance and is among the factors indicating an infant may be at risk for hearing loss and other problems.

Hypernasality (Rhinolalia aperta). Excessively nasal voice quality.

Hyponasality. Lack of sufficient nasality, as in the denasal or adenoidal voice.

Hypothyroidism. Insufficient production of hormone by thyroid gland; can produce fatigue and other symptoms; may cause voice problems, especially in women.

Iconic. Words, signs that resemble what they represent.

Idioglossia. Self-language with a vocabulary invented by the child.

Idiopathic. Of unknown etiology/causation.

Incidence. The rate at which a disease or other condition occurs, usually reported as the number of new occurrences per year.

Incisor. Any one of the four front teeth in the upper or lower jaws.

Incus. The second of three tiny bones in the middle ear.

Infantile swallow. A form of swallowing in which the tongue is usually protruded between the teeth.

Inflection. Upward or downward change in pitch of the voice during a continuous phonation.

Inner ear. Comprised of the cochlea, the semicircular canals, and the vestibule; important in balance as well as hearing.

Intensity. The power or pressure magnitude of sound; loudness.

Interdental. Between the teeth. An interdental lisp would show itself in the substitution of the *th* for the *s* as in *thoup* for *soup*.

Interiorized stuttering. A form of stuttering behavior in which no visible contortions or audible abnormalities are shown, but a hidden struggle usually in the larynx or breathing musculatures is present. Also characterized by clever disguise reactions.

Isolation techniques. Activities used to locate the defective sound in utterance.

Jargon. Continuous but unintelligible speech.

Jitter. Small perturbations/irregularities in the fundamental frequency of a voice; excessive jitter may be perceived as vocal "roughness."

Kernel sentences. The early primitive sentence forms from which other transformations later develop.

Kinesthesia. The perception of muscular contraction or movement.

Kinetic analysis. The analysis of error sounds in terms of their movement patterns.

Labial. Pertaining to the lips.

Lambdacism. Defective /l/ sound.

Laryngeal. Pertaining to the larynx.

Laryngectomee. Person whose larynx has been surgically removed, typically because of laryngeal cancer.

Laryngectomy. The surgical removal of the larynx.

Laryngologist. Physician specializing in diseases and pathology of the larynx; typically an *otorhinolaryngologist (ENT)*

Laryngoscopy. Viewing the larynx from above; may be done with illuminated mirror (indirect laryngoscopy), with a rigid fiberoptic oral endoscope or flexible nasendoscope, or with laryngoscope.

Larynx. Cartilaginous structure in neck between trachea and pharynx; includes vocal folds and muscles that control their tension and positioning; the "*voice box.*"

Lateral. A sound such as the /l/ in which the airflow courses around the side of the uplifted tongue. One variety of a lateral lisp is so produced.

Lesion. A wound; injured tissue.

Lexicon. The stock of terms in a vocabulary.

Lingual. Pertaining to the tongue. A lingual lisp is identical with an interdental lisp.

Lisp. An articulatory disorder characterized by defective sibilant sounds such as the /s/ and /z/.

Loudness. The perceptual correlate of intensity or amplitude.

Malingering. The conscious simulation of a disorder.

Malleus. The bone of the middle ear that rests against the eardrum.

Malocclusion. An abnormal bite.

Mandible. Lower jaw.

Maxilla. Upper jaw.

Mean length of utterance (MLU). A measure of average utterance length used in studying language development.

Medial. The occurrence of a sound within a word but not initiating or ending it.

Median. Midline, in the middle.

Minnesota Multiphasic Personality Inventory (MMPI). A test of personality problems.

Modal register. The manner of laryngeal adjustment and vocal fold vibration used to produce voice in normal speech; sometimes referred to as chest register in singing.

Monaural. Hearing with one ear.

Monopitch. Speaking in a very narrow pitch range, usually of one to four semitones.

Morpheme. Smallest meaningful combination of phonemes; may be a word, a prefix, a suffix.

Motokinesthetic method. A methods for teachings sounds and words in which the therapist directs the movements of the tongue, jaw, and lips by touch and manipulation.

Mucosa. The mouth and throat linings that secrete mucous.

Multiple sclerosis (MS). A progressive and deteriorating muscular disability produced by overgrowth of the connective tissue surrounding the nerve tracts.

Muscular dystrophy. A disease characterized by progressive deterioration in muscle functioning and also by withering of the muscles.

Mutism. Without speech. Voluntary mutism: refusal to speak.

Myasthenia. Muscular weakness.

Myasthenia gravis. Chronic neuromuscular disorder characterized by progressive weakening of musculature without atrophy.

Myelin. White fatty substance that encases some nerve fibers.

Myringotomy. Surgical perforation of the eardrum, usually accompanied by insertion of pressure-equalizing tube; used in treatment of persistent otitis media.

Nares. Nostrils.

Nasal emission. Airflow through the nose, especially during production of oral consonants.

Nasendoscopy. A technique for viewing velopharyngeal and/or laryngeal structures form above with a flexible fiberoptic instrument.

Nasopharynx. That part of the throat, pharynx, above the level of the base of the uvula.

Natural processes. Strategies used by children to simplify adult speech patterns.

Negative practice. Deliberate practice of the error or abnormal behavior.

Negative reinforcement. The cessation of unpleasantness when applied contingently.

Neurologist. Physician who specializes in diagnosis and treatment of disorders of the nervous system.

Neuron. Nerve cell; consists of cell body, dendrites, and axons.

Nonfluency. Pause, hesitation, repetition, or other behavior that interrupts the normal flow of utterance.

Obturator. An appliance used to close a cleft or gap.

Occluded lisp. The substitution of a /t/ or a /ts/ for the /s/, or the /d/ and /dz/ for the /z/.

Octave. Unit of measurement of frequency intervals; doubling or halving a fundamental frequency raises or lowers the sound by one octave; on the equal tempered music scale, one octave is equal to six tones or twelve semitones.

Omission. One of the four types of articulatory errors. The standard sound is replaced usually by a slight pause equal in duration to the sound omitted.

Operant conditioning. The differential reinforcement of desired responses through the systematic control of their contingencies.

Opposition breathing. Breathing in which the thorax (chest) and diaphragm work oppositely against each other in providing breath support for voice.

Optimal pitch level. The relatively narrow range of pitches, toward the low end of an individual's vocal pitch range, within which the individual may phonate most efficiently and effortlessly.

Organic. In the sense of causation, refers to an anatomic or physiologic etiology.

Organ of Corti. Organ in the cochlea containing sensory hairs that transform mechanical movements into electrical impulses capable of stimulating the auditory nerve; the "organ of hearing."

Orthodontist. A dentist who specializes in repositioning of the teeth.

Oscillations. Rhythmic repetitive movements, repetitions of a sound, syllable, or posture.

Ossicles. The three smallest bones in the body—the malleus, incus, and stapes; the ossicles convey vibrations of the eardrum to the oval window of the cochlea.

Otitis media. Inflammation of the middle ear; when accompanied by accumulation of fluid, called *serous otitis media.*

Otologist. Physician who specializes in hearing disorders and diseases; typically an *otorhinolaryngologist (ENT).*

Otosclerosis. Pathologic condition in which the footplate of the stapes becomes rigidly affixed to the oval window and is thus unable to transmit mechanical vibrations from the eardrum to the cochlea; common cause of hearing impairment in adults.

Outer ear. The auricles (pinnae) and external ear canal.

Palpation. Examining by tapping or touching.

Papilloma. Benign wart-like growth that can occur in the larynx; may create breathing difficulty as well as dysphonia.

Parallel talk. A technique in which the therapist provides a running commentary on what the client is doing, perceiving, or probably feeling.

Paraphasia. Aphasic behavior characterized by jumbled, inaccurate words.

Perinatal. During the birth process.

Period. In acoustics, the duration of one vibratory cycle.

Peripheral nervous system. The nerves outside the brain and spinal cord; carries messages to and from the central nervous system.

Perseveration. The automatic and often involuntary continuation of behavior.

PFAGH. An acronym representing penalty, frustration, anxiety, guilt, and hostility.

Pharyngeal flap. A tissue bridge between the soft palate and the back wall of the throat.

Pharynx. The throat cavity.

Phonation. Voice.

Phoneme. A "family" of speech sounds that may differ slightly from one another (allophones) with no effect on meaning; the smallest contrastive sound unit in a language.

Phonetic placement. A methods for teaching a new sound by the use of diagrams, mirrors, or manipulation whereby the essential motor features of the sound are made clear.

Phonology. The linguistic rule system dealing with speech sounds and their characteristics.

Phonosurgery. Specialized surgery on the larynx designed to restore or maintain good voicing; not all laryngologists are phonosurgeons.

Pitch. The perceptual correlate of fundamental frequency.

Pitch break. Sudden abnormal shift of pitch during speech.

Plosive. A speech sound characterized by the sudden release of a puff of air. Examples are /p/, /t/, and /g/.

Polyp. Tissue mass that may form on a vocal fold following abuse of the voice.

Pragmatics. How communication is used in a social context.

Prenatal. Before birth.

Preparatory set. An anticipatory readiness to perform an act.

Presbycusis. The hearing loss characteristic of old age.

Prevalence. The frequency with which a disease or other condition is found; the number of existing instances.

Primary reinforcer. A stimulus that satisfies a basic need and is not dependent upon learning. Examples are water, food, and sex.

Proboscis. Nose.

Prognosis. Prediction of progress or outcome.

Propositionality. The meaningfulness of a message or utterance; its information content.

Proprioception. Sense information from muscles, joints, or tendons.

Prosody. Linguistic stress patterns as reflected in pause, inflection, juncture; melody or cadence of speech.

Prosthesis. An appliance used to compensate for a missing or paralyzed structure.

Prosthodontist. A dental specialist who makes prostheses.

Psychogenic. Caused by underlying psychological or personality factors.

Pull-out. The voluntary release from a stuttering block.

Rarefaction. The phase during a vibratory cycle when molecules are spread more distantly from one another, creating a region of low pressure.

Receptive aphasia. Aphasia in which the major deficits are in comprehending.

Reciprocal inhibition. The mutual cancellation or inhibition produced by pairing incompatible response tendencies such as anxiety or anger.

Recurrent laryngeal nerve (RLN). Branch of the vagus nerve that innervates all but one of the intrinsic muscles of the larynx; also called the *inferior laryngeal nerve.*

Relaxation pressure. Passive forces, including gravity, untorquing of the ribs, and elastic recoil, which produce exhalation following an active inhalation.

Register. Manner of adjustment of the larynx for voice production (e.g., falsetto register, modal or chest register).

Resonance. Phenomenon whereby acoustic energy present at various frequencies in the complex laryngeal tone is selectively emphasized or suppressed by the vocal tract.

Resting lung volume (RLV). Amount of air remaining in lungs after a normal tidal expiration.

Retrocochlear. Behind (beyond) the cochlea, more central in the nervous system.

Rhinolalia. Excessive nasality.

Rorschach. A test of personality involving the use of ink blots.

Schwa vowel. The neutral vowel /ə/ as in the first phoneme in *above.*

Secondary reinforcer. A stimulus that has been previously associated with a primary reinforcer.

Secondary stuttering. Refers to the advanced forms of stuttering in which awareness, fear, avoidance, and struggle are shown.

Self-talk. An audible commentary by a person describing actions, perceptions, or feelings.

Semantics. Meaning; the relationship of symbols to objects and events.

Semitone. A half-tone, a half-step on the musical scale.

Sensorineural hearing loss. Impairment due to abnormality or disease of the inner ear or the cochlear portion of the auditory nerve.

Septum. The partition between the right and left nasal cavities formed of bone and cartilage.

Shadowing. Echo speech.

Shimmer. Small variations in vocal intensity from cycle to cycle.

Sibilant. A class of fricative consonant sounds characterized by high-pitched noise. Examples are /s/ and /z/.

Sigmatism. Lisping.

Sonant. A voiced sound.

Spasmodic dysphonia (SD). Uncontrolled spasmodic closures (adductor SD) or openings (abductor SD) of the glottis during phonation, causing voice interruption; now believed usually to reflect the presence of a focal laryngeal dystonia.

Spasticity. One of the varieties of cerebral palsy; characterized by highly tensed contractions of muscle groups.

Spastic dysphonia. Generally synonymous with *spasmodic dysphonia,* associated with great strain and effort in producing voice; has been referred to in the past as "laryngeal stuttering."

Spectrogram. Graphic display of the frequency components of a complex sound where time is shown on the horizontal axis, frequency on the vertical axis, and intensity is shown by relative darkness of the graph.

Speechreading. Perceiving the spoken word visually by observing the speaker's facial expressions, gestures, lip movements; also called *lipreading.*

Speech synthesis. Production of artificial speech signals by electronic or computerized means.

Stabilization. The process of making a response permanent and unfluctuating.

Stapedectomy. Surgical removal of the stapes and implantation of a prosthesis; used in treatment of otosclerosis.

Stapes. The innermost bone of the middle ear.

Stigma. A mark or a sign of defect or disgrace.

Stoma. Opening in the neck through which the person must breathe after a laryngectomy.

Stop consonant. A sound characterized by a momentary blocking of airflow. Examples are the /k/, /d/, and /p/.

Strident lisp. Sibilants characterized by piercing, whistling sounds.

Stroke. Stoppage of bloodflow to the brain, usually due to blood clot or hemorrhaging (see *cerebrovascular accident*).

Stuttering. Disrupted speech, characterized by prolongations, hesitations, and blockages.

Sulcus. Narrow furrow or groove.

Suprasegmental. Refers to *prosody:* pitch, loudness, and durational features of speech; features that extend beyond single segments or units of speech.

Surd. Unvoiced sound such as the *s* as opposed to its cognate *z,* which is voiced or sonant.

Synapse. The juncture where a neural impulse is transferred from one neuron to another.

Syndrome. Collection of signs and symptoms that together characterize a disease or other abnormal condition.

Synergy. Combined action of several components to produce a result greater than the sum of the parts.

Syntax. The grammatical structure of a language.

Tachylalia. Extremely rapid speech.

Teratogen. Any agent or substance that acts prenatally to cause a congenital abnormality.

Thorax. Chest.

Thrombosis. Blood clot formed in place that does not move.

Thyroid cartilage. The major cartilage of the larynx; notch of the thyroid is often called the "Adam's apple."

Tidal volume. The amount of air inhaled or exhaled during one cycle of quiet relaxed breathing.

Time-outs. Intervals of silence imposed contingently by the experimenter or clinician when an undesired response (e.g., stuttering) occurs.

Tinnitus. Ringing noises in the ears.

Tonsils. Lymphoid tissue at back edges of oral cavity; also known as palatine tonsils.

Toxemia. A condition in which toxins produced by infection are present in the blood.

Toxoplasmosis. Disease caused by parasites in the bloodstream; prenatal infection may cause death or severe brain damage.

Trachea. The windpipe.

Trauma. Shock or injury.

Traumatic brain injury (TBI). Damage to brain or nervous system caused by externally induced head injury; also called *closed head injury.*

Tremor. The rapid tremulous vibration of a muscle group.

Tympanic membrane. The eardrum.

Unilaterality. One-handedness; preference for one hand as contrasted with ambidexterity.

Uvula. The hanging portion of the soft palate.

Velopharyngeal closure. The more or less complete shutting off of the nasopharynx.

Velopharyngeal incompetence. Lack of sufficient closing off of the nasal cavity during speech.

Velum. Soft palate.

Ventilation. A process using a mechanical apparatus designed to maintain or assist respiration in patients unable to breathe or able to breathe only weakly due to respiratory paralysis or other medical conditions.

Ventricular folds. Folds of tissue immediately above the true vocal folds; also known as *false vocal folds.*

Ventricular phonation. Voice produced by the vibration of the false vocal folds.

Vestibular system. Portion of the inner ear that controls balance.

Vital capacity. Maximum amount of air that can be forcibly exhaled following a maximum inhalation.

Vocal fry. Low-pitched continuous clicking sound produced by the vocal folds; also known as *glottal fry* and as *pulse register.*

Vocal nodules. Small callus-like protuberances on medial edge of the vocal folds, usually bilateral; caused by misuse and abuse of the voice.

Vocal play. In the development of speech, the stage during which the child experiments with sounds and syllables.

Voice. Sound produced at the level of the larynx by rapid vibratory excursions of the adducted vocal folds; *phonation.*

Voice onset time (VOT). The amount of time between release of a plosive and the onset of voicing.

Voice prosthesis. Actually, any device used to produce voicing (such as an electrolarynx), the term now refers most often to a small valve that transports air from the trachea to the esophagus for producing tracheoesophageal voice.

Voluntary mutism. Refusal to speak.

Waveform. Graphic representation of sound pressure variations or vibratory amplitudes over time.

Wavelength. The distance in space between successive compressions (or successive rarefactions) in a sound wave.

INDEX